OBSTETRIC VIOLENCE AND SYSTEMIC DISPARITIES

The Anthropology of Obstetrics and Obstetricians:
The Practice, Maintenance, and Reproduction of a Biomedical Profession

Editors:
Robbie Davis-Floyd, Rice University
Ashish Premkumar, Northwestern University

Obstetricians are the primary drivers of the research on and the implementation of interventions in the birth process that have long been the subjects of anthropological critiques. In many countries, they are also primary drivers of violence, disrespect, and abuse during the perinatal period. Yet there is little social science literature on obstetricians themselves, their educational processes, and their personal rationales for their practices. Thus, this dearth of social science literature on obstetricians constitutes a huge gap waiting to be filled. These groundbreaking edited collections seek to fill that gap by officially creating an "anthropology of obstetrics and obstetricians" across countries and cultures—including biopolitical and professional cultures—so that a broad and deep understanding of these maternity care providers and their practices, ideologies, motivations, and diversities can be achieved.

Volume I
Obstetricians Speak:
On Training, Practice, Fear, and Transformation
Edited by Robbie Davis-Floyd and Ashish Premkumar

Volume II
Cognition, Risk, and Responsibility in Obstetrics:
Anthropological Analyses and Critiques of Obstetricians' Practices
Edited by Robbie Davis-Floyd and Ashish Premkumar

Volume III
Obstetric Violence and Systemic Disparities:
Can Obstetrics Be Humanized and Decolonized?
Edited by Robbie Davis-Floyd and Ashish Premkumar

Obstetric Violence and Systemic Disparities

Can Obstetrics Be Humanized and Decolonized?

Edited by
Robbie Davis-Floyd and Ashish Premkumar

berghahn
NEW YORK • OXFORD
www.berghahnbooks.com

First published in 2023 by
Berghahn Books
www.berghahnbooks.com

Library of Congress Cataloging-in-Publication Data

A C.I.P. cataloging record is available from the Library of Congress
Library of Congress Cataloging in Publication Control Number: 2023000966

British Library Cataloguing in Publication Data

A catalogue record for this book is available from the British Library

ISBN 978-1-80073-834-8 hardback
ISBN 978-1-80073-836-2 paperback
ISBN 978-1-80073-835-5 ebook

https://doi.org/10.3167/9781800738348

Robbie Davis-Floyd dedicates this book to her dear friend and colleague Debra Pascali Bonaro, who has worked long and tirelessly to train new generations of doulas in many countries in a heroic effort to humanize birth and will continue to do so for many years to come. She also thanks Debra for her intensive work as Chair of the International MotherBaby Childbirth Organization and on the ICI Executive Committee in developing and promoting the International Childbirth Initiative (ICI): 12 Steps to Safe and Respectful MotherBaby-Family Maternity Care, because the implementation of the ICI Principles and 12 Steps in hospitals and other birth facilities around the world is changing their maternity care practices for the better!

Ashish Premkumar dedicates this book to the people he was privileged enough to serve as an obstetrician and perinatologist. Their demands for safety, equity, and support echo throughout these chapters.

Contents

Illustrations

Figures

Tables

Acknowledgments

We thank our chapter authors for their dedication and perseverance in conducting and writing up the research projects on which their chapters are based and for sticking with us throughout our sometimes-extensive chapter editing processes. We also thank our Berghahn Books editors Tom Bonnington and Keara Hagerty for responding to our endless questions and for shepherding this book through to production. And profound thanks go to Charles D. Laughlin for taking the time and trouble to create the index for this volume.

The Darker and the Lighter Sides of Biomedical Maternity Care

Moving from Obstetric Violence, Disrespect, and Abuse to the Humanization and Decolonization of Birth

Robbie Davis-Floyd and Ashish Premkumar

This is the Introduction to Volume III of the three-part series *The Anthropology of Obstetrics and Obstetricians: The Practice, Maintenance, and Reproduction of a Biomedical Profession*, edited by reproductive anthropologist Robbie Davis-Floyd and by perinatologist and medical anthropologist Ashish Premkumar. The three volumes in this series are:

- Volume I. *Obstetricians Speak: On Training, Practice, Fear, and Transformation* (Davis-Floyd and Premkumar 2023a);
- Volume II. *Cognition, Risk, and Responsibility in Obstetrics: Anthropological Analyses and Critiques of Obstetricians' Practices* (Davis-Floyd and Premkumar 2023b);
- Volume III. *Obstetric Violence and Systemic Disparities: Can Obstetrics Be Humanized and Decolonized?* (Davis-Floyd and Premkumar 2023c).

An overview of the entire series (Premkumar and Davis-Floyd 2023d), which lays out its primary concepts and theoretical frameworks and provides an overview of each volume, can be found at the beginning of Volume I. This Introduction to Volume III mostly constitutes an overview of the chapters in this present volume, which focus on both the dark and the lighter sides of biomedical maternity care. The dark side is of course the obstetric disrespect, violence, and abuse that permeate much of maternity care globally. Jenna Murray de López (2018:61) has defined *obstetric violence* as "a specific form of violence against women that violates their reproductive health rights and results in physical or psychological harm during pregnancy, birth or puerperium," explaining that obstetric violence can include: "scolding, taunts, irony, insults, threats, humiliation, manipulation of information and denial of treatment; pain management during childbirth used a punishment; and coercion to obtain 'consent' for invasive procedures; and even acts of deliberate harm."

Part 1 of this book focuses on those darker topics. (The middle, shades-of-grey aspects of biomedical maternity care are addressed in multiple ways in Volume II of this series [Davis-Floyd and Premkumar 2023b]). Part 2 focuses on the lighter side of biomedical maternity care, which consists of the efforts being made, from both within and outside of the obstetric profession, to humanize and decolonize the biomedical treatment of birth. Part 3 takes a different tack: it consists of only one chapter, which presents the ethnographic challenges faced by our chapter authors in finding, surveying, interviewing, and observing obstetricians. We note here that the chapters in Parts 1 and 2 of this volume are based on ethnographic research conducted in Canada, the Dominican Republic, Mexico, Peru, the United States, the UK, Russia and other former Soviet countries, Turkey, South Africa, and Aotearoa New Zealand. We divide our overview of these chapters into the three Parts into which this book is organized.

Yet since some of these chapters utilize Robbie Davis-Floyd's (2001, 2018, 2022) delineations of "the technocratic, humanistic, and holistic paradigms of birth and health care" (described more fully in our Series Overview at the beginning of Volume I), we first present a brief overview of these paradigms, just as we did in the Introduction to our second volume. We also offer a brief overview of "the 4 Stages of Cognition" and "Substage," which Robbie describes in full in her Volume II chapter (Davis-Floyd 2023), and which are utilized in some of the chapters in this present volume. And we summarize the findings of an important article on which some of the chapters in this volume draw: "Obstetric Iatrogenesis in the United States: The Spectrum of Unintentional Harm, Disrespect, Violence, and Abuse" (Liese et al. 2021).

The Technocratic, Humanistic, and Holistic Paradigms of Birth and Health Care

The hegemonic technocratic model, based on the *principle of separation*—of mind and body, practitioner and patient—metaphorizes the human body as a machine, teaches practitioners to objectify their patients and their disorders, and relies on multiple technologies to manage, surveil, control, and intervene in the (usually) normal physiology of birth. This over-management and over-intervention exemplify the *obstetric paradox*: intervene in birth to keep it safe, thereby causing harm (Cheyney and Davis-Floyd 2019:8). These authors (Cheyney and Davis-Floyd 2020a, 2020b) have also argued for the replacement of TMTS (too much too soon) and TLTL (too little too late) forms of care (see Miller et al. 2016) with RARTRW care—the right amount at the right time *in the right way*—for *how* care is provided matters as much or more than what kind of care is provided and when.

The humanistic model, toward which many maternity care providers strive, is based on the *principle of connection*—the connections of mind to body, person to person. The humanistic paradigm heavily emphasizes this "right way," for it defines the body as what it is: an organism that responds well to kind and compassionate treatment, and poorly and defensively to what this organism perceives as unkind and hurtful treatment. A turtle retreats into its shell when threatened; a laboring woman can retreat into the "shell" of "learned helplessness" (Seligman 1972) when mistreated, in which she accepts that she is powerless, cognitively shuts down, and literally *learns to be helpless* when her agency and protagonism are completely denied and she sees no other option. This can easily result in severe, long-lasting trauma and postpartum depression (see Davis-Floyd 2022) as some of the chapters in this volume show.

Robbie (Davis-Floyd 2018, 2022) has been careful to distinguish between *superficial humanism*, in which compassionate treatment, including allowing the presence of a partner or doula, is just an overlay on multiple technocratic interventions in labor and birth, and *deep humanism*, in which the "deep physiology" (Davis-Floyd 2018, 2022) of birth is understood, honored, and facilitated. Because the differences between "superficial" and "deep" humanism are so essential to understand, Robbie (Davis-Floyd 2022) now considers that the paradigmatic spectrum should read: "technocratic—superficially humanistic—deeply humanistic—holistic." All childbearers want at least superficially humanistic treatment—they want to be treated kindly and with respect (see Davis-Floyd et al. 2009). Only some want deeply humanistic treatment, as many want epidurals, the administration of which de facto interferes with the physiologic processes of labor and birth (Davis-Floyd 2022).

On the "radical fringe" of this spectrum lies the holistic model, in which the body is defined as more than an organism but rather as an energy system in constant interaction with all other energy systems around it. This holistic model is based on the *principles of connection and integration*—of mind, body, and spirit; of "client" (a much more egalitarian word than "patient") and practitioner. Under this model, unlike in the other two, spirit and energy are brought into play, for example by having the parent(s) "call the spirit" of an unresponsive baby (before or while the practitioner performs neonatal resuscitation) to ask the baby's spirit to choose to come into its body, as many midwives (and some neonatologists) do, and/or by following the holistic maxim "Change the energy, change the outcome," which can mean keeping what Brazilian obstetrician Ricardo Jones (2009) has called the *psychosphere* of birth clear and clean, perhaps by asking people with fear-filled "negative energy" to leave the birthing room.

The 4 Stages of Cognition and "Substage"

In her chapter in Volume II, "Open and Closed Knowledge Systems, the 4 Stages of Cognition, and the Obstetric Management of Birth," Robbie (Davis-Floyd 2023) describes Stage 1, "closed" thinking in three categories: (1) naïve realism ("Our way is the only way, or the only way that matters"); (2) fundamentalism ("Our way is the only right way"); and (3) fanaticism ("Our way is so right that all who do not accept it should be assimilated or eliminated"). She codes Stage 2 thinkers as ethnocentrists ("Other ways are ok for others but our way is best"); and Stage 3 thinkers as cultural relativists ("All ways have value and human behavior should be understood within its sociocultural context"). She then codes Stage 4 thinkers as global humanists ("There must be higher, better ways that honor human rights, even when that goes against the sociocultural grain"), and describes some of the ongoing battles between Stage 1 fundamentalists and fanatics and Stage 4 global humanists, who are anathemas to each other. She goes on to show how many obstetricians are Stage 1 thinkers, often denigrating and persecuting Stage 4 humanistic obstetric practitioners who practice outside of the obstetric silo. She also describes "Substage"—a condition of cognitive regression, or "losing it," in which it is very easy for practitioners to take out their frustrations and stresses by mistreating or abusing others, most especially laboring people. And she describes how ritual can "stand as a barrier between cognition and chaos" by helping practitioners get out of Substage and cognitively stabilize themselves (see Table 0.1).

Table 0.1. The Stages of Cognition and Their Anthropological Equivalents. © Robbie Davis-Floyd and Charles D. Laughlin. This Table originally appeared in *The Power of Ritual* (2016), on which Charlie and Robbie hold the copyright, so we reprint it here with their permission. This Table also appears in the recently abridged version of that book, called *Ritual: What It Is, How It Works, and Why* (Davis-Floyd and Laughlin 2022).

Stages of Cognition	Anthropological Equivalents
Stage 4: Fluid, open thinking	**Global humanism**: All individuals have rights that should be honored, not violated.
Stage 3: Relative, open thinking	**Cultural relativism**: All ways have value; individual behavior should be understood within its sociocultural context.
Stage 2: Self- and culture-centered semi-closed thinking	**Ethnocentrism**: Other ways may be OK for others, but our way is best.
Stage 1: Rigid/concrete closed thinking, intolerance of other ways of thinking	**Naïve realism**: Our way is the only way, or the only way that matters; **Fundamentalism**: Our is way is the only *right* way; **Fanaticism**: Our way is so right that all others should be assimilated or eliminated.
Substage: Non-thinking; inability to process information; lack or loss of compassion for others	**Cognitive regression**: Intense egocentrism, irritability, inability to cope, burnout, breakdown, hysteria, panic, "losing it," abusing or mistreating others.

Obstetric Iatrogenesis: The Spectrum of Unintentional Harm, Disrespect, Violence, and Abuse

The article sharing the name of this section (Liese et al. 2021), on which some of the chapters in this volume draw, was written by practicing midwives Kylea Liese, Karie Stewart, and Melissa Cheyney, and was co-authored by medical/reproductive anthropologist Robbie Davis-Floyd. (We had originally planned to include that article in updated form as a chapter in this book, but were unable to obtain permission to do so; thus we summarize it here.) Taking off from Ivan Illich's (1976) term "medical iatrogenesis," and following Amali Lokugamage's (2011) original usage of the term *obstetric iatrogenesis*, these authors explore obstetric iatrogenesis along a spectrum that they acronymize as UHDVA.

This spectrum begins with the unintentional harm (UH) caused by interventions considered routine but are nevertheless harmful in that they interfere with the normal physiologic process of birth, exemplifying the "obstetric paradox" mentioned above (intervene to keep birth safe, thereby causing harm). This iatrogenic spectrum continues on to more intentional forms of disrespect, violence, and abuse (DVA), which can include utilizing demeaning words toward, yelling at, and even hitting the laboring person. This article also assesses how obstetric iatrogenesis disproportionately impacts Black, Indigenous, and People of Color (BIPOC), contributing to worse perinatal outcomes for BIPOC childbearers. Much of the work on obstetric violence that documents the most detrimental ends (violence and abuse) of the UHDVA spectrum has focused on low-to-middle income countries in Latin America and the Caribbean (see for examples Chapters 1, 2, and 5 of this volume). This article shows that significant UHDVA also occurs in high-income countries such as the United States.

One of this article's primary examples of the UHDVA spectrum is cervical exams during labor, which are often unnecessarily performed. The authors (Liese et al. 2021:5) state:

> The majority of U.S. births (69%) take place in teaching hospitals that train resident physicians (Fingar et al. 2018). Thus, much of the obstetric system is organized to facilitate physician education. Since cervical exams are a learned manual skill crucial to obstetrics, medical students and obstetric residents are encouraged to practice on patients . . . Cervical exams—which should be performed only when knowing the cervical dilation can impact care, such as before administering medications or at the patient's request—range from uncomfortable to excruciating . . . The pain is exacerbated when performed during contractions and/or on women with histories of sexual abuse; some childbearers experience or equate them to a form of rape . . . The practice moves from unnecessary to aggressive when exams are performed without provider introduction, consent, explanation, or heeding a patient's direct instruction to stop. Those who try to push the provider's hand away or yell "STOP!" may be responded to in ways disturbingly akin to the language used by rape perpetrators: "You're okay" and "I'm almost done."

Ashish Premkumar, maternal-fetal medicine specialist, co-editor of this volume and of this Book Series, and co-author of this Introduction, adds:

I distinctly remember having a woman come up from our triage bay who was completely dilated and pushing, unanesthetized. She was nulliparous [a first-time mother], and as such was getting the hang of pushing and was also dealing with the fact that she was rapidly progressing through the second stage of labor. She was actively trying to not be on her back as she had an uncontrollable urge to push constantly, given how low the baby's head was in her pelvis. The charge nurse in the room kept yelling at her to not push in between contractions and became visibly angry when she would grunt and continue to bear down.

I tried to pull the charge nurse aside to tell her that this was going to be uncontrollable, and that she should just let her push in any way that she felt comfortable doing so. The bedside nurse tried to auscultate heart tones with the electronic fetal monitor and noted that the fetal heart tones were low. Prior to getting a maternal pulse (which is standard to ensure that you're not picking up the maternal heart rate), the charge nurse immediately began to yell and snap at the patient, telling her to "get it together and PUSH." I began to raise my voice—something we do in emergency situations to have one clinician lead a situation where multiple voices might cause more disarray—and announced that she was already +3 and would have the baby in a matter of seconds. Sure enough, she had the baby, which came out crying and went right on mom! The fact that people lost it [went into Substage] because she was nulliparous, pushing uncontrollably, and that we couldn't really get heart tones despite her being five seconds from delivery, was completely unacceptable. This, sadly, is not the only time I've seen this scenario.

Premkumar's example, among many others (see Davis-Floyd 2022), shows that not only obstetricians (obs) but also labor and delivery nurses can be Stage 1 perpetrators of obstetric DVA.

Addressing other verbal forms of DVA, Liese et al. (2021:6) state:

In our experiences, the language used by obstetricians to convince/coerce consent from patients ranges from subtly to overtly abusive, with BIPOC and gender non-binary childbearers being especially affected . . . Most egregiously, pregnant mothers can be threatened with endangering the lives of their babies if they don't accept the doctor's advice. This tactic is observed in both in emergency and non-emergency situations, and pits the mother against her unborn baby, supporting a narrative of "good" motherhood in which the mother's needs are subservient to the child's.

For Robbie's revision and update of her first book, *Birth as an American Rite of Passage* (1992, 2003, 2022), Robbie, her colleague Melissa (Missy) Cheyney, and Missy's graduate students conducted interviews with 65 childbearers who had given birth since the year 2000. Here is a narrative from that dataset that exemplifies the UHDVA spectrum, in which Cate (a pseudonym), a white, heterosexual, cis-gendered women, describes:

> About six days past my due date, my water broke, and when I went into the hospital, I was only a fingertip dilated and my doctor was not on call—the other doctor came in and checked me—he didn't tell me his name—and he turned to the nurse and said, "Prep her, we're going to cut it out." I said, "Hold it, hold it—you're not doing anything until you tell me what is going on here." He said, "You're not dilating, you need a c-section." I said, "That will be fine as long as you can write down a medical reason why I need a section."

Knowing that, according to that hospital's protocols, she had 24 hours to deliver after her waters had broken, Cate "laid there all day" with the doctor repeatedly coming in to demand that she have a cesarean "because you need one." Just as repeatedly, Cate's response was the same. Later she found out that she was the only laboring patient in the maternity ward that day; apparently her ob just wanted to get her birth over with so that he could go home. (Of course doctors have lives too, but it is highly unethical to try to force an unnecessary cesarean on an unwilling laboring person.) Once Cate's labor picked up, she had the support of helpful nurses who kept saying "You're doing fine, the baby's fine, everything's fine," and of her Lamaze teacher Fran, who was acting as her doula, and she enjoyed her labor process when the obstetrician wasn't present. She said, "As long as I knew everything was fine, I could last forever." But:

> [the obstetrician] was very nasty. He would come in, send my husband out, check me, yell at me because I wasn't doing what he told me to do. He made my husband sign a form saying that we would take full responsibility for the death of my child. "You know," he said, "you're killing this baby because you won't have a section." I said, "I'll have one if you tell me why." He said, "Just because I say you need one," and I said, "That's not good enough."

> When she was born [at 5:36 a.m.], he cut a radical [unnecessarily large] episiotomy when her head was only 13 inches . . . and he didn't even say "It's a girl or it's a boy, it's a dog, it's a cat" . . . And he stitched me up with nothing. I kept telling him I could feel everything he was doing, and he kept saying "No, you can't feel that, you're crazy." I knew he did it just for spite. It was very enjoyable when he wasn't there, but he would come in and check me during a contraction and scare me to death . . . as soon as he would leave the room, my body would involuntarily tremble all over.

Cate's story, which also appears in *Birth as an American Rite of Passage* (Davis-Floyd 2022),

> illustrates many forms of UHDVA, including laboring in the supine position, verbal coercion and abuse, and physical violence via the unnecessary extensive episiotomy and stitching without local anesthetic. Cate stated that she was empowered to achieve a vaginal birth despite that doctor's demands because Fran was at her side, squeezing her hand while the doctor yelled at her, and her nurses were kind and supportive. Her positionality and social capital likely also facilitated her ability to resist. (Liese et al. 2021:8).

Citing various studies, Liese, Davis-Floyd, Stewart, and Cheyney (2021) state that *"The psychological cost to childbearers of overt DVA is high"* (italics in original). Interlocutors from Davis-Floyd's and Cheyney's dataset who had been subjected to such forms of DVA described themselves as deeply traumatized by their birth experiences. Like Cate, many suffered from postpartum depression and/or PTSD (as illustrated in Davis-Floyd 2022).

Having described the "technocratic—superficially humanistic—deeply humanistic—holistic" paradigms of birth and health care, the 4 Stages of Cognition and "Substage," and the UHDVA spectrum as background and context for the chapters in this book, we turn now to an overview of both Parts—the darker and the lighter—of this present volume.

Part 1. Obstetric Violence and Systemic Racial, Ethnic, Gendered, and Socio-Structural Disparities in Obstetricians' Practices

Chapter 1, co-authored by anthropologists Annie Preaux and Arachu Castro, provides an ethnographic account of obstetricians and the delivery of obstetric violence in the Dominican Republic. Arachu Castro and Virginia Savage (2018) have documented obstetric violence in public hospitals in the Dominican Republic; however, little has been known about this issue from the perspectives of obstetricians and of other hospital personnel. Thus Preaux and Castro conducted in-depth interviews with 97 obstetrician/gynecologists, attending physicians, residents, nurses, and administrative personnel in three public maternity hospitals in the Dominican Republic. These interviews addressed healthcare providers' perspectives on the concept of obstetric violence and their justifications for why it occurs. The interviews also included providers' reactions to past cases of maternal mortality in the Dominican Republic and their associations with obstetric violence. Through these interviews, Preaux and Castro saw how healthcare system constraints and long-standing traditions of discrimination based on gender, class, and race can both foment providers' acts of obstetric violence and serve as their justifications for women's complaints, complications, and sometimes even deaths. While some obstetricians and other personnel recognize and work against healthcare system limitations and ingrained biases that lead to obstetric violence, some deny any problems, and others use the limitations of the country's healthcare system to justify or rationalize their own harmful actions or those of their colleagues.

More "woman-blaming" is described in Chapter 2, "'Bad Pelvises': Mexican Obstetrics and the Re-Affirmation of Race in Labor and Delivery," in which anthropologist Sarah A. Williams links the historical development of gynecology and obstetrics in Mexico to contemporary patterns of cesarean overuse. In so doing, Williams unwinds racial myths about the smallness and inadequacies of Mexican women's pelvises and their inability to birth vaginally—myths that continue to influence Mexican obstetric decision-making. First, Williams traces the emergence of pelvimetry and gynecology in mid-1800s Mexico as a form of "race science," harnessed in service of the creation of a Mexican national identity predicated on a project of *mestizo* (mostly people of mixed Spanish and Indigenous descent) race-making and Indigenous erasure. Building on this historical analysis, Williams uses ethnographic data from fieldwork in the Yucatán peninsula to connect these race-making obstetric practices to the "hallmarks" of obstetric violence by both obstetricians and midwives in Mexico today—the routine use of techniques of obstetric management that manifest in burgeoning rates of cesareans and episiotomies and the continued use of "pelvimetric practices" (measuring the pelvis and usually concluding that it is "too small" for vaginal birth). As Williams's ethnographic research shows, obstetricians continue to draw on implicit and, at times, explicit theories of "race science" to justify often unnecessary birth interventions and to uphold normative racialized framings of maternal comportment, which this chapter describes.

In Chapter 3, sociologist Lauren Diamond-Brown points out that there are many accounts of obstetric violence, disrespect, and abuse in the United States, but we do not understand *obstetricians' perspectives* on why these events occur. In this chapter, Lauren seeks to understand obstetricians' thinking about the role of patients in birth and to shed light on the motivations of some obs for rejecting patient autonomy in labor and delivery. Lauren's chapter draws on in-depth interviews with 50 US obstetricians about decision-making in birth; she divides these interlocutors into Groups 1 and 2, which are close to equal in numbers. Group 1 members reject patient autonomy, often in the form of complete disregard of the wishes that childbearers express in their birth plans, whereas the members of Group 2 respect and support patient protagonism, welcome birth plans, and do their best to support the desires expressed in those plans. About these Group 2 interlocutors, Diamond-Brown notes that "scholars have focused on biomedical training as the primary agent of professional socialization for physicians, while missing the opportunity to examine *resocialization* throughout doctors' careers." The Group 2 ob interlocutors said that they "practice like a midwife"—meaning that they practice the humanistic and holistic midwifery model of care. Diamond-Brown found that for some, this was their training—showing what a difference the type of training can make in forming obstetric ideologies—whereas for others, it was exposure to a more humanistic model of birth later in their careers, often via watching midwives practice. (See also Davis-Floyd's [2023] chapter in Volume II of this series.)

Focusing primarily on the ob interlocutors in Group 1, Diamond-Brown explores three dominant gender tropes that these Group 1 interlocutors used to police "good patient" status: (1) women as control freaks; (2) women as misinformed; (3) and women as selfish. She analyzes these gendered tropes through a feminist lens and suggests that sexism and "misogyny" (broadly defined) continue to underpin obstetricians' interpretations of their patients—even when the obstetricians are female—and especially underpin her Group 1 ob interlocutors' approaches to dealing with self-advocating patients.

In Chapter 4, anthropologist Genevieve Ritchie-Ewing investigates "Implicit Racial Bias in Obstetrics: How US Obstetricians View and Treat Pregnant Women of Color." She begins by noting that persistent racism in US obstetric practices creates barriers to safe, quality health care for many pregnant women. As the vast majority of US women still receive prenatal and postnatal care from obstetricians, rather than from midwives, improving the relationships between pregnant Women of Color and their obstetricians is vital to empowering these women in making health-related decisions. In addition, as Ritchie-Ewing shows, the lack of quality prenatal care for minority women is one of the main reasons why the United States has extensive racial disparities in pregnancy and birth outcomes such as preterm birth and low birthweight rates. While much recent research explores the experiences of pregnant and laboring US Women of Color, no studies thus far have examined how obstetricians practicing in the United States view and react to their patients of various racial and ethnic backgrounds. Through an online survey and in-depth virtual interviews, Ritchie-Ewing investigates the racial and ethnic biases among obstetricians working in diverse biomedical settings, most of whom were unwilling to admit racial bias, preferring to talk in terms of "socioeconomic status" instead. She argues that recognizing how obstetricians view and treat childbearers of Color both subtly and overtly is essential to developing strategies for eliminating bias and increasing equality in healthcare interactions.

In Chapter 5, on "Censusing the Quechua: Peruvian State *Obstetras* in Light of Historic Sterilizations, Contemporary Accusations, and Biopolitical Statecraft Obligations," medical anthropologist Rebecca Irons begins by noting that, despite evidence that a Malthusian government health policy was to blame, individual healthcare workers, and particularly obstetricians, are increasingly being demonized in the ongoing case of Peru's more than 300,000 forced sterilizations of the 1990s—many of which were among the Quechua, an Indigenous group. Even before this blame, as Irons explains, the Peruvian profession of *obstetricia* (obstetrics) was in a position of precarity: it was, and remains, highly gendered, so female *obstetras* (obstetricians), who, unusually, are not allowed to perform cesareans, are subjugated to the authority of majority-male obstetrician/gynecologists and surgeons. Irons argues that while *obstetras* played a significant role in the condemnable forced sterilizations, even today the underlying push for "quota filling"—strongly recommending contraceptive use—as a condition of employment encourages similar coercive behaviors that seek to limit poor and Indigenous reproduction. Thus Irons suggests that a key role of Peruvian *obstetras* is to census and discipline the Indigenous Quechua population as a form of stratified biopolitical statecraft, resulting in health worker dissatisfaction, patient neglect, and obstetric violence. Only through exploring this situation from the perspective of the *obstetras* themselves does Irons find it possible to effectively understand how and why structural violence is perpetuated at a local level.

Part 2. Decolonizing and Humanizing Obstetric Training and Practice? Obstetricians, Midwives, and Their Battles against "the System"

Having exposed and sought to explain obstetrics' darkest aspects in this Introduction and in Part 1, in Part 2 our chapters turn toward positive efforts to decolonize and humanize obstetricians' practices via intentional changes in biomedical education and improved, more collegial relationships with midwives and the (humanistic/holistic) midwifery model of care, and with doulas and perinatal psychologists. These chapters in Part 2 address the struggles that this turn to decolonization and humanization often entail.

Chapter 6, by Amali Lokugamage, Tharanika Ahillan, and S. D. C. Pathberiya, addresses the crucial topic of *decolonizing medical education*, with a focus on that process in the UK. These authors begin by noting that the legacies of colonial rule have permeated into all aspects of life in multiple countries and have heavily contributed to healthcare inequities. They go on to explain that, in response to the increased interest in social justice, biomedical educators in the UK are thinking of ways to decolonize obstetric education—in other words, to replace its top-down colonialist hierarchy and produce obstetricians who can meet the complex needs of diverse populations. The authors investigate the implications of recentering displaced Indigenous healing systems and of *medical pluralism*, highlighting the concepts of "unconscious bias," "cultural competence," "cultural humility," and "Cultural Safety" in biomedical training. As Lokugamage, Ahillan, and Pathberiya describe, from a global health perspective, climate change debates and associated civil protests resonate with Indigenous ideas of *"planetary health,"* which focus on the harmonious interconnections of the planet, the environment, and human beings. Additionally, these authors look at implications for clinical practice, addressing the background of inequality in health care among the BAME (Black, Asian, and minority ethnic) populations of the UK and an increasing recognition of the role of intergenerational trauma originating from the legacy of slavery. By analyzing these theories and conversations that challenge the biomedical view of health, the authors conclude that encouraging healthcare educators and professionals to adopt a *"decolonizing attitude"* can address the complex power imbalances in health care and further improve person-centered, humanistic care.

In Chapter 7, on "Teaching Humanistic and Holistic Obstetrics: Triumphs and Failures," Beverley Chalmers, a psychologist, sociologist, and childbirth expert, explains that after decades of work striving toward the integration of humanistic and holistic approaches into peri-natal care alongside technological advances, the progress that has been made in this area is both significant and woefully insufficient. Varying approaches to obstetric education have resulted in both triumphs and failures in Chalmer's attempts to train obstetricians to provide optimal care. Her chapter describes some of the educational models she has used in her training efforts in Russia and in other post-Soviet countries, presents theories for why obstetricians continue to provide the least re-spectful care of any other maternal healthcare providers, and describes which models offer optimal paths to follow. She details these optimal models and addresses the challenges of assessing the effectiveness of such teaching models in terms of implementing humanistic and holistic approaches to perinatal caregiving.

Chapter 8, "The Inconsistent Path of Russian Obstetricians to the Humanization of Childbirth in Post-Soviet Russian Maternity Care," de-scribes the current situation in Russian obstetric care, almost 20 years after Chalmers' teaching and collaborative efforts in that country. The authors, anthropologist Anna Ozhiganova and sociologist Anna Tem-kina, consider the professional logics and strategies of Russian obstetri-cians. They conceptualize the post-Soviet system of maternity care as a "hybrid" of the legacy of Soviet bureaucratic paternalism and neoliberal reforms, which enhance managerialism and marketization in biomedical settings. On the one hand, from Soviet times to the present, the logics of bureaucratic control continue to play a decisive role in the Russian maternity care system. Russian obstetricians are not attributed the same power and autonomy as their counterparts in Western societies, and thus their knowledge often does not count as fully authoritative; bio-medical professional organizations do not have much influence; and the economic interests of doctors are largely ignored. On the other hand, due to the maternity care reforms carried out during the post-Soviet period, partly as a result of Chalmer's work, the practice of "soft" or "natural" childbirth and the honoring of the post-birth "golden hour" are becoming more widespread.

Temkina and Ozhiganova show that in Russia, State and market de-mands often contradict each other, necessitating special efforts from ob-stetricians to cope with both inconsistent regulations and the growth of childbearing women's consumer needs and complaints. Based on exten-sive ethnographic research and in-depth interviews with obstetricians, the authors explain this hybridization and the forces that created it, and place particular focus on the special invisible mechanism of "personal hands-on care," which is meant to compensate for the rigid and inflexi-ble regulation in the limited space of Russian obstetricians' professional autonomy. Ozhiganova and Temkina also describe and analyze the ways in which Russian obs have tried to fight the government's bureaucratic and paternalistic system of maternity care by engaging with doulas and cooperating with homebirth midwives—informally, because homebirth midwifery practice is illegal in Russia. The authors demonstrate how, through personal and professional efforts, some obstetricians "reimagine" the normative authoritative knowledge in favor of more humanistic care.

In Chapter 9, based on 32 interviews with Brazilian obstetricians who have made paradigm shifts from technocratic to humanistic, and sometimes holistic, practices, Robbie Davis-Floyd and Eugenia (Nia) Georges describe the "pivot points" for these paradigm shifts, explicate their processes, and detail their effects—both positive and negative— as these effects often involved professional ostracism and persecution, along with much greater satisfaction and pride in their work, and extremely satisfied and grateful clients. These 32 obs and their like-minded colleagues call themselves "the good guys and girls," as opposed to the "bad" obs who perform far too many cesareans (56% nationwide). Some of these good guys and girls had cesarean rates of 7%–10%, as they primarily attended the home births of women who were "10,000% committed" to "natural childbirth." Others who attended the births of anyone who came to them had higher rates, ranging from 13% to 30%, as they believe that all women—even those who want to schedule an elective cesarean—are entitled to the kind of care they provide. Robbie and Nia also highlight a particular Brazilian hospital—Hospital Sofia Feldman—as an exemplar of humanistic practice. And they describe the efforts of these "good guys and girls" to support professional midwives, who are few in Brazil while obs are many, and to effect humanistic policy changes in their respective institutions, which many of them have managed to do with high degrees of success.

Chapter 10 takes us to Aotearoa New Zealand (ANZ). ("Aotearoa" is the Māori—the Indigenous people—name for this country. Placing "Aotearoa" before "New Zealand" signifies recognition of Māori settlement long before British colonization.) In this chapter, ANZ anthropologist Rea Daellenbach, midwives Lorna Davies and Melanie Welfare, neonatal pediatrician Maggie Meeks, and obstetricians Coleen Caldwell and Judy Ormandy address interprofessional education for both medical and midwifery students. They begin by explaining that in Aotearoa New Zealand, community midwives are the primary providers of maternity care, chosen as such by 94% of ANZ childbearers and giving continuity of care to women and families throughout pregnancy, birth, and up to six weeks postnatally. If needed, midwives refer clients to obstetricians.

Midwives also work in hospitals, providing support for community midwives and working as part of the maternity care team. Thus, interprofessional collaboration is a key aspect of ANZ maternity services, and failure by midwives and obstetricians to effectively communicate leads to poorer outcomes for women and babies.

In an effort to aid interprofessional collaboration, a multidisciplinary team organized a project involving final-year midwifery and medical students who were planning to choose obstetrics as their specialty, in which they had the opportunity to learn about each other's roles and about perinatal interprofessional collaboration by participating in emergency simulation scenarios. The discussions among the students in these workshops demonstrated how widespread and ingrained are some negative views of each other's professions. Developing a good model for interprofessional education for midwifery and obstetric students highlights how important it is to ensure that each profession has familiarity with the professional skills and roles of others to negotiate, cooperate, and advocate as a team for the best possible outcomes, as this chapter describes.

In Chapter 11, obstetrician Deborah McNabb explores "The Changing Face of Obstetric Practice in the United States as the Percent of Women in the Specialty Has Grown." Her belief when she finished residency training in the 1990s was that increasing numbers of women in the field of obstetrics and gynecology would lead to better reproductive health care for women. She notes that those in training at a time when female faculty in obstetrics were uncommon and when women were just starting to enter ob/gyn residency programs in larger numbers too often followed the male obstetrician paradigm by maintaining some distance in the patient-provider relations, speaking with authoritative voices, and being "tougher than tough" to prove that they could be just as good as the men. In this chapter, through interviews with female obstetric faculty members who have been in those positions for the last 30 years, McNabb explores the question of whether or not female obstetricians have, over the decades, developed their own practice models, hoping that the field may have become less authoritarian and more patient-centered. She notes in her chapter Conclusion that:

> The three biggest contributions that I think female obstetricians have made, and continue to make, to women's health care are women-modeled empathy, strong communication skills, and patient-centered behavior—all of which have now become the standard of care . . . Though it has taken decades to make this progress, I believe that female physicians' contributions to obstetrics and gynecology

have been remarkable and deserve to be fostered, supported, and valued.

Part 3. The Ethnographic Challenges of Gaining Access to Obstetricians for Surveys, Interviews, and Observations

In Chapter 12—the only chapter in Part 3—we present descriptions provided to us (via emails) from the chapter authors of Volumes II (Davis-Floyd and Premkumar 2023b) and III (this present volume) of this series of the challenges they faced in finding, surveying, interviewing, and observing obstetricians. (We don't present descriptions of such challenges from the authors of Volume I, because they are all obstetricians [see Davis-Floyd and Premkumar 2023a.]) These challenges are multiple and complex; thus we often use these authors' own words to describe them. We also describe the equally complex and often clever ways in which these researchers managed to overcome many of these challenges.

In our Conclusions to this volume, we present some of the theoretical concepts and frameworks that our chapter authors found most helpful and primary lessons learned, and in our Series Conclusions, we present some reflections on the entire three-volume series, yet primarily focus on the suggestions for future research provided by ourselves and many of our chapter authors—one of which is included in Robbie's bio below.

Robbie Davis-Floyd, Adjunct Professor, Department of Anthropology, Rice University, Houston, Fellow of the Society for Applied Anthropology, and Senior Advisor to the Council on Anthropology and Reproduction, is a cultural/medical/reproductive anthropologist interested in transformational models of maternity care. She is also a Board member of the International MotherBaby Childbirth Organization (IMBCO), in which capacity she helped to wordsmith the *International Childbirth Initiative: 12 Steps to Safe and Respectful MotherBaby-Family Maternity Care* (www.ICIchildbirth.org). The ICI has been translated into more than 30 languages and has been implemented in more than 70 birth facilities, small and large, around the world, showing that transformative change is indeed possible. Researchers are needed to study the processes and effects of ICI implementation; if you are interested, please contact Robbie. E-mail: davis-floyd@outlook.com.

Ashish Premkumar is an Assistant Professor of Obstetrics and Gynecology at the Pritzker School of Medicine at The University of Chicago and a doctoral candidate in the Department of Anthropology at The Graduate School at Northwestern University. He is a practicing maternal-fetal medicine subspecialist. His research focus is on the intersections of the social sciences and obstetric practices, particularly surrounding the issues of risk, stigma, and quality of health care during the perinatal opioid use disorder epidemic of the 21st century. E-mail: premkumara@bsd.uchicago.edu.

References

Castro A, Savage V. 2019. "Obstetric Violence as Reproductive Governance in the Dominican Republic." *Medical Anthropology* 38(2): 123–136.

Cheyney M, Davis-Floyd R. 2019. "Birth as Culturally Marked and Shaped." In *Birth in Eight Cultures*, eds. Davis-Floyd R, Cheyney M, 1–16. Long Grove, Il: Waveland Press.

———. 2020a. "Birth and the Big Bad Wolf: A Biocultural, Co-Evolutionary Perspective, Part I." *International Journal of Childbirth* 09(4): 177–192.

———. 2020b "Birth and the Big Bad Wolf: A Biocultural, Co-Evolutionary Perspective, Part II." *International Journal of Childbirth* 10(2): 66–78.

Davis-Floyd R. 2001. "The Technocratic, Humanistic, and Holistic Paradigms of Childbirth." *International Journal of Gynecology & Obstetrics* 75, Supplement No. 1: S5–S23.

———. (1992) 2003. *Birth as an American Rite of Passage*, 2nd ed. Berkeley: University of California Press.

———. 2018. "The Technocratic, Humanistic, and Holistic Paradigms of Birth and Health Care." In *Ways of Knowing about Birth: Mothers, Midwives, Medicine, and Birth Activism*, Davis-Floyd R and Colleagues, 3–44. Long Grove IL: Waveland Press.

———. 2022. *Birth as an American Rite of Passage*, 3rd ed. Abingdon, Oxon: Routledge.

———. 2023. "Open and Closed Knowledge Systems, the 4 Stages of Cognition, and the Obstetric Management of Birth." In *Cognition, Risk, and Responsibility in Obstetrics: Anthropological Analyses and Critiques of Obstetricians Practices*, eds. Davis-Floyd R, Premkumar A, Chapter 1. New York: Berghahn Books.

Davis-Floyd R, Barclay L, Daviss BA, Tritten J, eds. 2009. *Birth Models That Work*. Berkeley: University of California Press.

Davis-Floyd R, Laughlin CD. 2016. *The Power of Ritual*. Brisbane, Australia: Daily Grail Press.

———. 2022. *Ritual: What It Is, How It Works, and Why*. New York: Berghahn Books.

Davis-Floyd R, Premkumar A, eds. 2023a. *Obstetricians Speak: On Training, Practice, Fear, and Transformation*. New York: Berghahn Books.

———, eds. 2023b. *Cognition, Risk, and Responsibility in Obstetrics: Anthropological Analyses and Critiques of Obstetricians' Practices*. New York: Berghahn Books.

———, eds. 2023c. *Obstetric Violence and Systemic Disparities: Can Obstetrics Be Humanized and Decolonized?* New York: Berghahn Books.

———. 2023d. "The Anthropology of Obstetrics and Obstetricians: The Practice, Maintenance, and Reproduction of a Biomedical Profession." In *Obstetricians Speak: On Training, Practice, Fear, and Transformation*, eds. Davis-Floyd R, Premkumar A, Series Overview. New York: Berghahn Books.

Fingar KF, Hambrick MM, Heslin KC, Moore JE. 2018. "Trends and Disparities in Delivery Hospitalizations Involving Severe Maternal Morbidity, 2006–2015." *HCUP Statistical Brief #243*. Agency for Healthcare Research and Quality, Rockville, MD. www. hcup-us.ahrq.gov/reports/statbriefs/sb243-Severe-Maternal-Morbidity-Delivery-Trends-Disparities.pdf.

Illich I. 1976. *Medical Nemesis: The Expropriation of Health*. New York: Bantam Books.

Jones R. 2009. "Teamwork: An Obstetrician, a Midwife, and a Doula in Brazil." In *Birth Models That Work*, eds. Davis-Floyd R, Barclay L, Daviss BA, Tritten J, 271–304. Berkeley: University of California Press.

Liese K, Davis-Floyd R, Stewart K, Cheyney M. 2021. "Obstetric Iatrogenesis: The Spectrum of Unintentional Harm, Disrespect, Violence, and Abuse." *Anthropology & Medicine* 28(2): 1–16.

Lokugamage A. 2011. "Fear of Home Birth in Doctors and Obstetric Iatrogenesis." *International Journal of Childbirth* 1(4): 263–272.

Miller S, Abalos E, Chamillard M, et al. 2016. "Beyond Too Little, Too Late and Too Much, Too Soon: A Pathway towards Evidence-Based, Respectful Maternity Care Worldwide." *Lancet* 388(10056): 2176–2192.

Murray de López, J. 2018. "When the Scars Begin to Heal: Narratives of Obstetric Violence in Chiapas, Mexico." *International Journal of Health Governance* 23(1): 60–69.

Seligman MEP. 1972. "Learned Helplessness." *Annual Review of Medicine* 23(1): 407–412.

Obstetric Violence and Systematic Racial, Ethnic, Gendered, and Socio-Structural Disparities in Obstetricians' Practices

CHAPTER 1

Obstetricians and the Delivery of Obstetric Violence

An Ethnographic Account from the Dominican Republic

Annie Preaux and Arachu Castro

Introduction: Maternal Health and Obstetric Violence in the Dominican Republic

In the Dominican Republic, 172 maternal deaths per 100,000 live births were reported in 2021 (Ministry of Public Health of the Dominican Republic 2022). This maternal mortality ratio (MMR) is among the highest in Latin America and the Caribbean, and above average for the region (WHO et al. 2019). Worldwide, most maternal deaths could be prevented with universal access to contraception and abortion and increased access to quality maternity care (Tulane University and UNICEF 2016; GTR Regional Task Force for the Reduction of Maternal Mortality 2017; United Nations 2019). Yet the Dominican Republic faces a unique paradox: in compliance with the international development push toward facility birth and away from births at home with midwives, almost all women (99.8%) give birth in healthcare facilities with a skilled attendant, yet the MMR remains high (Miller et al. 2003; UNICEF and WHO 2020). For comparison, Guatemala had the same MMR as the Dominican Republic in 2017 (WHO et al. 2019), but only 69.8% of women in Guatemala gave birth with a skilled attendant present (UNICEF and WHO 2020). In 2003, Suellen Miller and colleagues wrote about this paradox in the Dominican Republic, and 20 years later, the quality of maternity care in the country remains a major concern.

A central aspect of the maternity care services in that country is obstetric violence: "the appropriation of women's bodies and reproductive processes by healthcare personnel, which is expressed by a dehumanizing treatment, an abuse of medicalization and pathologization of natural processes, resulting in a loss of autonomy and ability to decide freely about their bodies and sexuality, negatively impacting their quality of life" (República Bolivariana de Venezuela 2007). More recently, Jenna Murray de López (2018:61) has defined obstetric violence as "a specific form of violence against women that violates their reproductive health rights and results in physical or psychological harm during pregnancy, birth or puerperium," explaining that obstetric violence can include: "scolding, taunts, irony, insults, threats, humiliation, manipulation of information and denial of treatment; pain management during childbirth used as punishment; and coercion to obtain 'consent' for invasive procedures, and even acts of deliberate harm." In 2019, Arachu Castro and Virginia Savage (2019:125–126) created six typologies of obstetric violence:

1. *Verbal abuse*, such as harsh and disrespectful language, patient blaming, public humiliation, scolding, and name-calling;
2. *Poor rapport with women*, such as miscommunication of procedures and processes and language and communication barriers;
3. *Sociocultural discrimination* based on socioeconomic position, cultural insensitivity, and lack of intercultural care;
4. *Physical abuse*, such as the performance of unconsented or unnecessary examinations and procedures, hitting, slapping, or touching women in painful or uncomfortable ways, refusal to administer pain medication, and sexual abuse;
5. *Failure to meet professional standards of care*, such as delays and purposeful neglect, denial of medical attention for both minor and life-threatening health concerns, lack of accountability to patients, lack of supportive care, and breaches of confidentiality; and
6. *Healthcare system conditions*, such as failure to ensure privacy, assigning multiple patients to a single hospital bed, lack of resources to provide more comfort to women, and refusal to allow visitors or family members to be present.

All these constitute forms of reproductive governance that lead women to lose control of their own reproductive processes. Reducing obstetric violence could improve both women's experiences of pregnancy and childbirth and maternal health outcomes.

In 2010–11, Arachu Castro led a study on the causes of maternal mortality in the Dominican Republic based on clinical observations, verbal autopsies, and clinical review discussions during a six-month period. Most deaths occurred inside a hospital, and often were due to the failure to meet professional standards of care. The story of one such death illustrates the abandonment of a woman with serious obstetric complications in the postpartum recovery room (A. Castro 2019:107):

> In February 2011, a 28-year-old woman in her 37th or 38th week of pregnancy and mother of four went to the emergency room of a public maternity hospital in Santo Domingo at 11:10 a.m. She was diagnosed with severe preeclampsia and was admitted to the prelabor room at 11:50 a.m. The staff contacted her family members by phone, urging them to bring blood. At 7:00 p.m., after the family brought the blood, the blood transfusion and cesarean section began under epidural anesthesia. The woman gave life to a newborn son and had her fallopian tubes and 200 cc of blood clots removed. She was transferred to the recovery room and was left alone until three hours later, when a second-year resident found her profusely bleeding and in respiratory distress. An attending doctor and a fourth-year resident evaluated the woman, diagnosed uterine atony, and conducted an emergency laparotomy, during which she lost 300 cc of blood and had her uterus removed. The woman went into cardiac arrest and died in the operating room at 1:00 a.m. The reported cause of death was preeclampsia. The maternal mortality review committee members determined, while I took notes, that her death could have been prevented if the woman had not been neglected in the recovery room.

Sadly, this narrative reflects the circumstances of many other maternal deaths in the Dominican Republic and elsewhere, as Arachu Castro described in her 2019 article.

Through interviews with women conducted in 2015, researchers Arachu Castro and Virginia Savage documented several forms of obstetric violence in public maternity hospitals in the Dominican Republic (Castro and Savage 2019; Castro 2019). Arachu Castro (2019:109) argued that:

> physicians and nurses learn to operate within the structural limitations of health care systems by not assuming the responsibility of the continuum of care that each woman needs, and . . . this discharge of accountability is at the heart of how health professionals can navigate, tolerate, and perpetuate the structure of the system and, in so doing, create the breeding ground for obstetric violence to occur.

In 2019, an observational study with a statistically representative sample of 275 births, conducted in two public Dominican hospitals, found 117 incidents of verbal violence and 24 incidents of physical violence (A. Castro 2020). The most frequent forms of verbal violence included: the pregnant or postpartum woman or girl received negative comments about her ethnicity, skin color, or other physical characteristics; was scolded or blamed for her or her newborn's health; was yelled at, made fun of, or was called names; and was threatened with physical violence, use of a procedure, or failure to care for her or the baby. The most frequent forms of physical violence included: the pregnant or puerperal woman or girl was pinched, gagged, pressed against the bed with force, or slapped, beaten, or pressed hard on her abdomen.

Based on this previous research, and due to the little we knew about the lived experiences of obstetrician/gynecologists (ob/gyns) and other hospital personnel in the Dominican Republic, we set out to understand their perspectives on the concept of obstetric violence and their justifications for why it occurs. In this chapter, we present these perspectives and discuss how they have been shaped and reinforced, and could be reshaped in the future.

Methods: Approaching Hospital Personnel about Obstetric Violence and Other Aspects of Mistreatment in Maternity Care

We conducted the qualitative study on which this chapter is based as part of a larger mixed-methods study, *Proyecto Mujer al Centro* (PMAC), or the "Women at the Center" project, named for the study's emphasis on patient-centered and humanized care. Arachu Castro initiated PMAC in 2015 in the Dominican Republic and is expanding the project to other Latin American countries in collaboration with the Health Equity Network of the Americas, with the goals of documenting, raising awareness about, and eliminating obstetric violence (A. Castro et al. 2021). In May 2019, we obtained approval from the Ministry of Public Health of the Dominican Republic and the Dominican National Health Service to conduct the study. In consultation with leaders from these institutions and from UNICEF Dominican Republic, we selected three public hospitals as study sites: the national reference maternity hospital and the regional reference maternity hospital in the capital city of Santo Domingo, and a public general hospital in San Cristobal—a town an hour west of Santo Domingo. In 2019, the two public maternity hospitals attended an average of 871 and 832 births per month respectively, and the public general hospital attended an average of 331 (Ministry of Public Health of the Dominican Republic 2019). All three hospitals serve primarily low-income women, as well as a mix of Dominican and Haitian women; 38%, 31%, and 8% of births respectively were among women of Haitian descent (Ministry of Public Health of the Dominican Republic 2019). The directors of the three hospitals authorized the study. In June 2019, Tulane University's Institutional Review Board approved the study.

We developed a semi-structured guide for the individual interviews based on the objective of understanding hospital personnel's perspectives on obstetric violence and why it occurs. The interviews began with short narratives that described cases of maternal mortality in Santo Domingo that had been previously collected by Arachu Castro (2019). We asked clinicians and hospital staff to read to themselves two to six narratives (depending on time) and answer follow-up questions about the cases. We then asked opened-ended questions about standard admissions, surgical and consent procedures, characteristics of positive and negative patient-provider relationships, characteristics of patient-centered care, forms of mistreatment, why mistreatment occurs, and how to define obstetric violence. Finally, we shared excerpts from a 2016 Dominican Ministry of Public Health guideline that called for preventing obstetric violence in maternity care for adolescents (Ministry of Public Health of the Dominican Republic 2016). We asked clinicians and hospital staff to discuss their thoughts about the guideline and why the Dominican health ministry was calling attention to this issue.

We strategically ordered our interview questions to promote candid discussions with the clinicians and hospital staff and to help them feel comfortable talking about mistreatment and obstetric violence, which can be sensitive topics for clinicians to discuss. To prevent the interviews from being interpreted as interrogations, we first asked about the issues that we perceived to be the most benign—such as admissions processes or common surgical procedures—and gradually led to the questions about obstetric violence toward the end of each interview.

We conducted these interviews during July and August 2019; Annie Preaux led the study's coordination and conducted most of the interviews. At each hospital, administrative personnel helped us identify and approach potential study participants. We selected participants to obtain representation from six groups: ob/gyns, residents in ob/gyn, physicians from other specialties, licensed nurses, auxiliary nurses, and administrative personnel. Administrative personnel included staff from human resources, security, reception, laundry services, and secretaries; we included them because they interact with patients even though they are not trained to interact and build rapport with patients. For example, without any training to do so, the *wachimán*, or security guard, conducts the first line of triage for women who arrive at public hospitals' emergency areas (Castro and Savage 2019). Unlike other countries, the Dominican Republic does not have professional nurse-midwives; the nursing specialty in maternal and neonatal health only began in 2020.

All participants received information about the PMAC study and provided verbal consent to participate in the interview and to record the audio of the interview. For participants who did not consent to be recorded, we wrote detailed notes about the interview. In total, we conducted 92 interviews across the three hospitals. We present the study sample by professional category and hospital in Table 1.1.

After each interview, we uploaded the recordings and transcribed them ourselves or used NVivo's automated transcription software. We listened to the interviews and read the transcripts several times to inform and develop a table to populate with data from each interview, creating a summary of each interview, including illustrative quotes. From these summary tables, we identified the key themes that emerged from the data.

How Clinicians and Hospital Staff Define Mistreatment and Obstetric Violence

We asked clinicians and hospital staff to describe mistreatment (*maltrato*) of women in maternity care before asking them about obstetric violence. Their responses were similar to the responses provided by women who had just given birth in two of the three public maternity hospitals in the Dominican Republic (Castro and Savage 2019). Health-

Table 1.1. Study Sample by Clinical and Staff Categories and Hospital. ©Annie Preaux and Arachu Castro.

	National Maternity Hospital	Regional Maternity Hospital	Provincial General Hospital	Total
Obstetrician-Gynecologists	5	4	7	16
Attending physicians from other specialties	0	0	2	2
Residents in obstetrics-gynecology	7	11	4	22
Licensed nurses	5	8	9	22
Auxiliary nurses	6	6	3	15
Administrative personnel	6	5	4	15
Total	29	34	29	92

care personnel's responses included engaging in physical and verbal abuse, conducting a medical procedure without consent, neglecting or ignoring patients, discriminating against them, showing lack of empathy, denying care, delaying the provision of care, and experiencing resource shortages. In Figure 1.1, we share example responses from clinicians and hospital staff who defined mistreatment.

Forty-eight clinicians and hospital staff said they were familiar with the term "obstetric violence" and were willing to discuss the concept and define what they thought it meant. Of the participants who were not familiar with the concept of obstetric violence, 27 were willing to try to define this concept. In general, they perceived "obstetric violence" to be the same as "mistreatment." Healthcare providers and staff who shared detailed definitions of obstetric violence commonly described physical abuse, verbal and psychological abuse, conducting a medical procedure without consent, neglecting or ignoring patients, discriminating against them, and denying care. Compared to responses about mistreatment, many clinicians and hospital staff also talked about obstetric violence in ways that were more abstract. These more abstract descriptions included obstetric violence as a violation of women's rights, a form of disrespect, the treatment of women as though they were not human,

---

The force that you use with her so that she can give birth in the event that she doesn't want to.

– Licensed nurse, female

Verbal mistreatment when sometimes you say bad words to her, even physical mistreatment…it's not that we hit patients here but sometimes they are placed in a bed that doesn't have sheets.

– Ob/gyn, female

Denying their rights is mistreatment…Talking to them in an unfriendly tone. Raising your voice. Touching them inappropriately. Swearing at them…When the woman complains and you say to her "Ok, now it's hurting you, but when you were making the baby, it didn't hurt you." That's mistreatment.

– Ob/gyn, female

When they leave you there, when they just tell you "Oh, no, you have not dilated anymore," and then they do not pay any more attention to you, they only tell you to be quiet. That is mistreatment, when they don't take care of you.

– Hospital secretary, female

Figure 1.1. Illustrative quotes from clinicians and hospital staff to the question "What would you say is mistreatment of a woman during pregnancy, labor, and the postpartum period?" ©Annie Preaux and Arachu Castro.

and not following clinical recommendations. Given that the Ministry of Public Health of the Dominican Republic has published numerous evidence-based clinical norms for prenatal, childbirth, and postpartum care, we argue that not following them equates to knowingly providing substandard care and lacking accountability to those women and girls. In Figure 1.2, we share quotes that are illustrative of clinicians' definitions of obstetric violence.

Although the majority of clinicians and hospital staff were willing to talk about obstetric violence to some extent, including those who were unfamiliar with the concept, 12 participants were apprehensive or unwilling to define or discuss the concept. As one ob/gyn explained: "Maybe it's like mistreatment? . . . I couldn't tell you anything with respect to obstetric violence." Some even rejected the need to discuss the issue and denied the possibility of mistreatment or violence occurring in healthcare facilities, most especially the ones in which they worked.

Clinicians and Hospital Staff Explain Why Mistreatment and Obstetric Violence Occur

I'd compare obstetric violence to gender-based violence. I imagine it would be the violence perpetrated against a patient in a maternity ward, against a pregnant patient as a result of her condition.

– Plastic surgeon, male

When a doctor wants the woman to give birth before she is ready, to force her to give birth.

– Ob/gyn in an administrative role, female

Any physical, verbal, or psychological abuse that a healthcare professional in obstetrics does to a patient during pregnancy or in the puerperal period.

– 4th year resident, male

When the doctor is attending, he takes the patient roughly, he doesn't speak to her correctly, he doesn't treat her gently. That is violence. To raise your voice at a patient to make her cooperate during the birth. That is violence.

– Auxiliary nurse, female

I think obstetric violence is when you don't comply with the rules, with the medical standards.

– Auxiliary nurse, female

Figure 1.2. Illustrative quotes from clinicians to the question "What is obstetric violence?" © Annie Preaux and Arachu Castro.

The clinicians and hospital staff who were willing to discuss and define mistreatment and obstetric violence also explained why these events occur in maternity wards. Even those who were unwilling to discuss these topics directly explained the characteristics of positive and negative patient-provider relationships. Their responses can be grouped into four categories to explain why mistreatment occurs: (1) blaming women for being uncooperative; (2) blaming women for misinterpreting clinicians' actions; (3) healthcare providers' lack of empathy, humanization, people-centeredness, and sense of vocation; and (4) institutional factors.

Blaming "Uncooperative" Women as the Primary Cause of Obstetric Violence

Clinicians and hospital staff frequently explained that negative patient-provider relationships, mistreatment, and obstetric violence were the results of women not collaborating with their care team or complying with their instructions and orders. Some blamed women for being violent and aggressive during labor or said that their colleagues blamed women for their inability to comply. Many healthcare providers also described women's noncompliance as an inconvenience for clinicians and a source of frustration:

> A good patient-provider relationship is when you communicate with the patient, and of course, the patient also listens and understands, because there are many rebellious patients who do not understand or do not like to listen to the doctor. That can bring a lot of inconvenience. (Second-year resident in obstetrics, female)

> There are patients who are so very irritating, really, very irritating, there is no way to reason with them, sometimes because of the language barrier, for cultural reasons, although that is not an excuse. (Ob/gyn, female)

"Noncompliance" and "aggression" were frequently attributed to women with certain sociodemographic characteristics, such as their socioeconomic position, education, age, parity, or being Haitian. As one female ob/gyn described:

> A good relationship could be when the patient speaks the same language, that the patient is interested in helping in everything that the doctor says. The same language because, as you will learn, almost all the Haitian patients do not speak Spanish. They have a different mentality. Many times, we indicate an analysis, sonography, all for

free here, and many times they do not do it . . . A patient who cares more about her checkups would be good. One where you indicate vitamins, some test, and she meets all the requirements. Here that is not the case. Here it is very difficult. First the difference in language, second that they do their part.

Other healthcare providers and staff said that although lack of collaboration or compliance was an important cause of mistreatment, clinicians were the ones who were responsible for fostering a positive relationship with their patients and creating an environment in which women trust their providers and feel safe during labor. As a female ob/gyn put it:

The patient is going to be safe, going to feel safe, she is not going to have that despair that occurs sometimes because they don't know what is happening, because they don't know what awaits them. The patient during labor will be more collaborative because if we have prepared her properly, the patient already knows what we are going to do and what she is going to face. The immediate postpartum period will also be more positive for the patient, she will be more receptive to her baby.

Many clinicians and hospital staff said that positive patient-provider relationships depended on clinicians' abilities to guide, educate, connect with, and communicate with patients to build rapport or increase women's confidence in their healthcare providers. Although establishing rapport, building a patient's trust, and preparing a patient for labor are positive and important responsibilities of clinicians, some of them still perceived women as uncooperative or non-collaborative during labor.

When educating the patient and connecting with the patient fail, some clinicians turn to physical and verbal abuse to force patients to comply during labor and birth. Some clinicians and hospital staff described women's lack of compliance as a source of frustration for healthcare providers, and others explained that the use of force or other forms of mistreatment when women do not cooperate was not merely an act of frustration, but a necessary action to save the woman and her child:

The doctor despairs, they don't know how to control the situation and can only say offensive things to [the woman]. (Third-year resident in obstetrics, female)

Women at this time are in a moment of stress, anxiety, and many times they behave in ways that you might not want them to. And if you don't know how to cope with that, you are going to attack them with words or actions or gestures. (Second-year resident in obstetrics, male)

Sometimes there are patients who do not want to open their legs . . . they don't cooperate . . . Because of this the doctor gets aggressive because what they want is to save them . . . A nurse has to grab her here, another nurse has to grab her to hold her . . . This is a negative action, but you have to do it because if you don't, they'll die. (Licensed nurse, female)

The clinicians and hospital staff who discussed this issue clarified that, even in these instances, mistreatment was inexcusable—yet it still occurs.

Women Misinterpret Clinicians' Actions as Violence

In addition to explaining how women's actions may lead to mistreatment and to justifying the acts that lead to obstetric violence in maternity wards to "save the life" of the woman or child, as previously noted, some clinicians and hospital staff denied the existence of obstetric violence in their hospitals. In these cases, obstetric violence was explained as a "misunderstanding" on the part of the women seeking care in these hospitals. As one female ob/gyn put it, "Here we almost never mistreat patients. Here we do not use mistreatment. Maybe if the patients feel mistreated it is because there was a large volume of patients and they had to wait. Do you understand? They could feel mistreated." Essentially, some clinicians and hospital staff believed that patients *felt* mistreated, but that no mistreatment had actually occurred:

One patient reported me for mistreatment and discrimination based on having HIV. I think the patients get a little sensitive if they think you are talking about them. If you say, "Don't put her in a bed with the others," she thinks it is because of her HIV status, and she feels mistreated. One or two patients have complained about me for this. (Ob/gyn, female)

That is, some clinicians tried to explain how women's complaints of mistreatment were a misunderstanding or an overreaction.

Lacking Empathy, Humanization, People-Centeredness, and Vocation

Many healthcare workers explained that negative patient-provider relationships and mistreatment result from a lack of empathy (an ability to "put yourself in the patient's shoes"), humanization, people-centered-ness, and vocation in the delivery of health care:

> You should look after the patient and with a good manner because you don't know what else they have going on. (Auxiliary nurse, female)

> Everything we do should be "pro-patient." For the benefit of the patient and her baby. Everything for her benefit. (Ob/gyn, female)

The clinicians and hospital staff explained that some providers do not know how to empathize with their patients' fears and stresses, resolve crises nonviolently, leave their own problems at home when they arrive at work, or provide people-centered care.

Several clinicians and hospital staff described colleagues who were trained to be doctors but simply did not have the vocation—the call-ing—necessary to do their work well: "They only work for money. Now there is no vocation, vocation to service. It's disappearing." Many of them used the word vocation (*vocación*) directly, while others described colleagues who had a "lack of love" or mistreated patients because of "who they are":

> The ones that have a vocation love their work and love what they do and love who they work with. If you have a vocation to work with people, you are going to love people . . . That is why there are good people who are good doctors, excellent doctors, and then there are others who are doctors or specialists in many areas, but nobody looks for them because of the way they speak, their way of treating patients. So, I think it is the vocation . . . if you do not have a voca-tion, you aren't going to love what you do. (Auxiliary nurse, female)

Lacking the vocation to be a doctor was a characteristic associated with obstetricians who disrespect or mistreat patients to maintain power and control.

Based on the interviews, we found that clinicians' quality of medi-cal training was another reason why they might mistreat patients. As a female licensed nurse explained: "They have the medical training, but as people, they lack maturity." However, there was some debate about whether vocation, training, or both affected mistreatment and the qual-ity of patient-provider relationships:

> It has a lot to do with how the person is. There was a case that I saw that they were mistreating a patient . . . I told them, "Don't talk to

them like that, that's a human being!" This has a lot do with the person, their upbringing as a person, and their training as a doctor. (Ob/gyn, female)

They don't know the Hippocratic Oath. They don't know it, or they know it, but they don't put it into practice. (Ob/gyn, female)

For some clinicians and hospital staff, the vocation to be a doctor was separate from biomedical training, while others suggested that both training and vocation were important factors determining whether or not patients were mistreated.

Institutional Factors

Several clinicians and hospital staff perceived that institutional factors and resource shortages such as a lack of beds, blood donations, and running water contributed to mistreatment. Healthcare providers explained that these issues caused them to be stressed and overworked. As a result of these shortages, some said that not only are women mistreated, but also they felt mistreated themselves.

The system for accessing blood in public hospitals in the Dominican Republic is symbolic of this issue. Even when a woman needs a lifesaving procedure that requires blood, clinicians may withhold care until her family brings a replacement blood donation (Castro 2019). Among the healthcare providers and staff who discussed blood donations, some identified the issue as a healthcare system problem. Others, however, blamed women and their families for not knowing that they need to bring blood or for not bringing it—disregarding the fact that families who bring blood need to pay the blood screening tests, which can be unaffordable for those living in poverty.

The Shaping and Reinforcement of Obstetric Violence

In public Dominican hospitals, clinicians can escape being held responsible for their actions with relative ease and can reconcile with the negative, and potentially fatal, consequences of perpetrating obstetric violence against women during pregnancy, childbirth, or the postpartum period (Castro 2019). One ob/gyn commented, "In the private sector, if you do certain things, you'll lose your patients. Here we don't lose patients. There's more impunity . . . It happens because there are no sanctions." Other healthcare providers and staff interviewed were aware of this issue. These characteristics of the healthcare system may discourage the sense of personal responsibility among clinicians to question and critique their own work.

All ob/gyns, residents, and nurses interviewed explained that it was highly uncommon for the ob/gyns or nurses to know the patients from prior prenatal visits, even though many women receive prenatal care in the same hospital where they give birth (Castro 2019). Clinicians explained that ob/gyns work in a rotation, sharing the responsibility of providing prenatal care by taking shifts for periods of time in the consultation area of the hospital. One female ob/gyn in an administrative role explained this system—and its consequences:

> Here, there are people that come, and they have been to eight prenatal visits, and it's never the same doctor. It's not the same one. I am saying that today I see them in a check-up and the next time someone else sees them, and the next. You see five, six different doctors. How can you have enough trust to tell them "I've had a fever for 15 days, I have a vaginal infection" . . . Today I see you, and I do your medical history, and I show empathy with you, but you are not ever going to see me again. And then another doctor comes and checks you in a month and I can't ask that they know you . . . She doesn't know you.

By chance, an ob/gyn may recognize a woman from prenatal care when she arrives to give birth, but that is unlikely. Additionally, her clinical history may be incomplete or filled with predetermined values (Castro 2019)—that is, with values for vital signs and other health indicators that are written down in the clinical history but that are invented because they have not actually been taken. These factors may preclude the provision of high-quality follow-up care.

Once a woman is admitted to the hospital to give birth, her care team continues to change. During her stay, she transfers between hospital departments—from the emergency department to delivery, to recovery, and sometimes to surgery or to the intensive care unit. Each time, new doctors, new residents, and new nurses attend to her care without having a designated provider who assumes responsibility for the continuum of care that each woman needs, and "the responsibility for the management of each woman is so diffused that nobody seems to be in charge" (Castro 2019:109), particularly in cases of maternal deaths, as illustrated in the narrative above. In truth, the public healthcare system and its institutions, as well as sexist constructs that assign inferior characteristics to women, hinder clinicians from feeling as though they have a duty to deliver high-quality respectful care to women and, when something goes wrong, from questioning what they could do differently to improve their practices.

Women themselves may unintentionally reinforce clinicians' beliefs that the quality of maternity care is good even when obstetric violence is present. Castro and Savage have identified this as an adaptive preference of women, who may downplay their negative experiences at the hospital and accept obstetric violence as part of routine care because they do not have the option to seek care elsewhere (Castro and Savage 2019). Sara Cohen Shabot (2019) has also identified this issue of women being made to doubt their own experiences with violence and has described it as a form of "gaslighting"—meaning to cause a person to doubt their sanity by using psychological manipulation. As women doubt their own experiences and accept obstetric violence, clinicians continue working and mistreating women with impunity.

Some providers see this "gaslighting" as women realizing that their clinicians were right all along, as a female third-year resident in ob/gyn explained:

> There are many patients that, at the end of labor, they thank their doctor because even though the pain stopped them from behaving their best, they understand that the doctor was there the whole time to support them and help them. In the end, they recognize that the doctor is good . . . They thank [the doctor] for their help.

Several obstetricians used the phrase *somos los que sabemos* ("we are the ones who know"). Through a process of gaslighting and stoking doubt in their patients, clinicians avoid holding themselves responsible for obstetric violence, and healthcare system administrators miss out on opportunities to improve the quality of care in maternity hospitals.

In the Dominican public hospitals where we conducted our study, clinicians are trained and work within a context that condones and perpetuates obstetric violence and poor relationships between women and their clinicians as part of their habitus (Bourdieu 1977). Their habitus represents "a cognitive space where group perceptions live, a space that they inhabit" (Premkumar 2023:16). In other words, structural aspects of the healthcare system are embedded in how healthcare providers think and act, often unconsciously. Ximena Briceño Morales, Laura Victoria Enciso Chaves, and Carlos Enrique Yepes Delgado (2018) have described this phenomenon through their work in Colombia, where clinicians are not "violent by nature," yet they perpetrate obstetric violence. In the field of nursing, Oscar Alberto Beltrán-Salazar, whose work also takes place in Colombia, has explained the process through which clinicians' behaviors are shaped by considering "the influence of three spheres: the first, the social and legislative context; the second, the regulations regulating the healthcare institutions; and finally, the relationships of patients and nurses. The first two establish the rules of the game for care; the third is actually the path for its undertaking." (2014:195).

Making the connection between the habitus of obstetric practitioners—the conceptual space in which they think and act—and obstetric violence, Briceño Morales, Enciso Chaves, and Yepes Delgado (2018:1308) explain how providers act in a social environment that promotes power relationships and in "healthcare [systems] whose political and economic foundations encourage inequality."

Engaging Clinicians and Hospital Staff to Eliminate Obstetric Violence

Eliminating obstetric violence requires policy and systems-level changes that address this issue as a form of structural violence (Castro, Savage, and Kaufman 2015; Sadler et al. 2016; Miller et al. 2016). Since the 1990s, activists in the Latin American and Caribbean region have been leaders in defining the concept of obstetric violence and in addressing the issue in the policy sphere (Bowser and Hill 2010; Savage and Castro 2017). Efforts exist to change the hegemonic biomedical model of care, promote humanized and rights-based care, and decrease obstetric violence, such as, for example, public policy for humanized care in Peru (Polo Campos et al. 2017). There are also efforts to promote humanized care among nurses in neonatal units in Brazil (Pontes Ferreira, Freitas do Amaral, and Oliveira Lopes 2016), and among Brazilian obstetricians and certain hospitals in that country (see Davis-Floyd and Georges, this volume).

However, despite policy level changes and institutional efforts, clinicians are ultimately responsible for delivering care (Moretti-Pires and Bueno 2009). Therefore, they need to take a central role in embarking on a process of becoming critical of their own work to reinvent maternity care to be equitable, just, and free from obstetric violence—even if they may at first be apprehensive to identify the issue (Ratcliffe et al. 2016), as to name something is to give it more power that it can otherwise hold.

Paulo Freire's (1970) and Robbie Davis-Floyd's (2018) concepts of "humanization" can support the education and training of clinicians to match the ideals and principles of humanized care (Moretti-Pires and Bueno 2009; Bowser and Hill 2010; Davis-Floyd 2018, 2022; see also the Introduction to this volume). Tying in the concept of "habitus," Freire's framework is an opportunity to create a much-needed consciousness-raising process among providers that could expand the medical habitus and transform it from what Roberto Castro (2014) calls the "authoritative medical habitus" to a habitus that is humanized and patient-centered. With this in mind, clinicians and hospital staff's comments about vocation, "lack of love," and providers who perpetrated obstetric violence because of "who they are" stand out as evidence that many clinicians are relatively unaware of their own medical habitus and how it has been shaped by the healthcare system and by institutional policies, biomedical training, and social beliefs that lead to discrimination against women for their ethnicity, age, class, education, parity, and for being women. In Davis-Floyd's terms (see Davis-Floyd's [2023] chapter on "Open and Closed Knowledge Systems, the 4 Stages of Cognition, and the Obstetric Management of Birth" in Volume II of this series [Davis-Floyd and Premkumar 2023] and the Introduction to this volume), such "unaware" clinicians are Stage 1 naïve realists who believe that "our way is the only way"—or "the only way that matters."

The clinicians and hospital staff whom we interviewed identified troubling examples of obstetric violence and other healthcare system flaws, and many of them were aware of the major problems for women who seek care in public maternity hospitals. Recognizing the issues that women face may be the first step for clinicians toward addressing obstetric violence in their own practices and within the systems in which they work and receive training. Although adminstrative personnel, security guards, and maintenance workers do not care for women directly, they may—and frequently do—come into contact with women during their pregnancies and births. Therefore, such non-clinical personnel also have opportunities to have meaningful impacts on the quality of women's care.

As we call for a consciousness-raising process among ob/gyns and other personnel to engage in self-critique and to reimagine their own practices, we also encourage researchers to engage with clinicians and hospital staff on the issue of obstetric violence. During our study, we contributed to this process through our conversations with clinicians and hospital staff, some of whom were introduced to the concept of obstetric violence for the very first time. Only awareness of a problem can lead to finding solutions to address it.

Acknowledgments

This research was funded by UNICEF Dominican Republic and by the Samuel Z. Stone Endowed Chair of Public Health in Latin America at Tulane University held by Arachu Castro. We thank Sarah Kington, Charyl Adams, Natalia Ramírez, and Yosarah Olivo for their help with conducting some of the interviews and Michaela Gerace for revising some of the transcripts.

Annie Preaux is a PhD candidate at the Tulane University School of Public Health and Tropical Medicine. She also has an MPH in International Health and Development from Tulane. Her main interests are maternal and child health and health equity, particularly in Latin America and the Caribbean. In addition to this work in the Dominican Republic, she has worked on projects related to COVID-19, and child marriage, community violence, and adolescent pregnancy in Ciudad Juarez, Mexico, and community-based health services in Indigenous communities in the Ecuadorian Amazon. She has also worked as a research assistant for the Collaborative Group for Health Equity in Latin America at Tulane and with the High Impact Practices in Family Planning team within the Office of Population and Reproductive Health at USAID through the STAR program.

Arachu Castro is the Samuel Z. Stone Chair of Public Health in Latin America and Director of the Collaborative Group for Health Equity in Latin America at the Tulane University School of Public Health and Tropical Medicine. She received a Guggenheim Fellowship in 2010 based on her work throughout Latin America and the Caribbean on reproductive and maternal health and infectious diseases. She is a member of the World Health Organization Strategic and Technical Advisory Group of Experts for Maternal, Newborn, Child, Adolescent Health & Nutrition; the Executive Committee of the Health Equity Network of the Americas; the Executive Committee of the Sustainable Health Equity Movement; and the International Advisory Panel of the International Professional Practices Framework (IPPF). She is the former President of the Society for Medical Anthropology.

References

Beltrán-Salazar OA. 2014. "Las Instituciones de Salud No Favorecen el Cuidado: Significado del Cuidado Humanizado para las Personas que Participan Directamente en él" [Healthcare Institutions Do Not Favor Care: Meaning of Humanized Care for People Directly Participating in It]. *Investigación y Educación en Enfermería* 32(2): 194–205.

Bourdieu P. 1977. *Outline of a Theory of Practice*. Translated by R. Nice, *Cambridge Studies in Social and Cultural Anthropology*. Cambridge: Cambridge University Press.

Bowser D, Hill K. 2010. *Exploring Evidence for Disrespect and Abuse in Facility-Based Childbirth: Report of a Landscape Analysis.* Boston: Harvard School of Public Health. https://cdn2.sph.harvard.edu/wp-content/uploads/sites/32/2014/05/Exploring-Evidence-RMC_Bowser_rep_2010.pdf.

Briceño Morales X, Enciso Chaves LV, Yepes Delgado CE. 2018. "Neither Medicine Nor Health Care Staff Members Are Violent by Nature: Obstetric Violence from an Interactionist Perspective." *Qualitative Health Research* 28(8): 1308–1319.

Castro A. 2019. "Witnessing Obstetric Violence during Fieldwork: Notes from Latin America." *Health and Human Rights* 21(1): 103–111.

———. 2020. *Violencia Obstétrica en la República Dominicana: Estudio Epidemiológico Observacional Realizado en Dos Hospitales Públicos* [Obstetric Violence in the Dominican Republic: Observational Epidemiological Study Conducted in Two Public Hospitals]. Santo Domingo: UNICEF.

Castro A, Sáenz R, Avellaneda X, et al. 2021. "The Health Equity Network of the Americas: Inclusion, Commitment, and Action." *Revista Panamerican Salud Publica* 45: e79. https://www.ncbi.nlm.nih.gov/pubmed/34220991.

Castro A, Savage V. 2019. "Obstetric Violence as Reproductive Governance in the Dominican Republic." *Medical Anthropology* 38(2): 123–136.

Castro A, Savage V, Kaufman H. 2015. "Assessing Equitable Care for Indigenous and Afrodescendant Women in Latin America." *Revista Panamericana de Salud Pública* 38: 96–109. https://pubmed.ncbi.nlm.nih.gov/26581050/.

Castro R. 2014. "Génesis y Práctica del Habitus Médico Autoritario en México." *Revista Mexicana de Sociología* 76(2): 167–197. https://www.jstor.org/stable/43495722.

Cohen Shabot S. 2019. "'Amigas, Sisters: We're Being Gaslighted': Obstetric Violence and Epistemic Injustice." In *Childbirth, Vulnerability and Law: Exploring Issues of Violence and Control*, eds. Pickles C, Herring J. Abingdon, Oxon: Routledge. https://www.taylorfrancis.com/chapters/edit/10.4324/9780429443718-2/amigas-sisters-re-being-gaslighted-sara-cohen-shabot

Davis-Floyd R. 2018. "The Technocratic, Humanistic, and Holistic Paradigms of Birth and Health Care." In *Ways of Knowing About Birth: Mothers, Midwives, Medicine, and Birth Activism*, Davis-Floyd R and Colleagues. Long Grove IL: Waveland Press, 3–44.

———. 2022. *Birth as an American Rite of Passage*, 3rd ed. Abingdon, Oxon: Routledge.

———. 2023. "Open and Closed Knowledge Systems, the 4 Stages of Cognition, and the Obstetric Management of Birth." In *Cognition, Risk, and Responsibility in Obstetrics: Anthropological Analyses and Critiques of Obstetricians Practices*, eds. Davis-Floyd R, Premkumar A, Chapter 1. New York: Berghahn Books.

Davis-Floyd R, Premkumar A, eds. 2023. *Cognition, Risk, and Responsibility in Obstetrics: Anthropological Analyses and Critiques of Obstetricians Practices*, eds. Davis-Floyd R, Premkumar A. New York: Berghahn Books.

Freire P. 1970. *Pedagogy of the Oppressed*. New York: Seabury Press.

GTR Regional Task Force for the Reduction of Maternal Mortality. 2017. *Overview of the Situation of Maternal Morbidity and Mortality: Latin America and the Caribbean*. Panama City: GTR Regional Task Force for the Reduction of Maternal Mortality. https://msh.org/wp-content/uploads/2018/09/msh-gtr-report-eng.pdf.

Miller S, Abalos E, Chamillard M, et al. 2016. "Beyond Too Little, Too Late and Too Much, Too Soon: A Pathway towards Evidence-Based, Respectful Maternity Care Worldwide." *Lancet* 388 (10056): 2176–2192.

Miller S, Cordero M, Coleman A, et al. 2003. "Quality of Care in Institutionalized Deliveries: The Paradox of the Dominican Republic." *International Journal of Gynecology & Obstetrics* 82(1): 89–103.

Ministry of Public Health of the Dominican Republic. 2016. *Protocolo de Atención para el Manejo Integral del Embarazo, sl Parto y el Puerperio en Adolescentes Menores de 15 Años* [Protocol of Attention for the Integral Management of Pregnancy, Childbirth, and Postpartum In Adolescents under the Age of 15]. Santo Domingo: Ministry of Public Health.

———. 2019. *Estadísticas de Producción de Servicios Hospitalarios de Enero-Diciembre 2019.* Santo Domingo: Ministry of Public Health. https://www.msp.gob.do/web/Transparencia/estadisticas-institucionales/#EIPSSS.

———. 2022. *Boletín Epidemiológico Semanal. Semana Epidemiológica Número 44.* Santo Domingo: Ministry of Public Health. https://digepi.gob.do/documentos-epidemiologicos/boletines-semanales/

Moretti-Pires RO, Bueno SMV. 2009. "Freire's Theoretical Framework and the Professional Capabilities of Nurses, Physicians, and Dentists for the Brazilian Universal Healthcare System." *Acta Paulista de Enfermagem* 22(4): 439–444.

Murray de López J. 2018. "When the Scars Begin to Heal: Narratives of Obstetric Violence in Chiapas, Mexico." *International Journal of Health Governance* 23(1): 60–69.

Polo Campos FH, Gollner Zeitoune RC, Rebaza Iparraguirre HA, et al. 2017. "Cuidado Humanizado como Política Pública: El Caso Peruano." *Escola Anna Nery* 21(2): 23–34.

Pontes Ferreira JH, Freitas do Amaral JJ, Oliveira Lopes MMC. 2016. "Nursing Team and Promotion of Humanized Care in a Neonatal Unit." *Revista da Rede de Enfermagem do Nordeste* 17(6): 741–749.

Premkumar A. 2023. "My Transformation from an Obstetrician to a Maternal-Fetal Medicine Subspecialist: Autoethnographic Thoughts on Situated Knowledges and Habitus." In *Obstetricians Speak: On Training, Practice, Fear, and Transformation,* eds. Davis-Floyd R, Premkumar A. Chapter 3. New York: Berghahn Books.

Ratcliffe HL, Sando D, Mwanyika-Sando M, et al. 2016. "Applying a Participatory Approach to the Promotion of a Culture of Respect during Childbirth." *Reproductive Health* 13(1): 80.

República Bolivariana de Venezuela. 2007. "Ley Orgánica Sobre el Derecho de las Mujeres a una Vida Libre de Violencia" [Organic Law on the Rights of Women to a Life Free of Violence]. Caracas, Venezuela: Gaceta Oficial de la República Boliviarana de Venezuela.

Sadler M, Santos MJDS, Ruiz-Berdún D, et al. 2016. "Moving beyond Disrespect and Abuse: Addressing the Structural Dimensions of Obstetric Violence." *Reproductive Health Matters* 24(47): 47–55.

Savage V, Castro A. 2017. "Measuring Mistreatment of Women During Childbirth: A Review of Terminology and Methodological Approaches." *Reproductive Health* 14(1): 138.

Tulane University and UNICEF. 2016. "Health Equity Report 2016: Analysis of Reproductive, Maternal, Newborn, Child and Adolescent Health Inequities in Latin America and the Caribbean to Inform Policymaking." Panama City, Panama. https://www.unicef.org/lac/media/386/file/Publication.pdf.

UNICEF, WHO. 2020. *UNICEF/WHO Joint Database on SDG 3.1.2 Skilled Attendance at Birth*. New York: UNICEF. https://data.unicef.org/topic/maternal-health/delivery-care/.

United Nations. 2019. Report of the Secretary-General on SDG Progress 2019: Special Edition. New York: United Nations. https://sustainabledevelopment.un.org/content/documents/24978Report_of_the_SG_on_SDG_Progress_2019.pdf.

WHO, UNICEF, UNFPA, World Bank Group, and UN Population Division. 2019. *Trends in Maternal Mortality*. Geneva: World Health Organization. https://data.unicef.org/resources/trends-maternal-mortality-2000-2017/.

CHAPTER 2

"Bad Pelvises"

Mexican Obstetricians and the Re-Affirmation of Race in Labor and Delivery

Sarah A. Williams

The "Too Small Pelvis"

"So I guess you'll want to hear about my births?" Malina asked, steering her rusted Toyota around the potholes in the dusty back streets of a small town in the Yucatán peninsula with a casual hand while rotating her heavily pregnant torso to give a piece of bread to her 18-month-old daughter. I was surprised to learn that Malina, a young Mexican woman who was dear friends with the midwives with whom I worked, and one of the birth clinic's strongest and most vocal supporters, had not always been a proponent of midwifery care and home births. Rather, she told me, when she first learned she was pregnant with her daughter, she and her husband had immediately started looking for an affordable and trustworthy doctor in a private clinic, as they preferred not to use public healthcare options.

They found their doctor in Cancun and began to attend prenatal appointments there each month. To their dismay, their doctor told them at 12 weeks that, due to her ancestry, Malina's hips were too narrow and the fetus too large to birth naturally, and he informed them that he would schedule her for a cesarean birth at 40 weeks. Malina and her husband were devastated, as they really wanted a vaginal birth and to avoid surgery. Where before they had been eagerly awaiting the arrival of their firstborn, now Malina was dreading the pending birth. As the weeks went by, she began to have nightmares about the surgery. At 37 weeks, she told her doctor that she wanted to cancel the cesarean and try to deliver vaginally. He convinced her to come in for another prenatal appointment, where he palpated her belly and told her that the baby was breech and that Mexican law required her to have a cesarean.[1]

Malina scowled, remembering how she had felt at that appointment. She pulled the car off the highway and put it into park, then turned to face me. "I was so scared and frustrated, and it seemed so clear that he was lying to make more money, but what could I do? I didn't know how to tell if she was breech or not on my own!" Malina and her husband debated what to do for the next two weeks. During that time, Malina began to ask around to friends and family to see if there were other options. One of those friends referred her to a local *partera empírica* (empirical midwife—one who learned midwifery in an apprenticeship with other midwives) and birth house (*casa de parto*—the Mexican term for "freestanding birth center"). She arrived at the gate the next day, without calling ahead, and was immensely relieved when the midwife finished examining her and pronounced the baby to be in perfect cephalic presentation. Malina skipped her scheduled cesarean without bothering to contact the doctor and went into labor a few days later. Her baby was born without complications or the need for any interventions. Malina has since come to consider herself a near-victim of obstetric violence and avoided visiting an ob/gyn during her second pregnancy and birth in favor of midwifery care.

Malina's experience of prenatal care is representative of many stories I have heard from pregnant women and mothers in Yucatán and Quintana Roo over the past ten years—this framing of their bodies, particularly their pelvises, as "too small," "malformed," or "too fragile" to birth vaginally. Obstetricians usually pair these criticisms with descriptions of the fetus as "too large," even at stages of pregnancy in which the fetus is still only the size of a nectarine. These diagnostic labels of the "malformed pelvis" or the "too-large fetus" are particularly important in light of broader patterns of obstetric interventions in Mexico.

Methodology

This chapter is based on ethnographic fieldwork conducted in the Mexican states of Quintana Roo, Yucatán, and Chiapas from 2009 to 2019 in seven fieldwork periods. I conducted interviews with professional and traditional midwives, obstetricians, clients and families, and nurses, and also conducted participant observations of Secretariat of Health Midwifery Program meetings, midwives' meetings and activist organizing, childbirth education classes at hospitals and birth houses, and home births and births in freestanding birth centers. This chapter draws on those observations, and on data collected from 15 interviews in 2009 and 2010, and 52 interviews in 2016–2019. This project was conducted under ethics approval from the University of Toronto (Protocol Reference #33164).

Cesarean Births in Mexico

Mexico is notable for its exceptionally high cesarean birth (CB) rate, which reached a pinnacle as the second highest in the world in 2010, sending waves of concern through the reproductive health community and government healthcare systems (Uribe-Leitz et al. 2019). A 2012 National Institute of Public Health survey found that between 2007 and 2012, 46% of the births in Mexico for which there were records were via cesarean—a statistic that is more than double the recommended rates set by the Official Mexican Standards (Secretaria de Salud 2012), which are themselves higher than the international standards set by the World Health Organization for that time period. Studies following the introduction of changes to the Official Mexican Standards in 2014 intended to curtail the use of medically unnecessary cesarean births (CBs) found that the CB rate dipped for approximately one year, but climbed steadily back up in the following years (Uribe-Leitz et al. 2019). Analyses of CBs in Mexico have found that, overall, private hospital facilities and urban hospitals have the highest percentages of CBs, with significant variation between states. For example, the cesarean birth (CB) rate in private hospitals in Nuevo Leon in 2017 was 83%, while in Chiapas, a much poorer and more rural state, it was 31% (Uribe-Leitz et al. 2019). Tarsicio Uribe-Leitz, Alejandra Barrero-Castillero, Arturo Cervantes-Trejo, and colleagues (2019) calculated the rates using birth certificates from 2014–2017, and found the national CB rate to be 45.3% on average in those years and increasing.

Thus, despite two decades of public and private mobilization, adjusted clinical recommendations, and NGO and governmental interventions, we can see that Mexico's CB rate remains extremely high. Scholarly and professional explanations for the perseverance of high rates of medically unnecessary cesarean births range from ob/gyn attempts to mitigate risk through interventions (Castro et al. 2003) to the financial incentives for both public and private sector ob/gyns (Vega et al. 2015) to the "hidden curriculum" of obstetric practice (Dixon, Smith-Oka, and El Kotni 2019) to institutional underfunding and physician overwork (FEMECOG 2015; Freyermuth, Muños, and Ochoa

2017). While all these explanations are indeed factors in a very complex situation, I propose that we can also read the culture of Mexican obstetric overreliance on cesareans through the lenses many ob/gyns apply to their clients' bodies: the perception of so many pregnant and birthing peoples' bodies as inherently and permanently unable to birth vaginally due to "malformations" of their pelvises.

In this chapter, I trace contemporary framings of Mexican women's pelvises as faulty back to the emergence of Mexican obstetrics and gynecology practice in the 1800s, and demonstrate their origins in the race-making discourses of eugenics and *mestizaje* (see below). I propose that these framings remain in part because Mexican biomedical obstetrics is heavily informed by eugenic philosophies passed down through the medical education system and informal mentorship. The "half-life" of eugenics is thus far longer than anticipated, and eugenics is the pool in which Mexican ob/gyns swim. Ultimately, I argue that the cesarean crisis in Mexico endures because legal and governmental interventions have not addressed the role of the "hidden curriculum" of clinical practice and mentorship in enculturating ob/gyns into attitudes and practices rooted in race science and eugenics.

The Emergence of Obstetric Violence in Mexico

Within the framing of obstetric violence, there are three main areas of abuse related to cesarean births. The first, of course, is the performance of a cesarean on a birthing person without consent. The second is the use of medically unnecessary cesareans, arguably the most common form of obstetric violence in Mexico. Third, I also consider cesareans to be intricately related to another form of obstetric violence—forced sterilizations. In Mexico, as in many other countries, CBs can provide the opportunity for ob/gyns and structurally racist biomedical institutions to perform sterilizations on Indigenous women, impoverished women, and other members of the population with little power. As scholars have noted (Smith-Oka 2009; Braff 2013), social, political, and medical pressures on all Mexican women, even the wealthy and privileged, to limit their fertility are intense and multifaceted. My own fieldwork in the states of Quintana Roo and Yucatán involved many interviews with Maya families who felt substantial pressure from their ob/gyns to be sterilized and to limit the number of children they had. These pressures are long-standing and have direct roots in the eugenics movement that began in the Porfiriato period (the period of time when Porfirio Díaz was President, 1876–1911), when the emerging disciplines of obstetrics and gynecology became intertwined with *Los Científicos*—privileged physician-researchers and scientists with connections to President Porfirio Díaz who worked for a vision of a modernized Mexico that was urban, non-Indigenous, and not held back by the supposed "burdens" of the poor, disabled, and non-white[2] (O'Brien 2012). Eugenicist ideologies were and, I argue, *are* integral to the practice of obstetrics and gynecology in Mexico, and provide ideological underpinnings to both the motivations and the justifications for pressuring women to have cesarean births or performing cesareans without consent.

By the late 1800s, Mexican ob/gyns were obsessed with the notion that the bodies—particularly the pelvises—of Indigenous women deviated significantly from those of their European-descendant peers (O'Brien 2012). Leaders in the emerging biomedical profession in Mexico City conducted case studies of women who birthed in public and teaching hospitals, arguing in dissertations and other publications that Indigenous women's pelvises were "backward and down-sloping"—failures of biological development that supposedly prevented such women from birthing successfully without physician intervention (O'Brien 2013). As Elizabeth O'Brien has noted, the terminology used to describe the pelvises of Indigenous women mirrors the disparaging language used by European-descendant Mexicans to describe Indigenous cultures as "unevolved" and "primitive."

While initially obstetricians claimed that they could identify "pure" Indigenous women by the shape of their pelvises, a short while later, obstetricians such as Florencio Flores and Francisco Flores argued that the miscegenation between Indigenous Mexicans and European colonists (and, though they are rarely acknowledged in Mexican writings or history, Africans and African descendants) had produced a uniquely Mexican "race": *mestizos* (people of mixed ethnic heritage, usually of both Spanish and Indigenous descent), identifiable through the "faults" in Mexican women's pelvises and cervixes, supposedly inherited from Indigenous ancestors. Conveniently for the budding profession of obstetrics, these uniquely Mexican physical "failures" necessitated careful management of birth by obstetricians, and surgical interventions to remove the baby from the inadequate body that refused to release it (Jaffary 2016:198). So integral to the newly emerging Mexican nation-state and identity was obstetrics—called *tocología Mexicana* (Mexican obstetrics) to distinguish it from other countries' emerging obstetric professions—that by 1880, obstetrics had its own separate school of medicine in Mexico City, distinct from other branches of medicine. Obstetricians were extremely powerful, not only for the usual reasons that they tended to come from upper-class urban families and were white, but also because obstetrics was viewed by politicians—including Porfirio Díaz—and the upper classes as critical to the development of a national identity based on race science. As Patricia Kelly (2008) observed in her ethnography of sex workers in the Mexican state of Chiapas, gynecologists in Mexico continue to wield an extraordinary amount of political and often juridical power, and frequently hold political positions that enable them to be the authors of legal codes governing the sexual and reproductive conduct of women in the contemporary era.

For all its founders' insistence that *tocología Mexicana* represented a distinct and uniquely Mexican form of obstetrics due to the supposedly distinct and uniquely Mexican female bodies it practiced upon, *tocología Mexicana* shared many key theoretical and ideological roots with emergent forms of gynecology in the United States and Europe. Like US gynecology, at its core, *tocología Mexicana* asserted that women's bodies—particularly the bodies of women of color—were inherently pathological, subject to unruly and chaotic (non-rational) functioning, and in dire need of upper-class white male medical management to ensure successful biological and cultural/national reproduction. In 1915, Mexico City obstetrician Dulque de Estrada asserted that all women who demonstrated "pelvic deficiency" should receive cesareans as a matter of course, even though at that time, cesarean survival was quite rare (O'Brien 2012). While early Mexican obstetricians were forbidden from experimenting on white upper-class women, and thus framed Indigenous and *mestiza* women as those particularly requiring interventions, as obstetric practice became more acceptable and less experimental in the early 1920s—while the "myth of *mestizaje*" (see below) simultaneously became more dominant—obstetricians eventually came to claim that virtually every birth required medical intervention due to the biological influence of Indigenous ancestry.

Even while *tocología Mexicana* was dependent on the national myth of *mestizaje* to provide the theoretical underpinning to the claim that Mexican women were different and more in need of birthing interventions, it was also co-constitutive and helped to create biological "proof" of the existence of supposedly mixed-race people, whom Spanish-descendant Mexican elites viewed as the "glorious" inheritors of both Indigenous civilizations and European culture; this is the "myth of *mestizaje*." Birth interventions, such as cesareans, not only were necessary due to the fragile, feminine, uniquely Mexican body that was evidence of one's relationship to power but also became the proof of that identity.

By the 1930s, it was fairly well-accepted that Mexican women, at least in metropolitan areas, required considerable birthing interventions (O'Brien 2012). As in the Porfiriato period, obstetric leaders in Mexico City were quite active in producing research publications rooted in their case studies of the impoverished women who sought care in their maternity wards (O'Brien 2012). However, in the post-Revolutionary era—from 1917 to the 1940s—it had become slightly less acceptable to directly name "race"—particularly Indigenous ancestry—as the reason for Mexican women's physical "faults." Instead, Mexican obstetricians such as Gustavo Rudulfo Trangay drew heavily from the eugenics movement that was then enjoying popularity in Europe and the United States (O'Brien 2012). In this adapted framing, "faulty" pelvises were interpreted as signs of mental, moral, and physical unfitness to reproduce—anatomical manifestations of poverty, non-whiteness, and criminality that not only required interventions such as cesareans, but also invited sterilizations to prevent the passing of these traits on to the next generation of Mexican citizens. Trangay and other practicing obstetricians, including his mentors, described in their writings knowingly and proudly violating the law in order to sterilize poor, generally Indigenous or mixed-heritage women without their consent, viewing such violations as a "sacrament" of their "noble" profession.

While O'Brien has suggested that the explicitly eugenicist beliefs and practices of this cohort of Mexican obstetricians fell out of fashion and subsided following the 1930s, the "hidden curriculum" of obstetric practice, highlighted by Lydia Dixon, Vania Smith-Oka, and Mounia El Kotni, is imbued with the eugenicist ideologies of the obstetric past. These authors explain:

> A large portion of knowledge can be transmitted in unintended ways, in what has been termed the "hidden curriculum" . . . defined as the gap between what people are *taught* (through direct means) and what they *learn* (through indirect means). In some cases what is transmitted is the opposite of what is intended. So, while clinicians might *speak about* patient-centeredness as important goals, their *actions* might emphasize measurable outcomes, cost-effectiveness . . . [and] authority, or even attitudes of contempt for patients. (2019:40; italics in original)

Though nearly a century has passed since the pinnacle of the eugenics movement, in terms of generational cohorts and obstetric mentorship, it is possible that Mexican obstetricians (obs) are only two generations removed from Trangay and his cohort's direct training of future obs, and only one generation removed from their students' possession of positions of power and influence in the Mexican biomedical community. Biomedicine is (in)famously slow to advance in clinical practice, and the profession of obstetrics has long been known by the unofficial motto of "It's an art, not a science"—a particularly relevant phrase when considering how long harmful or insufficiently researched practices have persisted in maternity wards.

Cephalopelvic Disproportion and Cesarean Births

Malina's experience with pelvimetrics and her near-miss of a medically unnecessary cesarean birth demonstrate a common chain of justifications that begins with an erroneous assumption of maternal anatomical deficiency and usually ends in a CB that *appears* necessary and inevitable, both for the birthing person and in medical documentation. Such a chain can often appear to be about "risk management"—a popular framing of obstetric iatrogenesis that focuses on obstetric decision-making, even when it leads to obstetric violence—as a partial means of compensating for obs' perceptions of laboring and birthing bodies as inherently risky and unstable, necessitating often aggressive interventions to avoid poor outcomes. However, in Malina's case, there was no legitimate risk to be managed. While Malina is a very tall, willowy woman, her pelvis is not pathologically small. Indeed, true cephalopelvic disproportion (CPD), commonly defined as a size mismatch between a pregnant person's pelvis and their fetus's head and, in the absence of a history of pelvic injury, most common in extremely short birthing people, is considered to be quite rare. While it is difficult to identify exact rates of CPD, obstetric studies of CPD generally note that it can be problematic to gather a robust sample size due to its rarity. For instance, a 1998 study in Dublin examining the outcomes of second births following a cesarean birth for CPD noted that only 84 out of 42,793 women in their sample had CPD—merely 0.196% (Impey and O'Herlihy 1998).

Despite the rarity of cephalopelvic disproportion, a 2017 study of cesarean births in four Mexican hospitals found that out of 604 CBs in the given period of time, 109 were indicated in the chart as necessary due to CPD. Upon review by the study authors, of those 109 births, only 24.8% were supported by evidence in the clinical chart indicating that CPD was indeed a possibility and could potentially be the cause of stalled labor (Aranda et al. 2017). The study authors concluded that the remaining 82 cesareans were medically unnecessary and were performed based on the faulty diagnosis of CPD, rather than on actual faults in the mother's pelvis. While this is only one study, it did include data from both public and private hospitals, and the finding that 18% of cesarean births were performed due to a diagnosis of cephalopelvic disproportion indicates that despite its actual rarity, contemporary Mexican ob/gyns readily reach for the "faulty pelvis" argument to justify stalled labor and to label a cesarean birth as "medically necessary."

Whereas Malina and her husband had the confidence and financial resources to seek out a second opinion and alternative to a planned CB that they doubted was needed, most pregnant and birthing people using public hospitals do not. And while private clinics and doctors are much more likely to perform cesarean births (in general, 80%–85% of births in private facilities are CBs), cephalopelvic disproportion is a convenient justification for CBs for ob/gyns working in public facilities as well. While maternal exhaustion, "failure to progress," and insufficient uterine contractions are much more common causes of stalled labor, they are also factors that can often be alleviated with the provision of rest, time, and occasionally, artificial labor augmentation. However, these resources are often in short supply in public facilities, and ob/gyns often report feeling overwhelmed and under pressure to turn over beds in labor and delivery wards as quickly as possible. The diagnosis of CPD makes a cesarean birth inevitable and necessary, and firmly the fault of a woman's anatomy and anatomical mismatch with her own child. It relieves healthcare staff of the obligation to try other options, and also helps to obscure the roles of structural barriers to vaginal birth.

The Pipeline from Cephalopelvic Disproportion to Sterilization

Many mothers whom I interviewed in Quintana Roo and Yucatán described stalled labors in public hospitals that became cesarean births due to the diagnosis of a "too big baby" or a "too small pelvis." For Maya women in a small rural village outside of Valladolid in Yucatán, where I have visited and conducted interviews for six years, doubts about their pelvises and reproductive abilities tend to proceed further, past their births. In interviews, many mothers described desiring a vaginal birth due to concerns about time to recover from cesarean births. However, their village has neither a doctor nor a *Centro de Salud* (Health Center), and they must take a taxi into Valladolid to give birth if they aren't using a midwife—and few do these days. There in the public hospital, the majority receive the *xoot*—the Yucatec Mayan word for "cut" that is used to refer to cesarean births. While "failure to progress" is a vague and common reason provided to the women for why a CB has become "necessary," women also report being told that their labors haven't progressed because their pelvises are "too small" to birth vaginally, leading to stalled labors. For many of these women, their supposed pelvic deficiencies also become the justification for another procedure that is commonly recommended and even urged by their ob/gyns—sterilization. Sterilization without consent and without informing patients that they have been sterilized is most common in situations where women are already in the hospital for surgery—often a cesarean birth—and the surgeon removes their uteruses while they are already under general anesthesia. General anesthesia was the most common anesthesia referenced by interlocutors who gave birth in public hospitals, perhaps because "emergency cesareans" are more common than elective or planned cesareans in the public healthcare system, which has implemented protocols discouraging nonindicated cesareans, and because epidurals are not as accessible to Maya women.

One afternoon, while traveling between interviews with obstetricians in Playa del Carmen, my Maya taxi driver asked why I was moving between two obstetric clinics when I didn't appear to be pregnant. I described my research to him, and he snapped to attention. I've found that there are few political topics that Mexican taxi drivers don't have an opinion on, but Salvador had personal experience in this arena. "You should interview my wife!" he suggested excitedly:

> The doctors just never stop pushing her to be sterilized. After the birth of our first child, when we refused to have the operation where they take out the uterus, they put in an IUD without telling her. We only discovered it six months later. Every time we go to the doctor, even for things like the flu or infections, they try to convince us to get the operation. They say, "You don't want to be like your grandmother, a peasant with too many children, do you?" But we've always wanted two children, and they made us feel like criminals for it.

Sterilization of Indigenous women—whether consensual or not—is extremely common in Quintana Roo and Yucatán. Most Maya mothers whom I knew had been sterilized during the cesarean births of their first or second child. Some, like Jesika, a friend's daughter, who received a hysterectomy during her youngest son's birth at the recommendation of her obstetrician, felt that the hysterectomy—and the cesareans for each of her births—were the proper, "modern" things to do. Doña Emelina, a woman in her 60s in a rural village in Yucatán who received a hysterectomy immediately after the cesarean birth of her second child in the mid-1990s, felt similarly:

The doctors here told all of us that to have more than one or two children was such an Indigenous thing, an anti-modern thing. And if you, as a woman, have more than one or two children, your health can go very bad, your uterus can fall out! So the hysterectomy is really the safest thing, to stop you from having too many children and to keep your health good.

In rural villages in Yucatán, many women over the age of 25 have had hysterectomies, and public health classes required for families' enrollment in welfare programs often feature units extolling the benefits of sterilization, both as a form of birth control and, rather dubiously, as preventative health care for uterine prolapse and sexual dysfunction. Like Doña Emelina, some Maya women felt that large families were unmodern and signaled reproductive irresponsibility—an association that researchers have noted in the broader Mexican population since the late 1990s. As Laura Braff's analysis of fertility clinics in Mexico City found, fertility clients frequently referenced the idea that Mexico's population was growing at an unsustainable rate, lamenting *Somos muchos!* (We are many!) even while grappling with their own infertility and desire to have a child (Braff 2013:121). However, by 2013, Mexico's birth rate was barely at replacement level[3]—hardly a crisis of over-fertility. Despite the reproductive realities in Mexico, government policies and public discourse emphasize the need to limit population growth and reward low fecundity. As Braff (2013) notes, the specter invoked by this discourse is of Indigenous, Brown (hyper)fertility that must be controlled for Mexico to "modernize." This discourse is, of course, not unique to Mexico, though it may be uniquely taken up there. Continued calls by Global North governments and NGOs to limit fertility and control population growth in Global South countries reinforce the normalization of the idea that the world's problems—climate change, poverty, epidemics—can all be solved by eliminating future generations of Indigenous and Brown people, rather than through resource redistribution or decolonized relations (Smith 2015; see also Lokumage, Ahillan, and Pathberiya, this volume). As Vania Smith-Oka's (2009) research has demonstrated, development programs such as *Oportunidades* often serve as channels for population policies intended to limit the fertility of Indigenous women, at which they are quite successful. In Maya communities in Yucatán and Quintana Roo, this message and the obstetric racism it accompanies, reinforced by public healthcare workers and ob/gyns, has been heard loud and clear.

While the clinical terminology currently used may be slightly more compelling than the overt race science and eugenics arguments put forth by Mexican ob/gyns a century ago, the justification and chain of events for birthing women, particularly Indigenous women, remains largely the same: deficient pelvis>>>surgical intervention required>>>sterilization. And just as 100 years ago, the clinical indications are often ambiguous, incomplete, or lacking altogether. But why is there such persistence of these ideologies, particularly in the face of increasing governmental policies designed to counteract and prevent unnecessary cesarean births?

An Obstetric Dilemma

As other chapters in this volume also explore, the hidden curriculum of obstetric training and practice exerts extreme pressure on early career ob/gyns to adopt the beliefs and practices of their mentors and peers. Trainee ob/gyns in Mexico generally learn how to attend births in high-volume labor and delivery wards primarily serving low-income patients—a context that usually features systemic underfunding, limited or unstable access to medical resources such as basic supplies and diagnostic equipment, and far more patients than there are beds and staff to attend them. As in the United States, teaching hospitals are also urban public hospitals, and trainee physicians learn on the bodies of those who cannot afford private health care. In these environments, ob/gyns rarely see vaginal births, and even more rarely witness unmedicated vaginal births without episiotomy. Beyond environmental barriers to humanized birth lies obs' adherence to the technocratic model of birth (described in the Introduction to this volume), which provides the ideological foundation for dismissing this large gap in ob/gyn education as unimportant. Within this framework, it is sufficient to learn how to manage and direct birth through the application of pharmaceutical and surgical interventions. Providing care that is "too much too soon" (TMTS) and avoiding care that is "too little too late" (TLTL) (Miller et al. 2016) become primary goals of healthcare staff, who are not incentivized to care about their patients' affective experiences. Nor are they incentivized to provide humanistic care in "the right amount at the right time in the right way" (RARTRW), as proposed by Melissa Cheyney and Robbie Davis-Floyd (2020). As a nurse-midwife who trained alongside ob/gyns in a large public hospital in southern Mexico described:

> There are just so many births each day—and you're told to get them out as quickly as you can. You start to feel like it's a train going by, and then you start to feel frustrated with patients for doing normal things like crying or screaming or asking for help. I learned mid-

wifery with my mom first so I had that foundation, but the ob/gyns think that this is normal, that it's okay to treat patients like that.

Changes to biomedical codes, such as the shift to policies in the mid-2010s intended to disincentivize and discourage unnecessary cesarean births in Mexican hospitals, have generally not been accompanied by the structural changes necessary to create an environment in which the time, space, and staffing resources are conducive to re-naturalizing vaginal births. Neither have these changed policies adequately addressed the culture of Mexican obstetrics and the social pressures that ob/gyns face when attempting to change obstetric practice.

For example, for many years, theories of the causes of obstetric violence in Mexico have tended to focus primarily on obstetric violence as a form of gender violence. While Mexican scholarship often references racial and class disparities in experiences of obstetric violence, the primary framing used to theorize it tends to be through the lens of gender, which positions biomedicine, and particularly obstetric practice, as patriarchal structures that midwives, as champions of women's rights, are fighting against (see, for example, Laako 2015). However, this form of analysis tends to collapse the very real class and racial disparities in access to quality, respectful, RARTRW care. It also does not account for the foundational roles of race science and eugenics in the formation of Mexican obstetric practices and orientations toward cesarean births and sterilizations. In addition, it presumes that the most important aspect of pregnant and birthing peoples' identities is gender/femininity/womanhood, and that this is an identity that is experienced and shared in the same ways between pregnant women and female healthcare providers.

However, just as the feminization of health care in the United States has not reduced obstetric violence nor gender abuses (see Liese et al. 2021), neither has the increased percentage (now a majority) of female ob/gyns in Mexico reduced abuses faced by obstetric patients. Indeed, as María Pozzio (2016) noted in her study of obstetric violence and obstetric practice in Mexico, it is women working in obstetrics and gynecology who most commonly exercise obstetric violence against patients, and the idea that female ob/gyns have more empathy for the suffering of their patients than male doctors is patently false (Pozzio 2014; for a contrasting view, see Deborah McNabb's chapter in this volume). Indeed, female ob/gyns may feel even less able to advocate for more humanized birthing practices than their male peers, as Teresa, an accomplished ob/gyn and former Director of a hospital Obstetrics and Gynecology Unit, explained: "If you're a woman in obstetrics, you have to be more macho than the men. You have to be the toughest, the strongest, the meanest. ven with patients. It's how you survive. You can't be soft." For Teresa, choosing not to use surgical interventions risks signaling to her colleagues that she lacks the skills or the mental resolve to use them. She continued:

> I'm a bit afraid of "natural" births—I don't like feeling out of control or as though something could go wrong at any time. But I do wish that I could do more humanized births (*partos humanizados*). I wish that I could allow the woman's family to be present and permit her to walk around and make decisions. I wish I could give her the time to let her body guide the birth. But public hospitals aren't built for that. The births must happen quickly . . . how could you not have poor outcomes in some of these maternity wards? There isn't enough space or staff. There is no space to trust the body or trust the birth . . . Humanized birth will never happen in public hospitals [in Mexico].

Teresa's colleague Jorge, another former Director of a hospital Obstetrics and Gynecology Unit, this one in Quintana Roo, described similar frustrations with the differences in care he was able to provide in public hospitals versus in his own private practice, where most of his clients were able to have successful home births without complications or interventions:

> I was trained in the technocratic model, where we had to intervene as much as possible, and told that medicine had to make up for nature's faults. But my wife became a doula, and it opened up a new world to me. And then I started working with [a local homebirth midwife] and she taught me how to pause, to wait, to trust the process and trust women. And I loved it. And the outcomes were better. But I can't practice that way in the hospitals. They won't let you.

Jorge's use of Davis-Floyd's term "the technocratic model" indicates his familiarity with her work on "the technocratic, humanistic, and holistic models of birth" (Davis-Floyd 2001, 2018, 2022; see also the Introduction to this volume). I mention this here as a demonstration of how anthropological work can impact practitioners by giving them terminology that is "good to think with" (Levi-Strauss 1962). Though Jorge was fairly young (in his late 30s), when I interviewed him in 2017, he had already achieved a relatively high position within the public hospital system in his state. He had also opened a birth center (in Mexico called a *casa de parto*—a birth house) and was in the process of transitioning out of the public system entirely, partially due to how disenchanted he was with hospital birthing practices and the beliefs and actions of his colleagues. Jorge had tried to use his position to effect change and lower the incidences of medically unnecessary CBs in his unit, but found it almost impossible, in part due to the challenges of changing his colleagues' technocratic ideology about birth and about the (dysfunctional) bodies of the women they attended.[4]

A couple of months after interviewing Teresa and Jorge, I accompanied Teresa and a group of midwives to the grand opening of a private hospital in the town in Quintana Roo, where I was living. Although this hospital was modestly sized, it was packed with the latest in diagnostic equipment, state-of-the-art medical supplies, and units intended to handle emergencies, births, and primary care appointments. As the hospital director described in his welcoming speech, the hope of the investors was that the hospital would serve as a local catchment for tourists and wealthy Mexicans who preferred not to use the local *Cruz Roja* (Red Cross) station or drive the two hours to the nearest city with a tertiary-level hospital. This hospital included a small labor and delivery unit, in recognition of an opportunity to divert some local residents who would otherwise drive to Cancun to hire private doctors for prenatal care and birth; the ob/gyn in charge of this unit was on hand at the party to circulate with guests and provide tours. I introduced myself to this ob/gyn, Dr. Lorentz, and he offered to give me a tour of the labor and delivery unit. Throughout, he emphasized the technological resources available to birthing mothers—the newest monitors and gleaming surgical suites ready to "keep things under control." "This is the safest place to birth in town," he said proudly. "We have everything we need to step in when things go wrong."

Jorge and Teresa's experiences, and that of Dr. Lorentz, illustrate the great difficulties of changing obstetrics from within, even from positions of considerable power. They also indicate something else that is concerning for the profession and for the country's poorest patients—a brain drain (or perhaps a "heart" drain) of obstetricians who want to practice humanized birth and decrease cesarean births away from public hospitals and into private practices. The culture of obstetrics is not only conservative and slow to change but is also reactive against humanistic conceptions of birth that challenge long-standing beliefs about the deficiencies of Mexican women's bodies and their ability to birth without intervention. According to the humanistic model as Davis-Floyd defines it in the Introduction to this volume (see also Davis-Floyd 2018, 2022), the body is not a machine (as it is viewed under the technocratic model), but rather the organism that it actually is, and women's birthing bodies are not defective machines in need of constant surveillance and intervention, but rather are organic systems fully equipped for normal, physiologic birth in the vast majority of cases. Their pelvises are only very rarely too small. I, and the series editors Robbie Davis-Floyd and Ashish Premkumar, argue that TLTL and TMTS interventions must give way to humanistic, RARTRW care. That is what such obstetricians strive to achieve—but can only achieve it in private practices that generally cannot afford to provide free care for the poor. Thus, as Davis-Floyd (2018) points out, humanism in maternity care, while not stratified by gender or ethnicity, is often economically stratified.

Conclusions: Remembering the Past While Shaping the Future of Cesareans

Attempts to identify and correct barriers to the reduction of unnecessary cesareans in Mexico continue to have limited success, and overly high rates of cesarean births persist despite decades of protests against them and efforts to lower them. While policy interventions beginning in 2002 (Ministry of Health) and updated more aggressively in 2014 (IMSS) and 2016 (Consejo de Salubridad General) intended to dissuade ob/gyns in the public healthcare sector from conducting unnecessary cesareans temporarily reduced percentages of cesarean births, as previously noted, ob/gyns quickly returned to their habitual levels (Uribe-Leitz et al. 2019). Structural factors such as underfunding and oversaturation of maternal healthcare services certainly play a role in creating environments where CBs have utility for alleviating pressures on obstetric staff. However, as this chapter has demonstrated, early obstetricians in Mexico created a race science and eugenics-based ideological foundation for cesareans that persists to this day through the faulty diagnosis of cephalopelvic disproportion. The chain of interventions that begins with claims of CPD and moves to cesarean births, and often, for Indigenous women, leads to sterilization, has remained largely the same since it was proposed by obstetrician Gustavo Rudolfo Trangay in the 1930s as a means of "improving" the Mexican population. Its persistence is a marker of the enduring traditions of obstetric practices and ideologies, even long after biomedical school curricula have evolved. If Mexico's cesarean rate is ever to be permanently and significantly lowered, obstetricians and hospitals must account for the role of eugenics-based ideologies and racist treatment of patients, and must adjust the hidden curriculum so that obstetricians who wish to practice in more humanized ways are not driven out of public practice.

Sarah A. Williams holds a PhD in Medical Anthropology from the University of Toronto and is currently the Louise Lamphere Visiting Assistant Professor of Anthropology and Gender Studies at Brown University.

Notes

1. The 2014 Guide for Clinical Practice published by the *Consejo de Salubridad General* to reduce unnecessary cesareans notes that breech presentation is an absolute indication for cesarean. This is slightly more strict than global obstetric recommendations, which generally note breech presentation as a *possible* indication for cesarean.
2. My use of the term "non-white" is informed by an understanding of whiteness not as necessarily a phenotypic manifestation of European ancestry per se, but by an understanding of whiteness as indexing a relationship to power. In the Mexican context, despite a century of the propaganda of *mestizaje*, descendants of colonists and European settlers continue to wield disproportionate amounts of wealth and power, and the eugenics movement there was generally an ideology focused on "whitening" the Black and Indigenous populations. Early obstetricians drew a clear line between women who were available for experimentation (Black, Brown, and Indigenous women) and women who were off-limits as subjects of medical investigation and research (white women, the descendants of European and especially Spanish colonists) (O'Brien 2012). Eventually this delineation relaxed, not because the client population had become mixed-race and whiteness had disappeared, but because obstetrics became more generally accepted and elite.
3. Replacement level fertility is approximately 2.1 children per birthing person. This is considered to be the birth rate at which the population can reproduce itself from one generation to the next without lowering the total population number.
4. For the stories of other obs who have made a paradigm shift from technocratic to humanistic or holistic practice, see Jones (2009); Davis-Floyd and Georges (this volume); Çoker et al. (2021); and several of the chapters in Volume I of this series (Davis-Floyd and Premkumar 2023), which are autoethnographically written by obstetricians themselves (Çoker 2023; Cooper 2023; Fernandez 2023; Fontes 2023; Jones 2023; Handlon-Lundberg 2023).

References

Aranda N, Carlos J, Suárez-López L, et al. 2017. "Indications for Cesarean Delivery in Mexico: Evaluation of Appropriate Use and Justification." *Birth* 44(1): 78–85.

Braff L. 2013. "'*Somos Muchos*' ['We Are Many']: Population Politics and 'Reproductive Othering' in Mexican Fertility Clinics." *Medical Anthropology Quarterly* 27(1): 121–138.

Castro A, Heimburger A, Langer A. 2003. "Iatrogenic Epidemic: How Health Care Professionals Contribute to the High Proportion of Cesarean Births in Mexico." Paper No. 02/03-3. David Rockefeller Center for Latin American Studies at Harvard University.

Cheyney M, Davis-Floyd R. 2020. "Birth and the Big Bad Wolf: A Biocultural, Co-Evolutionary Perspective, Part 2." *International Journal of Childbirth* 10(2): 66–78.

Çoker H. 2023. "'Birth with No Regret' in Turkey: The Natural Childbirth of the 21st Century." In *Obstetricians Speak: On Training, Practice, Fear, and Transformation,* eds. Davis-Floyd R, Premkumar A, Chapter 10. New York: Berghahn Books.

Çoker H, Karabekir N, Varlik S. 2021. "'Birth with No Regret' in Turkey." In *Birthing Models on the Human Rights Frontier: Speaking Truth to Power,* eds. Daviss BA, Davis-Floyd R, 348–358. Abingdon, Oxon: Routledge.

Cooper J. 2023. "An Awakening." In *Obstetricians Speak: On Training, Practice, Fear, and Transformation,* eds. Davis-Floyd R, Premkumar A, Chapter 5. New York: Berghahn Books.

Davis-Floyd R. 2001. "The Technocratic, Humanistic, and Holistic Paradigms of Childbirth." *International Journal of Gynecology & Obstetrics* 75, Supplement No. 1: S5–S23.

———. 2018. "The Technocratic, Humanistic, and Holistic Paradigms of Birth and Health Care." In *Ways of Knowing about Birth: Mothers, Midwives, Medicine, and Birth Activism,* Davis-Floyd R and Colleagues, 3–44. Long Grove IL: Waveland Press.

———. 2022. *Birth as an American Rite of Passage,* 3rd ed. Abingdon, Oxon: Routledge.

Davis-Floyd R, Georges E. 2023. "The Paradigm Shifts of Humanistic and Holistic Obstetricians: The 'Good Guys and Girls' of Brazil." In *Obstetric Violence and Systemic Disparities: Can Obstetrics Be Humanized and De-Colonized?* eds. Davis-Floyd R, Premkumar A, Chapter 9. New York: Berghahn Books.

Davis-Floyd R, Premkumar A, eds. 2023. *Obstetricians Speak: On Training, Practice, Fear, and Transformation.* New York: Berghahn Books.

Dixon LZ, Smith-Oka V, El Kotni M. 2019. "Teaching about Childbirth in Mexico: Working across Birth Models." In *Birth in Eight Cultures,* eds. Davis-Floyd R, Cheyney M, 17–48. Long Grove IL: Waveland Press.

FEMECOG. 2015. "Pronunciamiento." https://drive.google.com/file/d/0B_Wsl17n COpWd0d0d3ZFUnNEdUk/view.

Fernandez E. 2023. "Adopting Midwifery Care in India." In *Obstetricians Speak: On Training, Practice, Fear, and Transformation,* eds. Davis-Floyd R, Premkumar A, Chapter 9. New York: Berghahn Books.

Fontes R. 2023. "Repercussions of a Paradigm Shift in the Professional and Personal Life of a Brazilian Obstetrician." In *Obstetricians Speak: On Training, Practice, Fear, and Transformation,* eds. Davis-Floyd R, Premkumar A, Chapter 6. New York: Berghahn Books.

Freyermuth MG, Muños JA, Ochoa MDP. 2017. "From Therapeutic to Elective Cesarean Deliveries: Factors Associated with the Increase in Cesarean Deliveries in Chiapas." *International Journal of Equity in Health* 16(1): 88.

Handlon-Lundberg K. 2023. "Cold Steel and Sunshine: Autoethnographic Perspectives on Two Obstetric Careers in the United States from across the Chasm." In *Obstetricians Speak: On Training, Practice, Fear, and Transformation,* eds. Davis-Floyd R, Premkumar A, Chapter 4. New York: Berghahn Books.

Impey L, O'Herlihy C. 1998. "First Delivery after Cesarean Delivery for Strictly Defined Cephalopelvic Disproportion." *Obstetrics & Gynecology* 92(5): 799–803.

Jaffary N. 2016. *Reproduction and Its Discontents in Mexico: Childbirth and Contraception from 1750 to 1905*. Chapel Hill, NC: UNC Press Books.

Jones R. 2009. "Teamwork: An Obstetrician, a Midwife, and a Doula in Brazil." In *Birth Models That Work*, eds. Davis-Floyd R, Barclay L, Daviss BA, Tritten J, 271–304. Berkeley: University of California Press.

———. 2023. "The Bullying and Persecution of a Humanistic/Holistic Obstetrician in Brazil: The Benefits and Costs of My Paradigm Shift." In *Obstetricians Speak: On Training, Practice, Fear, and Transformation*, eds. Davis-Floyd R, Premkumar A, Chapter 7. New York: Berghahn Books.

Kelly P. 2008. *Lydia's Open Door*. Berkeley: University of California Press.

Laako H. 2015. "La Política del Nacimiento, La Política de la Transformación: Los Casos del Movimiento de Parteras en México y Finlandia." In *Imagen Instantánea de la Partería*, ed. Sánchez Ramírez R, 85–110. México: ECOSUR & Asociación Mexicana de Partería.

Levi-Strauss C. 1962. *Le Totémisme Aujourd'hui*. Paris: Presses Universitaires de France.

Liese K, Davis-Floyd R, Stewart K, Cheyney M. 2021. "Obstetric Iatrogenesis in the United States: The Spectrum of Unintentional Harm, Disrespect, Violence, and Abuse." *Anthropology & Medicine* 28(2): 1–16.

Miller S, Abalos E, Chamillard M, *et al.* 2016. "Beyond Too Little, Too Late and Too Much, Too Soon: A Pathway Towards Evidence-Based, Respectful Maternity Care Worldwide." *Lancet* 388(10056): 2176–2192.

O'Brien E. 2012. "Measuring Maternal Worth: Racial Science in Mexican Obstetrics, 1869–1936." PhD dissertation. The University of Texas at Austin.

———. 2013. "Pelvimetry and the Persistence of Racial Science in Obstetrics." *Endeavour* 37(1): 21–28.

Pozzio M. 2014. "El Hecho de que Sean Más Mujeres, No Garantiza Nada: 'Feminización' y Experiencias de las Mujeres en la Ginecobstetricia en México." *Salud Colectiva* 10: 325–337.

———. 2016. "La Gineco-Obstetricia en México: Entre el 'Parto Humanizado' y la 'Violencia Obstetrica.'" *Revista Estudos Feministas* 24: 101–117.

Secretaria de Salud. 2012. *Programa Nacional de Salud 2007–2012*. Mexico City: Secretaria de Salud, Mexico.

Smith A. 2015. *Conquest: Sexual Violence and American Indian Genocide*. Durham NC: Duke University Press.

Smith-Oka V. 2009. "Unintended Consequences: Exploring the Tensions Between Development Programs and Indigenous Women in Mexico in the Context of Reproductive Health." *Social Science & Medicine* 68(11): 2069–2077.

Uribe-Leitz T, Barrero-Castillero A, Cervantes-Trejo A, et al. 2019. "Trends of Caesarean Delivery from 2008 to 2017, Mexico." *Bulletin of the World Health Organization* 97(7): 502–512.

Vega ES, Urrutia-Osorio M, Arellano-Valdez F, et al. 2015. "The Epidemic of the Cesarean Birth in a Private Hospital in Puebla, Mexico." *Obstetrics & Gynecology International Journal* 2(6): 184–187.

CHAPTER 3

"Selfish Mothers," "Misinformed" Childbearers, and "Control Freaks"

Gendered Tropes in US Obstetricians' Justifications for Delegitimizing Patient Autonomy in Childbirth

Lauren Diamond-Brown

Introduction

There is a joke in obstetrics that goes something like this: "The longer the birth plan, the quicker to the OR [operating room]!" I heard this joke repeated many times during the interviews I conducted with obstetricians (obs) in the United States about decision-making in birth between 2013–2015. The joke was not an off-the-wall remark; it was told because it captured a certain attitude in the shared social reality among some obs. Throughout my interviews, I discovered a common negative characterization of birth plans and patients who use them as "overcontrolling women." This characterization and the narratives that demonstrate it are the foci of this chapter. Stories reflect the taken-for-granted in our socially constructed realities. They help us to make sense of our experiences and to reproduce the social structure. In this chapter, the obstetricians' narratives that I provide offer insights into certain strains of obstetric ideology in the United States that shape biomedical practice.

Not all the obs I interviewed in the scope of this project spoke negatively about birth plans; in fact, some passionately promoted their use. Only 22 out of my 50 interviews contained negative commentary about childbearers' plans for their births. Although the technocratic model

(Davis-Floyd [1992] 2003, 2018a, 2022; see also the Introduction to this volume, in which the "technocratic, humanistic, and holistic para-digms of birth and health care" are described) heavily shapes obstetric care in the United States, I found wide variations in obstetric ideologies and birth practices. These variations suggest that the field of obstetrics is in flux. Norms are unsettled, and there is competition over the funda-mental tenets of practice. The stories obs tell about childbearing patients can be understood as attempts to assert a particular version of reality: a subculture of obs who do not value patient autonomy.

Although respect for patient autonomy is a core indicator of qual-ity maternity care, many childbearers are denied this respect. There is growing global concern over acts of obstetric violence such as disre-spect, non-consented care, intimidation, abandonment, and abuse in labor and delivery (see Sadler et al. 2016; Quattrocchi 2020; and the other chapters in Part 1 of this volume). These behaviors can be linked to obstetric culture, whereby culture transmitted in everyday interac-tions reproduces ideas about what is expected of patients and providers, and, to some extent, normalizes patient mistreatment during labor and birth. Although obstetric violence was not the focus of my research, obs often discussed how they felt about and interacted with patients whose preferences about care conflicted with their own, and some of their treatment of those patients falls on the spectrum of unintentional harm, disrespect, violence, and abuse (UHDVA) identified by Kylea Liese and colleagues (2021), as also described in the Introduction to this volume. Some interlocutors tried to convince me of the illegitimacy of certain women's choices. As these obs characterized certain women as "bad" women/mothers/patients, they did so by drawing on gender tropes.

Obs' characterizations of "problem patients" framed these women as "overcontrolling," "naïve," "miseducated," "superficial," and/or "selfish." Gender tropes such as these are symbolic representations that obs can rely on as being present in their birth practitioner colleagues' minds. I analyze these characterizations of problematic patients at the intersec-tion of gender and patient norms. In the current unsettled context of obstetric culture, these norms influence obstetricians' expectations for how to interact with patients. Drawing on Kate Manne's (2018) femi-nist conception of *misogyny*, I examine these stories as rhetorical devices that function as a form of norm policing for women/mothers/patients).

Methods

The interviews analyzed in this chapter come from a study of obstetric decision-making that I conducted based on 50 in-depth interviews with obstetricians/gynecologists from a wide range of practices in Massachusetts, Louisiana, and Vermont between 2013 and 2015. The obs varied in years of practice and gender, and their practices varied in ownership, size, and hospital affiliation. (See Table 3.1 for physician and practice characteristics.) To conduct these in-person interviews, I met with the interlocutors wherever they chose, including their homes, offices, callrooms, and local coffee shops. I transcribed and analyzed the interviews using thematic coding. All interlocutor names used are pseudonyms.

As their differences emerged from the data, I divided these ob interlocutors into two groups: in Robbie Davis-Floyd's (2023) terms in Chapter 1 of Volume II of this series (Davis-Floyd and Premkumar 2023b) (see also the Introduction to this volume, in which Davis-Floyd's chapter is summarized), the 22 members of Group 1 expressed narratives that reflect Stage 1 fundamentalist thinking, in which they are convinced that their way is the only right way, whereas the 28 members of Group 2 expressed narratives that fall somewhere along a continuum of cognition from Stage 2 to Stage 4 (closed and ethnocentric to open, fluid, and humanistic) thinking. Of the interlocutors in Group 1, 12 are women and 10 are men. In Group 2, 13 are female and 15 are male (see Table 3.1). Paradoxically, I have found that women obs seem just as

Table 3.1. Obstetrician and Practice Characteristics. © Lauren Diamond-Brown.

	Group 1 Obs	Group 2 Obs	Entire Sample
State of Practice	N (22)	N (28)	N (50)
Massachusetts	19	4	23
Louisiana	3	13	16
Vermont	0	11	11
Years in Practice			
Fewer than 10	3	9	12
11–20	6	7	13
More than 21	13	12	25
Gender			
Male	10	15	25
Female	12	13	25
Hospital Type			
Academic Medical Center	9	11	20
Non-Academic Tertiary Care Center	0	4	4
Community Hospital	14	13	27

*One Group 1 OB worked in both settings

likely to adopt controlling, paternalistic attitudes as male obs (but see McNabb, this volume, for an opposing view).

Gender and Authority over Decision-Making in Birth

There are many aspects of difference among competing obstetric ideologies; of particular focus in this chapter are obs' varying attitudes about who has authority over decision-making in birth. In Davis-Floyd's (2018a, 2022) typology of obstetric ideologies, under the technocratic model, authority is owned exclusively by the practitioner; in the humanistic model, authority is shared between patient and practitioner; and in the holistic model, the client has ultimate authority within the healing team (again, see also the Introduction to this volume). Although patient-centered care and shared decision-making have become new standards of practice across biomedicine in general, obs, like other biomedical practitioners, have not universally accepted the humanistic approach (Charles et al. 1997, 1999). There is also evidence to suggest that obstetricians may shift their decision-making approach based on their judgments of *patient worth* (Diamond-Brown 2018).

"Cultural health capital" theory offers insights into the kind of differential decision-making power that doctors are willing to share with patients based on the patient's social capital. Cultural health capital theory is rooted in Pierre Bourdieu's field theory, in which "cultural capital" functions as a form of capital that confers social status and promotes social mobility. In the field of health care, capital is shaped by a range of individual (e.g., healthcare providers and administrators) and institutional actors (e.g., hospital systems, insurance systems, public health systems). Janet Shim (2010:1) defines cultural health capital as "the cultural skills, verbal and nonverbal competencies, attitudes and behaviors, and interactional styles" that function to earn better healthcare relationships for certain patients. In doctor-patient interactions, patients' cultural health capital signals to healthcare providers a sense of patient worth that can give patients an advantage in accessing decision-making partnership, better treatment, and higher quality of care. Self-efficacy, self-control, self-esteem, and health literacy are traits that have been identified as positive attributes in cultural health capital research. In general, the possession of these traits is held by the well-educated middle- and upper-classes (Shim 2010). However, Leslie Dubbin, Jamie Suki Chang, and Janet Shim (2013) have highlighted that health capital is contextual, and that the efficacy of a patient's cultural health capital depends on what specific qualities doctors seek in a "good" patient. How cultural health capital works is complex in relation to the intersectionality of power relations. While middle-class patients may be favored in a system that rewards self-efficacy and control, could a gender hierarchy that favors passive females punish women for self-efficacy and control in labor and delivery?

Outside of providers' expectations about authority over decisions in birth, women who seek authority and power in popular culture are framed negatively as "overly controlling." For instance, scholars have highlighted representations of Hillary Clinton as "overly controlling and aggressive" as focal points for the struggle over gender norms in US society (Templin 1999; Carlin and Winfrey 2009). There are also gendered social pressures placed on the pregnant woman regarding maternity care decision-making. The cultural expectation of intensive motherhood demands that women be competent consumers of health care, showing self-awareness, careful research, and savviness to qualify as "good mothers" (Song et al. 2012). Yet the social construction of femininity teaches women to be submissive, to defer to authority, and to be self-sacrificial (Choi et al. 2005; Malacrida and Boulton 2012). As Lisa Wade and Myra Ferree remind us, "Power is gendered, the requirement to do femininity is also the requirement to do powerlessness: passivity, deference, submission, fragility, and weakness" (2018:146).

In an environment in which the social norms that guide decision-making expectations for the obstetrician and childbearer are unsettled, how do social constructions of gender and the patient role intersect in these interactions? There is a clear tension between the expectations of many women to be active agents in the maternity care process and the fact that some obs are not interested in sharing decision-making authority with their patients. This tension is highly visible in maternity care, where women's health movements have worked for decades to empower women to be active participants in their care. The birth plan is a tool that is created for the purposes of encouraging childbearing people to educate themselves about birth, create a plan for care that reflects their values, and communicate that plan to maternity care providers. The birth plan is ubiquitous in pregnancy self-help literature, but research—and close to half of my interviews—suggest that many maternity care providers have negative views of birth plans (Afshar et al. 2019).

What happens when a self-advocating childbearer is paired with a paternalistic obstetrician, whether male or female? Mimi Niles and colleagues (2021) have shown that when women challenge the routine use of interventions and assert their autonomy, they may face disrespect and abuse from care providers. In analyzing the experiences of childbearers who declined persistent care recommendations, these researchers found that gender-based oppression is at the root of providers' refusals to support informed consent. We lack an understanding from the perspectives of obstetricians on how they handle situations with patients whose expectations for decision-making in birth or specific choices about care do not align with their own (but see Volume I of this series, in which obstetricians tell their own stories: Davis-Floyd and Premkumar 2023a).

This chapter addresses a group of obstetricians whose narratives reflect a paternalistic approach to decision-making and also includes, for comparison, some quotations from obs who do not take such an approach. I analyze how my ob interlocutors talked about "problem patients" who wanted "too much control" over their births. The interlocutors wove their negative characterizations of patients and birth plans together with gender tropes such as women as "control freaks," women as "naïve," and women as "selfish." I suggest that these narratives function as discursive techniques to spread and reproduce particular ideas and ideologies about "acceptable" women/mothers/patients.

"Control Freaks": The Overcontrolling Childbearer

One of the consistent messages communicated by Group 1 obs was that some women "want too much control over their births." A particular stereotype about such women emerged in my interviews of a woman who has control over her life and thus falsely expects, in a way that is problematic for these obs, to have control over her birth. The following quote from a midcareer male ob working in a major academic medical center illustrates this characterization:

> It's all about control—you know we're not so good at not having control over our lives anymore . . . And a lot of people have high powered jobs where they're well educated, and they have the illusion that they can have some control over what's going on around them, and I think the birth plan is just another extension of that.

Women who want too much control were stereotyped as upper-middle-class, educated professionals (see Davis-Floyd 2018b). The following vignette illustrates these layers of characterization found in obs' narratives.

I sat with obstetrician Mark Tanner in a closet turned into an on-call room in the hospital. The call room was tiny and there was barely enough space for the two of us to sit together for our interview. Tanner was currently employed by one of the largest hospitals in the city that serves primarily low-income residents, though he had previously worked in private practice settings serving a high-income population. He was noticeably calmer than other doctors, who raced around the hospital. He had been practicing for many years and had a sweet demeanor. We were well into the hour-long interview when we began discussing birth plans, and the following conversation took place.

Tanner: There are people who have thought about every aspect of their prenatal care and what they want to do. And they have a birth plan, and they want skin-to-skin right away, and not to have the vitamin K injection right away, and they don't want the ointment in the eyes, and they want their partner's, their husband's hand on the baby as it comes out, and they want some special music for the moment of delivery. I mean there are people that have pictured this. It doesn't always work out exactly how they've pictured it. When someone comes to me, I try to accommodate all those things. But a sign of good mental health is being flexible and knowing that you can't control all the things that you'd like to control. But what I find is that this population is less likely to be like that than other places where I've worked.

Lauren: Interesting, why is that?

Tanner: I think that the upper-middle class [is] where people tend to have these idealized notions of what the delivery is supposed to be like and put a lot of energy into accessing prenatal care and thinking about, like, figuring out what is the best thing to do. And it's a very sort of calculated, contrived notion. And their biggest burden is . . . finding the right doula, not feeding their kids . . . And so, when you're [a lower socioeconomic status person] working with basic survival issues, crafting the perfect birth experience isn't as high up on your set of needs. That doesn't mean they're not having a good birth experience.

Lauren: Right, do you think they're having a different birth experience?

Tanner: Usually better, I think.

Lauren: Yeah?

Tanner: You know there was a funny article that you might want to look up from the *Journal of Irreproducible Results* in Colorado. For years, people have tried to do these scales where people come up with aspects of the clinical scenario that predict what their chances are of ending up with a cesarean section . . . So, it's like, what's their pelvis? And how many babies they've had before? Their cervix at the time they arrived? And all sorts of different things. And they are notoriously bad at predicting who is going to end up with a cesarean section. And so, the University of Colorado came up with one where everything is worth five points and if you have more than 30 when someone shows up, you should just do a section right off the bat. And the first is driving a late model Volvo, and having a hyphenated last name, five points for each page of your birth plan, five points if your cervix was checked before you got to the hospital, and an extra five if you'd checked it yourself somehow. I mean, it's a good joke!

This narrative captures many aspects of the characterizations of over-controlling women that I discovered in the obstetric imagination. The "late model Volvo" is a reference to upper-middle-class status; the hyphenated name a marker of feminist power; the long birth plan, a sign of the desire for control and the entitlement of expectations; the cervix checked—and especially if by the woman herself—a reference to embodied knowledge and empowerment.

Obstetricians whose stories drew on these characterizations argued that privileged women are too controlling, and that the "good" patients are those who are too poor or inexperienced to challenge biomedical authority. As one late-career female ob, Susan Crane, who works in a major academic medical center, explained, "The younger teenagers would do great in labor because they just, they weren't as controlling as say a 30-something career woman." When this ob says that the younger women "do great in labor," she is communicating an idea repeated across Group 1 interviews that a "good patient" or a "good birth" is one where the woman does not have firm expectations about how her labor will proceed and trusts the experts to take care of her (see Davis-Floyd 2022 for examples). A good patient defers to the paternalistic obstetrician, male or female, as, again, the women obs I have interviewed are often just as paternalistic in their attitudes as the men (once more, for an opposing view, see McNabb, this volume). Mark Tanner's extended vignette even questions the mental health of women who seek control over their maternity care.

These Group 1 obstetricians argued that birth is unpredictable, and therefore women should not enter it with expectations. It is true that the course of labor and delivery is unpredictable, but that does not necessitate that childbearers should have no expectations for how their birth experiences will take shape. Obs have all sorts of expectations and routines for how to "manage" labor, though none of them identified their *own* desire for control as problematic. Kevin Rollins, a midcareer male ob who works in a private practice at a community hospital, refers to the joke above when he states: "We have a saying in ob that 'The longer the birth plan, the more likely they are not going to get what they want.' We can't guarantee anything in birth." This statement misses the point that maternity care providers *could* guarantee to listen to their patients and to respect their directions for care to the best of their abilities. Should they wish, they could guarantee patient autonomy at every step of the labor and delivery process. These are the bottom-line desires communicated in a birth plan. Instead, the interlocutors drew on the trope of the "overcontrolling woman" to delegitimize her choices about how to give birth, because this trope resonates in the cultural consciousness and distracts from real debates about best practices in labor and delivery.

The obs in Group 1 criticized these patients for their desire to take control, and argued that these patients are the least likely to have the kind of birth they want because they are too specific about what they want, and so are bound to be disappointed when they don't get it. The stories told about this group of women were that their plans get in the way of having a good birth. As Shauna Cowan, an early career female ob in solo private practice at a community hospital, put it, "It's like a jinx. If they have a birth plan in the chart, it's going to end up in a c-section." This narrative says that women want too much control, and that their overcontrolling tendencies are to blame for bad outcomes.

One of the ways in which Group 1 obs sought to delegitimize women's attempts to control decision-making in birth was to articulate that women's specific demands were illegitimate. The next section connects the "overcontrolling woman" trope to women's choices being framed as naïve, misinformed, and/or selfish.

The Childbearer as "Naïve," "Misinformed", and/or "Selfish"

Mark Tanner, who provided the extended vignette above, used the words "idealized," "calculated," "contrived," and "esoteric" to describe patients' birth plans. To this obstetrician and others in Group 1, these adjectives suggest naïveté about birth, as well as a kind of irrelevant superficiality. Group 1 doctors spoke about women's birth plans as "unrealistic," using language like "idealized," "perfect," and "magical," such as the late-career female ob who works in a large academic medical center, Carly Dockins, who said:

> If you've never been in labor and you have no idea how painful it can potentially be, you have no idea how tired you are, how hungry you are, you don't know what might go wrong, you can't imagine your child might have a tracing that's bad or that you're not going to progress normally. And so, then if you've created this dream that "I will only be happy if I meet this dream idea of what labor should be"—no, I mean you're still giving birth to a child, you need to be . . . some people just are very rigid. And I find that very difficult, because they're going to be crushed. No matter what you do to try to support them, only a few are going to really easily have that perfect magical delivery, not because we have to intervene or anything—it's just, if you've never done it before, how are you going to imagine it perfectly? You're not.

Framing birth plans as "naïve" frees medical staff from feeling that they should respect the document—rather, it is tossed aside as "unrealistic."

Another way in which Group 1 obstetricians disavowed birth plans was to state that the act of creating a birth plan itself was superficial and irrelevant to the work of delivering a baby. For instance, one late-career ob in private practice at a community hospital, Max Fields, dismissed his patient's birth plan because he felt that she only wrote one because it was "trendy"; as he said, "because they read about it, and it's cool." And consider the comment of this late-career female obstetrician, Heather Grana, who has a private practice in a small community hospital: "Five years later nobody cares about your experience. You know I have high school kids, and everyone is talking about what college you're going to, nobody cares if you . . . had a vaginal delivery, people move on pretty quickly, it's just not a big life altering thing."

Grana's statement discredits birth plans by suggesting that the prioritization of the birth experience itself is inappropriate. Yet according to Davis-Floyd's data (2022), all the 165 interlocutors in her studies said that their birth experiences stayed with them vividly throughout their lives, for better or for worse. Wealthy or poor, high social capital or low, their major complaint, highly relevant here, is that *their care providers did not listen to them*; their voices were not heard.

Other obs similarly reject the emphasis on the childbearer's experience as they critique the specific choices in the birth plan as misinformed and/or selfish. Consider the following explanation. The ob quoted below, Henry Smith, is a late-career male physician who works as an employee of a community hospital; he stated:

> A lot of women want to go natural and water birth and music and angels and everybody singing and all the Indian chants and all that kind of stuff. The baby doesn't give a rat's ass about all that stuff, he just wants to be born. Most of their thoughts before were about the style of birth experience they were going to have, and I usually try to explain that a fetus inside your uterus doesn't give a crap about the music or the candlelight or whether you're in a tub or not, or any of that. The baby just cares about getting enough oxygen. And as long as you're going to be making these decisions, just understand whose agenda you're making them for, you know—yours or your baby's? And I'm not trying to be judgmental about people who have a sort of self-centered view of it, I'm just trying to open their eyes a bit about what's truly going on.

There is a palpable sense of resentment articulated in this quotation and in others like it, as these Group 1 ob criticize models of birth that do not align with their own and in which the experience of the childbearing person is centered. Clearly, such obs do not respect the choices of the birthing woman and disavow her perspective. The comments they made during my interviews with them reflect a clear separation between the needs of the fetus and the birthing person and a prioritization of the fetus. The ethics of this kind of fetocentric thinking are being actively discussed in the field of obstetrics as concepts of fetal personhood and patienthood have become more normative (McCollough and Chervenak 2008; Lyerly, Little, and Faden 2008). In his quote above, Smith explicitly labels the patient with the birth plan as "self-centered," drawing on cultural expectations of maternal sacrifice to further delegitimize the patient's choices. Rather than trying to understand the meanings of these patients' requests to them, these Group 1 obs judge them as problematic and irrelevant to their job of delivering a healthy baby. By drawing on fetocentric thinking and broader cultural expectations that mothers should be selfless, they label the woman with a birth plan as a "bad mother" with illegitimate demands. In dramatic contrast, in the holistic model of care, what is good for the mother is good for the baby (Davis-Floyd [1992] 2003, 2018a, 2022). A birthing ambience that relaxes the mother will make for an easier birth for both mother and child.

Part of dismissing women's choices in birth as irrelevant and illegitimate is to double down on paternalism and pronounce that biomedical professionals have exclusive ownership of the authoritative knowledge (Jordan 1997) to be used in labor and delivery. In the 22 interviews in which Group 1 obs delegitimized birth plans, they also sometimes told me how they explained to their patients that it was inappropriate for them to expect to participate in decision-making. I heard variations of the following saying, told to me by obstetrician Henry Smith: "You know sometimes I would say to them [patients with birth plans], 'If you don't like how the ride is in an airliner, are you going to go into the cockpit and tell the guy how to drive the airplane?'" Doctors' re-tellings of these interactions with patients further delegitimize women's birth plans by asserting the obs' exclusive ownership of authoritative knowledge—the knowledge that counts (but is not necessarily correct; see Jordan 1997)—about labor and birth. As some Group 1 obs narrated their disrespect of patient choice, they justified the rejection of patient decision-making by debasing women's knowledge as based on faulty information from the internet, other women, or lived experience. For example, consider the following quote from ob George Fields:

> Patients get information in various ways. They read, they talk to friends, they go on the computer, and very often the material they read puts a big chip on their shoulder, develops a certain hostility toward the medical establishment. They feel that or they have read that people are trying to do things to them. They're trying to give them medicines they don't want, operate on them when they don't want, do a cesarean section they don't want, do an instrumental vaginal delivery they don't want . . . And I find it amazing that a patient that I've had a wonderful relationship with for seven months of prenatal care will often still feel that they have to protect themselves against our mechanizations. That, I find very discouraging. In fact, sometimes in frustration I will say, "So let me think about this, I've had 35 years of experience doing this and you've been working with me for seven months, but something that you read for two minutes on the web makes you think that your decision in this instance is going to be more likely correct than mine?" And they sometimes get the point and sometimes they don't. So that's the second big area—working with patients, convincing them that what we're doing is in their best interest, based on our experience. And this is probably not politically correct, but in these instances, we are better at deciding these things.

This Stage 1, fundamentalist ob suggests that a lot of his work is spent convincing patients of his exclusive decision-making authority. His patients are met with clear resistance when they present choices in birth that do not align with his.

Obstetricians on the Other End of the Spectrum

Unlike the Group 1 obs who spoke negatively about birth plans and, in Davis-Floyd's (2023) terms (see also the Introduction to this volume) expressed narratives that reflect Stage 1, fundamentalist thinking, Group 2 obs did not speak negatively about women who sought control over their birth experiences. As previously noted, the narratives from the 28 members of Group 2 fall somewhere along a continuum of cognition from Stage 2 (ethnocentric) to Stage 4 (humanistic) thinking, and embraced women's self-determination in birth with varying levels of enthusiasm. For comparison's sake, consider this comment from Sandra Collins, a late-career female ob in private practice who passionately promotes the use of birth plans.

> I think . . . the management of labor . . . should be very personalized. I always, like from the very first visit, and especially later on in the third trimester, I go over what their expectations are of labor, how they want to approach it, whether they want totally medicated labor or if they want it as natural as possible . . . We go through a very detailed birth plan with them. They actually bring it in in writing and then I sign it . . . I'm a big believer in personalizing birth plans.

This Stage 4 ob prioritizes the childbearer's experience and centers her values in decision-making with the routine use of birth plans. Obs in Group 2 like Collins were highly attuned to the power dynamics in the doctor-patient relationship and actively sought to empower their patients. For example, Andrea Ford, a late-career female ob in private practice at a community hospital, spent a good deal of our interview talking about the importance of empowering patients. She explained:

> I assume that you as the patient want to know everything I know, and you want to share my decision-making . . . Patient autonomy and individual rights are *really* important to me . . . I've been saying it for years: "I can't do anything to you without your permission." You know when you say, "Well, how far overdue will you let me go?" I will let you do whatever you do. I'm not going to send people to your house to bring you to the hospital—that's not the way this works. I will beg, plead, borrow, enlist your friends, enlist your

family supports if I think you're really doing something unsafe. But my job is to explain to you what is going on, what the risks and benefits are of any of these approaches, and help you choose which one you want ... If there is something that is really outside the boundaries of standard care, I can't make you do something, but I can tell you, "We are now in a place where we don't usually go in Western medicine."

Ford's emphasis on patient empowerment is reflected in her choice of language. She acknowledges that by saying whether or not an ob will "let" a patient do something reflects a paternalistic approach and rejects this way of thinking. For example, when discussing how she handles decision-making in relation to the standards of care for labor induction at term outlined by ACOG (American College of Obstetricians and Gynecologists), Ford explained:

ACOG has a position saying that most experts would recommend inducing the labor right away. But patients always have the right to refuse that or decline. And doesn't it sound different if I say, "She declined induction" versus "She refused." You decline an offer, you refuse advice.

By positioning the option to induce as an "offer," Ford emphasizes that her role is to educate patients and encourage them to be the decision-makers as opposed to assuming a position of authority and directing the patient about what to do.

Ford's level of reflexivity and attention to language reflects the far end of the spectrum of obs who support patient autonomy. The Group 2 obs on this end of the spectrum value patient experience in birth, unlike those in Group 1, who argued that it is irrelevant. As Paul Lister, a late-career male ob who practices in a small community hospital, stated: "My objective is to say, 'This is your experience. Your birth. What's going to make you happy with this?' And I am there. And I will help."

Obstetricians like Ford and Lister embody a Stage 4 type of cognition that, in Davis-Floyd's terms, is "globally humanistic." They are open to many ways of approaching birth, and are committed to honoring women's informed choices and human rights in childbirth. For example, Lister explains that he is willing to practice outside of his comfort zone to follow the patient's preferences for care. He said, "If a patient says to me, 'You know what . . . I'd like to do a water birth if possible' . . . I let people do it. I'm not a big fan of water births . . . but a lot of women like it, so, you know, it's fine." Although Lister does not favor water birth, he is openminded and willing to attend such births because his patients enjoy the water birth experience. (For descriptions of the many benefits of water birth, see Kara and Miller 2021).

Andrea Ford exhibits her open-mindedness and informed consent in the following quote about vaginal breech deliveries, a practice that falls outside the normative standards for obs in the United States:

> I will do vaginal breech deliveries . . . when people call and ask me that, I say, "Yes, I will do them. You may or may not want to have one after we talk about it, because there is definitely more risk involved." But it's that woman's risk to take . . . That feels very different than having it imposed on you, "No, you can't do that, nobody will do that for you." That's blatantly untrue.

Rates of vaginal breech births decreased after the Term Breech Trial was published in 2000 and showed worse outcomes for breech babies born vaginally than those born by cesarean delivery (Hannah et al. 2000). The study's methodology and findings have been heavily criticized and refuted, but its findings nevertheless have shaped the standard of care, which has entailed a dramatic lowering of vaginal breech births, in which many obs have by now become de-skilled (Morris 2013; Daviss and Bisits 2021; see also Bisit's [2023] chapter in Volume I of this series [Davis-Floyd and Premkumar 2023a]. Ford's willingness to attend such births is now a rarity in US obstetrics; most US obs will only deliver breech babies by cesarean (Morris 2013; Daviss and Bisits 2021). The narratives from these obs in Group 2 starkly contrast with those in Group 1 by centering patient experience, supporting patient autonomy, and encouraging an informed and shared Stage 4 model of decision-making. This comparison illustrates the wide range of attitudes among US obstetricians and the importance of the possibility of *resocialization*. Scholars have focused on biomedical training as the primary agent of professional socialization for physicians, while missing the opportunity to examine resocialization throughout doctors' careers. Some of the ob interlocutors in Group 2 said that they "practice like a midwife"—meaning that they practice the Stage 4 humanistic and holistic midwifery model of care. For some, this was their training—showing what a difference the type of training can make in forming obstetric ideologies—whereas for others, it was exposure to a more humanistic model of birth later in their careers, often via watching midwives practice (for examples, see Davis-Floyd 2023 and the chapter by Davis-Floyd and Georges, this volume).

Obstetric Misogyny:
Enforcing Gendered Patient Norms in Childbirth

In the continuously shifting landscape of biomedical practice, doctors' narratives reproduce their versions of reality and support their practices, expressing frustration with women who don't accept those versions of reality. I stress again that the circulation of narratives that delegitimize certain patient choices by claiming that some women are overcontrolling, naïve, miseducated, superficial, selfish, or control freaks reflects a deeply paternalistic and sexist attitude. That sexism and gender discrimination play significant roles in maternity care is not a new understanding, but how this works is less clear today when there are more female than male ob residents (AAMC 2020; see also McNabb, this volume), and subsequently more women in practice, and when patient-centered care is a growing expectation in biomedicine. The blatant paternalism of earlier eras is less socially acceptable now. Indeed, as previously noted, the Group 2 obs were highly supportive of birth plans and were actively working to empower patients. Yet the Group 1 obs repeated the same lines about overcontrolling patients in such a ritualized fashion that their normative power is clear. These doctors were narrating ideologies that communicate the expectations of a subset of their field—ideologies that set limits around a patient's rights to autonomy in birth.

Because the vast majority of childbearing people are women, the assessment and reproduction of health capital in this context is also a space where obstetrician/gynecologists police patients' femininity. "Good patient" status is co-constructed with "good women/mothers." The expectations embedded in these Group 1 obs' narratives are that childbearers should be passive as opposed to agentic, have no or low expectations about the birth experience, trust in medical expertise, have a narrow focus of concern on health as defined by providers, and be selfless in the interest of protecting their babies. Women are labeled as "deviant" for breaking these norms. The storytelling about "bad" women/mother/patients stigmatizes women who challenge gendered patient norms.

We see examples of this kind of gender policing across many social institutions. As women push boundaries and challenge patriarchal social norms, they face backlash as a form of gender policing. Wade and Ferree explain, "When we are policed, we are being taught that we should learn the rules, that these rules warrant conformity, and that we can expect consequences for breaking them" (2018:71). Kate Manne's feminist philosophical examination of misogyny argues that "misogyny is the system that operates within a patriarchal social order to police and enforce women's subordination and to uphold male dominance" (2018:33).

Drawing on the sociological concept of "gender policing," Manne argues that misogyny—which can be perpetrated by both male and female obstetricians—is the act of putting a woman in her place when she deviates from socially acceptable gender norms. Rather than a general hatred of women, it is a reactive phenomenon that negatively sanctions certain women who break norms set by patriarchal environments. Women obs learn in those environments and tend to internalize those norms, even when they are disempowering to their patients (again, for a contrasting view, see McNabb, this volume).

The narratives recounted in these Group 1 interviews put women "in their place" when they deviate from socially acceptable norms of woman/mother/patient. What is paradoxical about the way this kind of misogyny works is that obstetricians can operate under this assumption and still believe wholeheartedly that they are there to serve women and that they are patient-centered, even as, in the same breath, they delegitimize women's rights to autonomy. They can argue that women deserve a say in their care—except for those women who step out of line—and then it is their fault for causing problems in the birthing process. Consequently, obs can joke in such a cavalier fashion about women with birth plans getting unwanted cesareans, all the while blaming the women for having specific expectations in the first place.

The class dynamics present in this collection of Group 1 interviews are noteworthy, as they contradict theoretical assumptions about social capital in healthcare interactions. A higher socioeconomic level is generally understood to boost a person's cultural health capital, but this chapter demonstrates that for those obstetricians who want to maintain authority, too much self-efficacy on the childbearer's part may place her in the role of a "bad" patient. It is unclear in this data if wealthy or educated patients really do present birth plans more often, or if this is simply part of the classed and gendered stereotype. Either way, because this view is part of the obstetric imagination, it can reduce the benefits otherwise associated with socioeconomic privilege, turning them into disadvantages.

An interesting observation about this subset of interviews is that 19 out of the 22 Group 1 interviews I have described herein come from obstetricians working in Massachusetts. The concentration of these similar stories told in one geographical location, and the absence of these stories in Louisiana and Vermont, are worthy of future investigation. For example, I repeatedly heard from doctors in Louisiana that it is rare for a patient to present a birth plan, and that patients did not challenge the doctor as much as patients in other areas. In Vermont, it seemed that there was more of an openness among obstetricians to accommodate patient values into clinical practice. The areas I sampled from in Massachusetts do have a high concentration of highly educated women, a strong history of the women's health movement, and a vibrant maternal health advocacy scene. These factors could produce a local gender/patient/parenting culture to which these ob interlocutors are (negatively) responding.

Again, the Group 1 narratives recounted above reproduce a version of obstetric ideology that is misogynistic. As social scientists understand culture to be the baseline for practice, misogynistic ideology often foregrounds and underlies obstetric violence. Misogynistic obstetric culture provides the frame of categories in which the self-advocating patient is out of line and must be corrected by actions that police her violations of gendered patient norms. The narratives and jokes told about bad patients/women/mothers serve the rhetorical purpose of de-legitimizing patient autonomy for those childbearers who want it most, and at the same time reinforce patriarchy, paternalism, and biomedical authority. Advocates for birth justice can work toward changing this subculture within obstetrics and also toward strengthening competing ideologies that support autonomy for all childbearing people.

Lauren Diamond-Brown is an Assistant Professor of Sociology at SUNY Potsdam. Her research, published in *Social Science & Medicine* (2016, 2018) examines how obstetricians negotiate patient choice, clinical experience, and standards of care during birth, as well as how doctors use interactions with patients to manage uncertain clinical decisions. Her research on unassisted birth, published in *Advances in Medical Sociology* (2019), challenges the notion of choice for women who have unassisted births and instead suggests that these are enacted as a compromise of ideals and structural barriers. She teaches reproductive justice and advocates for improving birth in her community.

References

AAMC. 2020. "Report on Residents: Table B3. Number of Active Residents, by Type of Medical School, GME Specialty, and Sex." *AAMC.org*, 13 August 2020. Retrieved 12 December 2022 from https://www.aamc.org/data-reports/students-residents/interactive-data/report-residents/2020/table-b3-number-active-residents-type-medical-school-gme-specialty-and-sex.

Afshar Y, Mei J, Fahey J, Gregory KD. 2019. "Birth Plans and Childbirth Education: What Are Provider Attitudes, Beliefs, and Practices?" *Journal of Perinatal Education* 28(1): 10–18.

Bisits A. 2023. "Attempting to Maintain a Positive Awareness about Vaginal Breech Birth in Australia." In *Obstetricians Speak: On Training, Practice, Fear, and Trans-*

formation, eds. Davis-Floyd R, Premkumar A, 210-227. New York: Berghahn Books.

Carlin DB, Winfrey KL. 2009. "Have You Come a Long Way, Baby? Hillary Clinton, Sarah Palin, and Sexism in 2008 Campaign Coverage." *Communication Studies* 60(44): 326–43.

Charles C, Gafni A, Whelan T. 1997. "Shared Decision-Making in the Medical Encounter: What Does It Mean?" (Or "It Takes At Least Two to Tango"). *Social Science & Medicine* 44(5): 681–692.

———. 1999. "Decision-Making in the Physician-Patient Encounter: Revisiting the Shared Treatment Decision-Making Model." *Social Science & Medicine* 49(5): 651–661.

Choi P, Henshaw C, Baker S, Tree J. 2005. "Supermum, Superwife, Supereverything: Performing Femininity in the Transition to Motherhood." *Journal of Reproductive and Infant Psychology* 23(2): 167–180.

Davis-Floyd R. (1992) 2003. *Birth as an American Rite of Passage*, 2nd ed. Berkeley: University of California Press.

———. 2018a. "The Technocratic, Humanistic, and Holistic Paradigms of Birth and Health Care." In *Ways of Knowing about Birth: Mothers, Midwives, Medicine, and Birth Activism*, Davis-Floyd R and Colleagues, 3–44. Long Grove IL: Waveland Press.

———. 2018b. "The Technocratic Body and the Organic Body: Hegemony and Heresy in Women's Birth Choices." In *Ways of Knowing about Birth: Mothers, Midwives, Medicine, and Birth Activism*, Davis-Floyd R and Colleagues, 71–106. Long Grove IL: Waveland Press.

———. 2022. *Birth as an American Rite of Passage*, 3rd ed. Abingdon, Oxon: Routledge.

———. 2023. "Open and Closed Knowledge Systems, The 4 Stages of Cognition, and the Obstetric Management of Birth." In *Cognition, Risk, and Responsibility in Obstetrics: Anthropological Analyses and Critiques of Obstetricians' Practices*, eds. Davis-Floyd R, Premkumar A, Chapter 1. New York: Berghahn Books.

Davis-Floyd R, Premkumar A, eds. 2023a. *Obstetricians Speak: On Training, Practice, Fear, and Transformation*. New York: Berghahn Books.

———. 2023b. *Cognition, Risk, and Responsibility in Obstetrics: Anthropological Analyses and Critiques of Obstetricians' Practices*. New York: Berghahn Books.

Daviss BA, Bisits A. 2021. "Bringing Back Breech: Dismantling Hierarchies and Re-Skilling Practitioners." In *Birthing Models on the Human Rights Frontier: Speaking Truth to Power*, eds. Daviss BA, Davis-Floyd R, 145–183. Abingdon, Oxon: Routledge.

Diamond-Brown L. 2016. "The Doctor-Patient Relationship as a Toolkit for Uncertain Clinical Decisions." *Social Science & Medicine* 159: 108–115.

———. 2018. "'It Can Be Challenging, It Can Be Scary, It Can Be Gratifying'": Obstetricians' Narratives of Negotiating Patient Choice, Clinical Experience, and Standards of Care in Decision-Making." *Social Science & Medicine* 205: 48–54.

———. 2019. "Women's Motivations for 'Choosing' Unassisted Childbirth: A Compromise of Ideals and Structural Barriers." In *Reproduction, Health, and Medicine: Advances in Medical Sociology*, Vol. 20, eds. Armstrong EM, Markens S, Waggoner MR, 85–106. Bingley UK: Emerald Publishing Limited.

Dubbin LA, Suki C, Shim JK. 2013. "Cultural Health Capital and the Interactional Dynamics of Patient-Centered Care." *Social Science & Medicine* 93: 113–120.

Hannah ME, Hannah WJ, Henson SA, Hodnett ED, Saigal S, Willan AR. 2000. "Planned Ceasarean Section versus Planned Vaginal Birth for Breech Presentation at Term: A Randomized Trial." *Lancet* 356: 1375–1383.

Jordan B. 1997. "Authoritative Knowledge and Its Construction." In *Childbirth and Authoritative Knowledge: Cross-Cultural Perspectives*, 55–79. Berkeley: University of California Press.

Kara K, Miller S. 2021. "Water as a Technology to Support Embodied Autonomous Birthing." In *Birthing Techno-Sapiens: Human-Technology Co-Evolution and the Future of Reproduction*, ed. Davis-Floyd R, 179-192. Abingdon, Oxon: Routledge.

Liese K, Davis-Floyd R, Stewart K, Cheyney M. 2021. "Obstetric Iatrogenesis in the United States: The Spectrum of Unintentional Harm, Disrespect, Violence, and Abuse." *Anthropology & Medicine* 28(2): 1–17.

Lyerly AD, Little MO, Faden RR. 2008. "A Critique of the 'Fetus as Patient.'" *American Journal of Bioethics* 8(7): 42–44.

Malacrida C, Boulton T. 2012. "Women's Perceptions of Childbirth 'Choices': Competing Discourses of Motherhood, Sexuality, and Selflessness." *Gender & Society* 26(5): 748–772.

Manne K. 2018. *Down Girl: The Logic of Misogyny*. New York: Oxford University Press.

McCullough LB, Chervenak FA. 2008. "A Critical Analysis of the Concept and Discourse of the 'Unborn Child.'" *American Journal of Bioethics* 8(7): 34–39.

Morris T. 2013. *Cut It Out: The C-Section Epidemic in America*. New York: New York University Press.

Niles PM, Stoll K, Wang JJ, et al. 2021. "'I Fought My Entire Way': Experiences of Declining Maternity Care Services in British Columbia." *PLoSOne* 16(6): eO25645.

Quattrocchi P. 2020. "The Platform on Obstetric Violence." *Obstetric Violence Project*. Retrieved 12 December 2022 from https://www.obstetricviolence-project .com/.

Sadler M, Santos MJ, Ruiz-Berdún D et al. 2016. "Moving Beyond Disrespect and Abuse: Addressing the Structural Dimensions of Obstetric Violence." *Reproductive Health Matters* 24(47): 47–55.

Shim J. 2010. "Cultural Health Capital: A Theoretical Approach to Understanding Health Care Interactions and the Dynamics of Unequal Treatment." *Journal of Health and Social Behavior* 51(1): 1–15.

Song FW, West JE, Lundy L, Smith Dahmen N. 2012. "Women, Pregnancy, and Health Information Online: The Making of Informed Patients and Ideal Mothers." *Gender & Society* 26(5): 773–798.

Templin C. 1999. "Hillary Clinton as Threat to Gender Norms: Cartoon Images of the First Lady." *Journal of Communication Inquiry* 23(1): 20–36.

Wade L, Feree, M. 2018. *Gender: Ideas, Interactions, Institutions*. 2nd edn. New York: W.W. Norton & Company.

CHAPTER 4

Implicit Racial Bias in Obstetrics

How US Obstetricians View Pregnant Women of Color

Genevieve Ritchie-Ewing

Introduction

Racism in US society is systemic (systematic and endemic). This persistent racism affects how biomedicine is practiced in the United States in multiple ways, including by lowering the quality of patient-physician interactions, particularly when the patient and physician are of different races and/or ethnicities (Hagiwara et al. 2016). In obstetrics, US women of any race/ethnicity may experience the UHDVA (unintentional harm, disrespect, violence, and abuse) spectrum of obstetric iatrogenesis described by Kylea Liese and colleagues (2021) (whose findings are also described in the Introduction to this volume). On one end of this spectrum is the *unintentional* harm originating from routine interventions that are meant to keep birth safe, but actually cause harm, in what Melissa Cheyney and Robbie Davis-Floyd (2019:8) term "the obstetric paradox." On the other side of the UHDVA spectrum lie *intentional* disrespect and discrimination, such as demeaning behaviors and insults to childbearers by healthcare workers. In the United States, Black, Indigenous, and other People of Color experience intentional disrespect and abuse during pregnancy and childbirth more often than white women, due to the systemic racism in US society (Altman et al. 2019; Davis 2019; Vedam et al. 2019; Liese et al. 2021).

In fact, Women of Color report that disrespect, abuse, and discrimination *dominate* their interactions with healthcare providers, making sharing information and establishing trust in the patient/provider relationship extremely difficult (Altman et al. 2019; Davis 2019; Vedam et al. 2019). This creates barriers to safe, quality health care for many pregnant women (McLemore et al. 2018; Altman et al. 2019; Vedam et al. 2019). Building trust in the patient/provider relationship is essential for open communication (Cuevas, O'Brien, and Saha 2016; Altman et al. 2019; McNabb, this volume). Without open communication, patients do not have access to all available options, and are much less likely to follow provider advice (Hagiwara et al. 2016; Altman et al. 2019). Patients also may not give providers important information about their symptoms, feelings, and circumstances, thereby limiting the ability of a provider to make correct diagnoses and offer appropriate assistance. As most women in the United States receive pre- and postnatal care from obstetricians, improving this provider/patient relationship for pregnant Women of Color is vital to empowering them to make decisions about their pregnancies and childbirth experiences (Altman et al. 2019; Vedam et al. 2019).

Research also shows that open communication and informed decision-making between women and their healthcare providers enhance women's positive emotions about their pregnancies and childbirth experiences and decrease adverse birth outcomes (Vedam et al. 2019). In addition, the lack of quality health care for minority women due to racism and discrimination is one of the main reasons why the United States has extensive racial and ethnic disparities in pregnancy and birth outcomes such as preterm birth and low birthweight rates (Giurgescu et al. 2011; Alhusen et al. 2016; Braveman et al. 2017). For example, in 2018, non-Hispanic Black women in the United States had a significantly higher preterm birth rate (14.13%) compared to non-Hispanic white women (9.09%) (Martin et al. 2019). This disparity in preterm birth rates persists even among Black women in higher socioeconomic status groups (Alhusen et al. 2016; Braveman et al. 2017; Sacks 2018; Fryer, Vines, and Stuebe 2020). Several studies have attributed this significantly higher preterm birth rate to chronic stress from pervasive, institutionalized, systemic racial discrimination experienced every day by Women of Color, particularly women who are Black (Alhusen et al. 2016, Braveman et al. 2017). Stress from everyday racial discrimination is exacerbated when minority women are discriminated against by their healthcare providers (McLemore et al. 2018).

While recent research has begun to explore the experiences of pregnant and laboring US Women of Color, few studies have examined how obstetricians practicing in the United States view their patients of various racial and ethnic backgrounds (Hagiwara et al. 2016; Davis 2019; Vedam et al. 2019). Most of these studies test obstetricians or other physicians for implicit bias, but do not gather ethnographic data from the physicians themselves (Green et al. 2007; Maina et al. 2018; Saluja and Bryant 2021). Recognizing how obstetricians perceive racial and ethnic minorities is essential to developing strategies for reducing bias and increasing equality in healthcare interactions (Cuevas et al. 2016; Sacks 2018; Parsons 2020). Adding an understanding of obstetricians' views to the emerging ethnographic work on minority woman's experiences provides a more comprehensive picture of the long-standing tradition of obstetric violence in US maternity care (McGregor 1998; Parker-Benfield 2000; Bridges 2011; Diaz-Tello 2016; Altman et al. 2019; Davis 2019; Liese et al. 2021).

Specifically, my objective for this study is to address the following three research questions (RQs):

RQ1: Do US obstetricians have implicit racial bias toward darker-skinned individuals and/or Black persons?

RQ2: How do US obstetricians view patients of various races/ethnicities?

RQ3: What challenges do US obstetricians experience in establishing relationships with their patients of different races and ethnicities?

Methods

I conducted a cross-sectional, descriptive study of obstetricians who are currently practicing or have practiced in the United States between July and December 2021. I collected both quantitative and qualitative data with an online, anonymous survey and semi-structured virtual interviews.

Participants

I recruited eight obstetricians through emails to doctor's offices, clinics, and medical schools in Ohio. I also reached out to contacts in biomedicine and in my field of anthropology to assist with recruitment. I had extensive difficulties finding willing participants due to several factors, including strict COVID-19 restrictions in my local area of Dayton, Ohio, at the time of my research in 2021; the exhaustion and overwork of healthcare providers; and the general reluctance of obstetricians to participate in social science research. (See Chapter 12, this volume, for detailed descriptions of the ethnographic challenges of gaining access to obstetricians). While my sample size was small, the participants were diverse in many areas, including age, race/ethnicity, work environment, and years they began practicing as an ob (Table 4.1). All participants were married except one, and all participants had children. They came from three different states: Ohio, Texas, and Illinois. All eight obstetricians responded to the anonymous online survey, although not all completed all sections of the survey. Five of these obstetricians also participated in a virtual, semi-structured interview conducted by myself—a white medical anthropologist who identifies as a cisgender woman.

Study Procedures

I created and administered the survey instrument using Qualtrics.[1] Qualtrics is a well-known, trusted program for creating and administering online surveys in academic, research, and business settings with strict protocols to maintain the confidentiality of participant data. The online survey instrument consisted of 36 close-ended questions and 10 open-ended questions. These questions asked about the sociodemographics of the participants and about work experience and setting. The other questions on the survey were designed to explore both explicit

Table 4.1. Selected Participant Characteristics. © Genevieve Ritchie-Ewing.

Participant	Gender	Race/Ethnicity	Age Range (Years)	Work Environment	Year Began Practicing as OB
A1	Woman	White or European American	40–44	Government health clinic	2019
A2	Man	White or European American	60–64	Hospital	1982
A3	Man	Asian American	30–34	Hospital	2013
A4 (Diane)	Woman	White or European American	60–64	Private doctor's office	1984
A5	Man	White or European American	55–59	Academic health care office	1993
A6	Woman	Black or African American	40–44	Private doctor's office	2007
A7	Woman	White or European American	50–55	Hospital	1987
A8	Woman	Asian American	50–54	Private doctor's office	1995

and implicit bias. *Explicit bias* is bias of which people are aware, while *implicit bias* is unconscious bias. Expressions of explicit bias are strongly discouraged among healthcare providers, but implicit bias is harder to self-regulate (Green et al. 2007; Hagiwara et al. 2016). Implicit bias can influence nonverbal behaviors such as eye contact and posture, as well as how speech is delivered (Dovidio et al. 2002; Hagiwara et al. 2016). A growing body of literature indicates that higher levels of implicit bias among physicians adversely impact their medical interactions with their patients (Cooper et al. 2012; Hagiwara et al. 2016).

To address my first research question, participants completed two implicit association tests (IATs) developed for online research by a collaborative research group from several universities.[2] In IATs, participants respond to items that are classified into four categories: two social or physical categories (white versus Black or light-skinned versus dark-skinned) and two valence categories (positive versus negative words) (Greenwald, McGhee, and Schwartz 1998). The categories are presented in pairs, and participants are asked to respond to an original pairing and then to the opposite of the original pairing (i.e., white-positive word or Black-negative word, then white-negative word or Black-positive word). Response times are compared for the first set of pairs and the second set of pairs. Negative scores further from zero indicate more implicit bias. For the Race IAT, this means more pro-white, anti-Black implicit bias. For the Skin Tone IAT, negative scores further from zero indicate more pro-light-skinned, anti-dark-skinned bias (Xu, Nosek, and Greenwald 2014). IATs have been validated for use in research and utilized by numerous researchers to examine implicit bias in different groups of healthcare professionals (Maina et al. 2018).

To address my second research question, the survey contained open-ended questions about participants' experiences with Black or African American patients, white or European American patients, Latina patients, and patients of any other race or ethnicity. I asked participants for their overall impressions of each category of women and for information about some of their experiences with patients in each category. I also included a set of Likert-style statements about racial stereotypes that Black and African American women report facing in healthcare situations (Cooper et al. 2012; Sacks 2018; Altman et al. 2019; Vedam et al. 2019). I designed the Likert-style statements based on similar studies of people's perceptions about sensitive topics (Brigham 1993; Payne et al. 1999; Brewis and Wutich 2012; Hagiwara et al. 2016; Martinez et al. 2018; Cullin 2021).

Given that many people in the United States think that "Black" and "African American" index the same people, I here explain that: (1) in the United States, people often assume that anyone who has dark skin is African American and treat them as such, when in reality, someone can be Black, but not African American. I have many Bahamian students in my classes who experience this phenomenon. (2) Some of my Black students actively embrace being African American as part of their identity, but others don't; they say that they have no connection to Africa and don't want to be viewed as African American.

All participants were given the opportunity to participate in a single semi-structured, personal interview lasting 30–45 minutes. As previously noted, five participants agreed to the interview. These participants were given pseudonyms to protect their anonymity. I was only able to connect one participant's survey data to her interview data, as the survey was anonymous. This one participant, Diane, had added her email address at the end of her survey responses. All other participants agreed to the interview through direct emails. I asked participants about their work environment and history, and about their experiences with patients of various races and ethnicities. To address my third research question, we also discussed challenges participants face in building relationships with their patients and the challenges their patients face in maintaining their own health. I conducted and recorded the interviews via my professional Zoom account. I also wrote interviewer notes after each interview. I then transcribed each interview and deleted any contact information for the participant and the Zoom recording to maintain their anonymity. Participants completed an online informed consent form before answering questions on the survey, but I did not collect names on the form. Participants who agreed to the interview completed a separate online informed consent form. The Central State University Institutional Review Board (IRB) approved the study procedures.

Data Analysis

IATs measure the strength of association between concepts by comparing response times when participants match groups to positive versus negative words. The assumption is that a response is easier (and faster) when closely related items share the same response key.[3] In other words, if a person has implicit bias for white over Black people, they will match positive words to images of white people faster than images of Black people. They will match negative words faster to images of Black people than to images of white people. The response time scores were calculated within the code taken from Project Implicit's IATs that I installed into the Qualtrics survey.[4]

My original plan for analysis of the qualitative data included identifying themes from the survey instrument and interview transcripts (Bernard 2011). However, as my sample size was small, I was not able make generalizations about how obstetricians view their patients of Color. Instead, I focused on in-depth insights into each participant's own perceptions and experience revealed in the qualitative data. Similarly, I was not able to perform statistical analyses on the Likert-style set of statements also due to the small sample size. Instead, I report general tendencies in the data without generalizing the results to the broader population of US obstetricians.

Results and Discussion

RQ1: Do US Obstetricians Have Implicit Racial Bias toward Darker-Skinned Individuals and/or Black Persons?

Only six of eight participants completed the two IATs that I included in the online survey (Table 4.2). Three of the participants (A1, A2, and A5) who self-identified as white or European American showed a slight preference for white over Black individuals and a moderate preference for light-skinned individuals. One participant (A4) who self-identified as white or European American showed no preference for white over Black individuals and a slight preference for light-skinned individuals. This participant revealed to me during the interview that she had completed IATs before and was disappointed with her results, which had shown a preference for white individuals. This previous experience may have impacted her IAT results for this study. No other participant mentioned completing an IAT before. The two participants (A3 and A8) who self-identified as Asian American showed a moderate preference for white over Black individuals and a moderate preference for light-skinned individuals. The two participants who did not complete the IATs self-identified as Black or African American and white or European American.

While, again, I cannot make generalizations about implicit

Table 4.2. Race and Skin Tone IAT Scores for Participants Who Completed the IATs. © Genevieve Ritchie-Ewing.

Participant	Race IAT Scores	Skin Tone IAT Scores
A1	–0.21	–0.44
A2	–0.43	–0.41
A3	–0.62	–0.48
A4	–0.09	–0.20
A5	–0.24	–0.38
A8	–0.45	–0.52

biases among obstetricians in the United States from these results, the tendency shown in Table 4.2 of white or European American persons to have a slight to moderate preference for individuals within their own social group or who look more like them is supported by results from other data collected on the Project Implicit website and other research studies[5] (Green et al. 2007; Hall et al. 2015; Hagiwara et al. 2016). Negative scores further from zero indicate more implicit bias.

RQ2: How Do US Obstetricians View Patients of Various Races/Ethnicities?

All participants saw a variety of races and ethnicities in their work (Table 4.3). One participant did not estimate the approximate percentage of patients in each category, but rather stated that the percentages varied by work location.

Two of the eight participants did not respond to my open-ended survey questions about their impressions and experiences with patients of different races and ethnicities. Furthermore, five of the eight participants did not provide full answers to these questions. These five participants wrote that their impressions of and experiences with African American/Black, European American/white, and Latina patients were no different from each other or from any other patient interactions. I see two possible explanations for obstetricians' reluctance to discuss how their patient interactions may be dissimilar between various racial/ethnic groups. (Both explanations require further research.)

First, as mentioned in my Introduction to this chapter, physicians are strongly dissuaded from expressing explicit bias (Green et al. 2007;

Table **4.3.** Approximate Percentage of Patients Seen by Participants in Each Racial/Ethnic Category. © Genevieve Ritchie-Ewing.

| Participant | Approximate Percent of Patients | | | |
	Black or African American	White or European American	Latina	Other Races or Ethnicities
A1	40–54%	10–24%	70–84%	1–9%
A2	25–39%	40–54%	25–39%	10–24%
A3	70–84%	10–24%	25–39%	10–24%
A4—Diane	10–24%	70–84%	25–39%	1–9%
A5	25–39%	55–69%	10–24%	1–9%
A6	10–24%	70–84%	1–9%	1–9%
A8	25–39%	55–69%	10–24%	1–9%

Hagiwara et al. 2016). Obstetricians, like other physicians, state a lack of preference for any race or ethnicity, despite the abundance of research showing implicit bias among physicians similar to the implicit bias found in the general US population (Green et al. 2007; Hall et al. 2015; Hagiwara et al. 2016). In addition, several studies show that patients of some races and ethnicities routinely experience disrespect and discrimination in healthcare settings (Cooper et al. 2012; Sacks 2018; Altman et al. 2019; Vedam et al. 2019). While I did not ask specifically for poor impressions or difficult experiences with each category of patients, participants may not have wanted to risk showing explicit bias in answering these questions.

Participants' answers to the Likert-style questions may be further evidence of their desire to avoid explicit bias. In response to questions such as "Black or African American women are more difficult to communicate with compared to white or European American women" and "Black or African American women are more likely to be addicted to drugs compared to white or European American women," almost all participants marked "Strongly disagree." I drew the statements used in this section of the survey from Black and African American women's experiences in biomedical settings (Cooper et al. 2012; Sacks 2018; Altman et al. 2019; Vedam et al. 2019). Black and African American women reported having more difficulties communicating with healthcare providers, often due to assumptions about addictions to drugs and their inability to parent (McLemore et al. 2018; Sacks 2018). The statements that elicited a more neutral response were related to socioeconomic status (i.e., making less money or living in more dangerous areas). Later, I discuss this tendency to focus on income level rather than race in describing the challenges the participants face in building relationships with their patients.

Second, it may have been challenging for obstetricians to summarize their impressions and experiences of any one group over the course of their careers. One participant illustrated this struggle. In response to the question, "Tell me about some of your experiences with Black and/or African American patients," the participant wrote, "wonderful and terrible, sad and happy, obnoxious and thoughtful, just as with any large group of persons." Asking about a recent specific set of experiences or impressions might have prompted more responses, but I would not have been able to explore overall impressions or experiences. Again, however, the obstetricians' overall reluctance to discuss how their interactions with childbearers of some races and ethnicities might be different than others may have been connected to their desire to avoid explicitly biased statements, in which case asking about specific experiences or impressions would not have produced better results.

In contrast, one participant (A4—Diane) wrote extensively about her impressions and experiences with women of various races and ethnicities over the course of her career. Diane worked in private practice with mostly white middle-class patients, but she also practiced at a Planned Parenthood clinic where she saw a more diverse set of patients in both race/ethnicity and income levels. She described her initial impressions and how those impressions changed over time. In response to the question about her impressions of Black or African American patients, she wrote:

> I treated many more Black patients when I was in medical school at the County Hospital. At the time, my impression was that they were more typically angry in their first encounter with me. I found that intimidating, and I didn't understand, thinking, "Why are they angry at me? I'm a good, friendly person, and we just met." I later realized that they had every reason to be angry and distrustful of any County Hospital and those of us working within said institution. If I had understood this at the time, I would not have taken it personally, and I think that I would have been better able to establish a trustful relationship.

This quote illustrates several possible avenues to explore regarding relationships between racially discordant providers and patients. First, Diane's place in society at the time of her residency as a middle-class, white, cisgender woman created certain expectations about how medical interactions with patients should take place. As with many white, middle-class women, Diane expected patients to be respectful and friendly toward their doctors and accepting of doctors' advice. She, therefore, did not understand why her Black patients entered the doctor/patient relationship with a different mindset. Diane demonstrated further insight about her expectations and level of comfort in her comments about her white patients: "I had far more white patients in private practice (and they made up the majority of my private patients) than in my training. I realize now that I entered these relationships in a more relaxed fashion than I did with my Black patients. In most of these relationships, it was like looking in a mirror."

While there is a higher percentage of underrepresented minorities among US ob/gyns compared to other adult biomedical specialists, the majority still are white (Rayburn et al. 2016; AAMC 2019). According to the Association of American Medical Colleges (AAMC 2019), in 2018, 56.2% of active ob/gyns were white, 17.1% were Black, and 5.8% were Hispanic. Other active ob/gyns fall into different racial and ethnic categories, although 13.7% of the ob/gyns listed in the data collected by AAMC (2019) did not report race or ethnicity. In addition, most doctors, including ob/gyns, come from middle to upper socioeconomic status families (Jolly 2008; Le 2017). In 2019, approximately 56% of medical students came from the top income quintile, whereas only 4% came from the bottom quintile (Youngclaus and Fresne 2020). Undergraduate university and medical school tuitions are expensive, and the time to complete this education is lengthy. In 2019, the median education debt for medical school graduates was $200,000, and 73% of graduates had education debt (Youngclaus and Fresne 2020). Grants and scholarships rarely cover the entire cost of attending medical school, making graduating from medical school difficult for many who do not have family or other support (ibid.). Most obstetricians have life experiences that differ strongly from those of underrepresented minorities, particularly if their minority patients are of lower socioeconomic status.

During our interview, Diane further discussed the lack of experience many obstetricians have with low-income patients of Color, and provided some reasoning for why many obstetricians do not choose to work with underserved populations:

> Here's what I would really like to change about public policy, but it probably will never happen. I wish that we had public funding for medical education and in exchange for that all students did public service. You know, to go to a rural area, to go to an urban area, take care of patients for less money than you would make in private practice. The problem is that we all graduate with a lot of debt . . . which makes it nearly impossible to go work at a clinic for underserved people because you cannot pay that debt if you want to have a house, a car, and kids. I would have loved to stay in the county system, but it wasn't financially possible.

Second, Diane recognizes that she was not taught about the history of abuse that Black and African American patients have faced in the biomedical community, and that this lack of knowledge influenced her reactions to such patients. W. Michael Byrd and Linda Clayton (2001) and Cynthia Prather and colleagues (2018) have summarized some of the historical abuses experienced by Black and African American people from slavery through the 20th century (see also Chapter 6, this volume, in which some of these historical abuses are also summarized). These abuses and others also are prominent in the history of reproductive health practices for Black and African American women (Roberts 1998; Washington 2006; Cooper Owens 2017). This history is only recently becoming more widely recognized among healthcare providers (see Prather et al. 2018; Lokugamage, Ahillan, and Pathberiya, this volume). Later, when Diane learned of that history, she recognized how it could have impacted how Black and African American patients may feel upon entering a healthcare setting. Prather and colleagues (2018) also discussed how this history, combined with contemporary experiences of racism, make Black and African American women more vulnerable to adverse reproductive health outcomes.

When asked about her Latina patients, Diane compared her interactions with Latina and Black patients in the following way:

> My city, where I also did my residency, is a majority minority town, with the largest group of People of Color being Latina. Though I cared for a significant number of Latinas in my private practice, I cared for more at the County Hospital where I trained. The Latina patients who I encountered in training were friendly, but afraid. I later realized that Black patients were also afraid, but exhibited their fear with anger. Their fear, I believe, caused them to express more pain. Also, looking back, there was probably a sense of subservience in [Latinas'] friendliness, i.e., "be nice so that the doctor will treat you well."

Again, Diane's insights changed over the course of her career after she gained more knowledge about the challenges faced by minority groups. Whether or not her patients felt the ways she believed they felt later is less important than her ability to adjust her expectations and insights from the beginning of her career to the present.

The other interviewed participants touched on these same issues in their interview responses, although they highlighted socioeconomic differences rather than race. One of these participants, Jackson, had recently made a transition from a well-known hospital with a mixed demographic in which 20–30% of his patients were Women of Color to a hospital in which he treats 80–90% Women of Color. While he had worked with some women of lower socioeconomic status in his previous hospital, some of his patients were extremely wealthy. The women he cares for in the new environment come from a considerably lower average socioeconomic status. In talking about his interactions with patients, Jackson highlighted how those interactions changed with his work transition:

> Patients, for example, don't necessarily when I'm in the hospital . . . ask my name. And my take on that, I don't know if this is exactly right, I haven't asked anybody this, but . . . it never occurred to them

that they could have a personal relationship, like a patient/physician relationship. And, while they're happy that I'm nice and kind and thoughtful and seem to be responsive to their needs . . . I sort of fit this slot of "healthcare provider." And that is a radical departure from the way I've practiced for a long time. That was not my experience prior to this transition for me.

Jackson also talked about examining his own reactions and questioning his own motives, much as Diane spoke regarding her experiences as a resident; Jackson said:

My daughter who is a gender studies person, she's like, "Well Dad, why would anybody listen to like an old, fat, white, Jewish doctor talking about their health?" I've been forced to put the mirror up more thinking about that question. One sort of anecdote. My first week working at the [new hospital], I was [doing] postpartum rounding, and there was a patient who looked sad. She wasn't making eye contact. She just didn't feel, I didn't get a sense that she was engaged in the conversation. Although she was polite. There was nothing explicitly or overtly angry. And I said, you know, I was sort of overwhelmed by my transition and I said [to myself], "Oh let me do the stuff I'm sort of good at." I sat down and I said, "You know, it looks like that maybe there is a lot going on. Tell me something you're excited about bringing the baby home. Tell me something you're nervous about" . . . And she was polite, but she kind of looked at me and said, "What are you talking about?"

And I got kind of . . . embarrassed for myself because I think I had embarrassed her. And it became clear that I was doing it for me because I wanted to feel comfortable . . . it was unsettling for me because I was used to dealing with a population that was excited to have a baby that I wasn't sure that she was. And I felt like I needed to somehow fix that, but again that was my, in some ways, my own narcissism of wanting obstetrics to be happy . . . I am more humble than I was before I switched my job to know that I really don't know what they are feeling and what they are thinking.

While Jackson was not sure if these interactions were due to racial/ethnic and cultural differences or to diverse life experiences due to family socioeconomic status, he was struck by how different his patient interactions were in each work environment. Those differences made him rethink his own reactions to his patients and consider new ways to approach his work.

Abdul is a specialist in Maternal-Fetal Medicine who handles patients with high-risk pregnancies. He works almost exclusively at a safety net hospital that caters to women who are uninsured or underinsured. As a result, his patients are almost all low-income Women of Color. He has had better experiences with Women of Color because, as a high-risk doctor, he was able to build relationships with his patients that many residents cannot. (I will cover this issue in more detail in the next section [RQ3]). Abdul described this phenomenon as follows:

> Most of the time they are coming to see me precisely because something is wrong. So by definition, it's a little bit of a different interaction more so because they were already told by someone, there is something going on and you need to see a high-risk doctor. So many times, people are coming in worried, with questions or have no idea. *And part of this has to do with a referring provider and sometimes they just say, you have to go see a high-risk doctor and don't actually give a context of what the issue is or why these individuals come to see me.* A lot of it is just sort of playing catch-up. Having a conversation about why they're seeing me and what their goals are for the pregnancy. Many times it's obviously, it's a little bit different as well because . . . by the very nature of having a high-risk pregnancy, it's much more of an intimate and close follow-up with patients. [Italics mine]

The italicized part of this quote shows the disrespect by some providers that Abdul's patients face. Abdul often has to explain the issues with his patients' pregnancies because their regular obstetricians did not provide that information.

Abdul is a Person of Color himself who self-identifies as Indian American. When asked if he thought the way he looks impacts his interactions with his patients, he said:

> I think so. I think some of it is misrecognition. Full disclosure, I self-identify as a cis male of South Asian descent, but I shave my head, I have a beard. So many times, individuals can't really figure out where I'm from. So sometimes they may not hear my name or they may not have the background to know what that is traditionally. I have a very South Indian name . . . But when they see me, you know, individuals have thought that I passed as Black, West Indian, Middle Eastern . . . I think that has done a lot for people because people I think, more often than not when they see someone who is not white, I think they automatically feel a little different.

As I mentioned earlier, all interview participants stated that they believed that socioeconomic status was a more important influence on their interactions with patients than race or ethnicity. They also were more comfortable discussing socioeconomic status. However, each participant recognized that race correlates strongly with socioeconomic status in the United States due to systemic racism. This makes it hard to determine whether or not the challenges they faced in creating relationships with their patients of Color were due to race/ethnicity, socioeconomic status, or a combination of both (Becker and Newsom 2003). Yet Saraswathi Vedam and colleagues (2019) found that among low-income women, Women of Color reported mistreatment significantly more often than white women. Therefore, race likely still impacts medical interactions among women in lower socioeconomic categories, but many obstetricians may be reluctant to discuss how race affects their exchanges with patients, as these participants were. While their experiences are not necessarily indicative of other obstetricians' experiences, their stories correlate in several ways with how Women of Color categorize interactions with healthcare providers (Sacks 2018; McLemore et al. 2018; Altman et al. 2019; Parsons 2020). For example, in their study of the healthcare experiences of pregnant, birthing, and postnatal Women of Color, McLemore and colleagues (2018) reported that participants categorized many of their interactions with all levels of healthcare staff as disrespectful and stressful. The level of discomfort on both sides likely creates these kinds of interactions, particularly when implicit or even explicit bias is present among healthcare workers.

RQ3: What Challenges Do US Obstetricians Experience in Establishing Relationships with Their Patients of Different Races and Ethnicities?

Interview participants spoke about two main types of challenges that they and other obstetricians face in establishing relationships with their patients. Participants first discussed the challenges that their patients of low-income families must tackle, such as food insecurity, transportation issues, job and time constraints, strained relationships, and financial difficulties (Crimmins et al. 2004; Chang et al. 2015). Again, participants focused on challenges created by socioeconomic status rather than race, with the caveat that People of Color, particularly Black or African American women, are more likely to come from lower income families (Crimmins et al. 2004; Noël 2018).

Abdul discussed some of the challenges his patients deal with during labor and delivery with anecdotes illustrating his points:

A lot of the issues that get brought up on labor and delivery have less to do with the laboring process and more to do with the life outside the hospital. So, for example, I've had patients who need to leave in the middle of their laboring process because they lose childcare or something else happens. Or they get preeclampsia, and we're recommending induction, but they have children at home or a partner that, you know, they're the sole person who can drive their partner to work.

Sara is an obstetrician working in an urban county hospital who sees mostly underrepresented minorities from low-income families. She also mentioned several ways in which her patients struggle to survive in poverty and how that struggle impacts these patients' desires to build a relationship with her:

Many of my patients are trying to feed their families or have no one to watch their children or no way to get to the hospital—taking several buses over hours to reach a hospital just doesn't work. They're tired. Being alone and stressed is hard, for anyone. When they get to me, they just want to be done and move on. I'm a means to an end. I'm sure they would prefer that I don't treat them badly, but they aren't looking for a friend, they want a doctor.

Whereas Abdul and Sara recognized how these challenges could influence building relationships with their clients, many clinic and hospital policies regarding booking and keeping appointments reveal a lack of understanding of the patients' realities. Diane described the policies of the clinics in her area:

So, I think it's still the case here, but when I was in residency, so there's a high rate of people not showing up for their appointments so they double and triple-booked appointments. Well, what do you do if everybody shows up? And they would book everybody to come in first thing in the morning. So, if you saw a patient at 11:00 a.m., they had been waiting there at least since 8:00 a.m.

These practices not only affect how minority patients feel about going to a doctor, but also create barriers to receiving care. Patients of Color may also view these practices as disrespectful and discriminatory, which could make building trust even more difficult.

The other set of challenges participants discussed were related to obstetricians' training. In particular, Diane and Jackson, as obstetricians who had been working for decades, mentioned the lack of medical school training they received for working with diverse populations. Jackson described the training and atmosphere in the medical school he attended:

I went to a public medical school that had the largest—term that they used was the "urban health program." It was the largest urban health program in the country. I not only didn't get any cultural sensitivity training, but—and you know, I'm 55—but there was real resentment. I didn't feel it particularly in the class because kids who were part of the urban health program received a key to a room that had old exams and sort of special things for them purely by virtue of their ethnicity or race . . . I wasn't intellectually bothered by it and . . . I remember being emotionally bothered by the people who were bothered by it, but also by the institution for not doing a good enough job on explaining it . . . In residency, it wasn't so formal, but there was strong mentorship. These were issues that were talked about.

Abdul, Sara, and Makayla each reported having training in diversity and inclusion in their medical schools. The issue, however, is that many training practices, including mandatory diversity and inclusion training, are not consistent across the United States. Sharon Parsons (2020) found that racism was apparent at many levels within medical schools, including school curricula and climates. Few programs directly addressed healthcare disparities, partly because students showed little interest in practicing in underserved or primarily minority areas (ibid.). In an earlier quotation, Diane discussed the lack of interest (or ability) to work with underserved populations, stating that the amount of debt most medical students have upon completing their degrees prevents them from practicing in underserved areas.

Diane also described the situation in many clinics that treat patients of Color from low-income areas, and how that situation, combined with the history of abuse that patients of Color have faced, impacts the potential for a lasting patient/physician relationship:

They walk in the door and they get assigned to a medical student who is using them for practice, which is pretty much the case across the country. Medical students and residents use poor patients for practicing. So, they get a medical student that doesn't know that much. They try to explain what's going on. The medical student does the best they can. Then the intern comes in. Then the upper-level resident comes in. And if it's a bad enough situation, the attending comes in. So, they have no choices in who is taking care of them. Some of the people taking care of them will be exhausted. The nurses can be indifferent to their suffering because the nurses are overworked . . . so, they have no choice, and they are totally at the mercy of the system. And they've seen that bad things have happened to their grandparents and their parents and their aunts and uncles, and they have no reason to trust us.

In addition, Diane mentioned another phenomenon in medical training that increases exhaustion and overwork among medical residents, reducing the quality of care that patients receive:

So in residency programs in ob/gyn, everybody has to finish that program with a certain degree of proficiency in gynecologic surgery. So, you have to limit the number of residents, so that everybody can get enough cases to be proficient. In a county program or a public hospital program, that's never enough to cover the obstetric population. So, in public programs, residents are stretched thin in obstetrics.

Makayla and Sara reported similar policies in their workplaces. Makayla and Diane also discussed how the location of a hospital can contribute to making getting care difficult. Makayla explained it this way:

The new hospital was built on the north side of the city because they could surround it with businesses there and make money. The poorer residents live on the south side, though, which means they have to take a bus to get to the hospital. When the bus arrives, people just flood off all at once. There aren't enough staff to take care of everyone at once, so people wait. Sometimes, they can't wait because someone needs to pick up their kids or go to work, so they leave and try to reschedule.

The challenges that low-income patients, particularly patients of Color, and healthcare providers face work together to create an atmosphere that is not conducive to building relationships. Most participants recognized this problem, but were unsure how to make structural changes to the healthcare system. Nevertheless, each participant continued to search for ways to connect with their patients and to acknowledge their patients' struggles. Overall, these efforts increased the longer a participant was in practice. However, as previously noted, many patients of Color from low-income areas see medical students, interns, and residents instead of providers who have been practicing for years. Physicians early in their careers are more likely to be overwhelmed and overworked, which affects their ability to show empathy, as Diane discussed (see also McNabb, this volume).

Conclusions: A "Perfect Storm"

In the United States, there is a "perfect storm" of mistrust and misunderstanding and personal and structural roadblocks that prevent many physicians and patients from building the patient/physician relationship necessary for reducing healthcare disparities. While, as previously noted, I cannot make general conclusions about US obstetricians from the impressions and experiences of the eight participants in this study, their responses do reveal several avenues for future research. First, many of these participants were uncomfortable discussing the effects that race and ethnicity may have had on their interactions with patients. More learning about these issues in medical schools could not only reveal minority patients' realities to physicians earlier in their careers but also could stimulate important discussions. Second, there are many structural factors in how medical schools train their students that can affect the students' ability to show empathy and understanding. Shifting priorities to reduce overwhelm and overwork would encourage students to treat patients more humanely. Third, the policies of many hospitals and clinics that serve low-income individuals create more misunderstanding and make people less likely to seek out care. Again, increasing awareness and changing policies could begin to build trust between the biomedical community and patients of Color, particularly those from lower socioeconomic categories.

Genevieve Ritchie-Ewing is a biocultural and medical anthropologist working as an Assistant Professor in the Department of Social and Behavioral Sciences at Central State University in Ohio. Her research interests include how cultural expectations and social structures affect maternal experiences during pregnancy and childbirth in the United States. She also explores how the racial biases of US obstetricians create racial and ethnic health disparities.

Notes

1. Qualtrics XMos. n.d. Landing page. Retrieved 12 December 2022 from https://www.qualtrics.com/.
2. Project Implicit. n.d. Landing page. Retrieved 12 December 2022 from https://www.projectimplicit.net/.

3. Project Implicit. n.d. "About the IAT." Retrieved 12 December 2022 from https://www.projectimplicit.net/resources/about-the-iat/.
4. Project Implicit. n.d. "Social Attitudes." Retrieved 12 December 2022 from Project Implicit (harvard.edu)
5. Project Implicit. n.d. "Frequently Asked Questions." Retrieved 12 December 2022 from https://implicit.harvard.edu/implicit/faqs.html#faq10.

References

Alhusen, JL, Bower KM, Epstein E, Sharps P. 2016. "Racial Discrimination and Adverse Birth Outcomes: An Integrative Review." *Journal of Midwifery and Women's Health* 61: 707–720.

Altman MR, Oseguera T, McLemore MR, et al. 2019. "Information and Power: Women of Color's Experiences Interacting with Health Care Providers in Pregnancy and Birth." *Social Science and Medicine* 238: 112491.

Association of American Medical Colleges (AAMC). 2019. "Diversity in Medicine: Facts and Figures 2019." Retrieved 15 December 2021 from https://www.aamc.org/data-reports/workforce/report/diversity-medicine-facts-and-figures-2019.

Becker G, Newsom E. 2003. "Socioeconomic Status and Dissatisfaction with Health Care among Chronically Ill African Americans." *American Journal of Public Health* 93(5): 742–748.

Bernard HR. 2011. *Research Methods in Anthropology: Qualitative and Quantitative Approaches*, 5th edn. Lanham MD: AltaMira Press.

Braveman P, Heck K, Egerter S, et al. 2017. "Worry about Racial Discrimination: A Missing Piece of the Puzzle of Black-White Disparities in Preterm Birth?" *PLoS ONE* 12(10): e0186151.

Brewis AA, Wutich A. 2012. "Explicit versus Implicit Fat-stigma." *American Journal of Human Biology* 24(3): 332-338.

Bridges K. 2011. *Reproducing Race: An Ethnography of Pregnancy as a Site of Racialization*. Berkeley: University of California Press.

Brigham JC. 1993. "College Students' Racial Attitudes." *Journal of Applied Social Psychology* 23: 1933-1967.

Byrd WM, Clayton LA. 2001. "Race, Medicine, and Health Care in the United States: A Historical Survey." *Journal of the National Medical Association* 93(suppl): 11S–34S.

Chang MW, Nitzke S, Buist D, et al. 2015. "'I Am Pregnant and Want To Do Better But I Can't': Focus Groups with Low-Income Overweight and Obese Pregnant Women." *Maternal and Child Health Journal* 19: 1060–1070.

Cheyney M, Davis-Floyd R. 2019. "Birth as Culturally Marked and Shaped." In *Birth in Eight Cultures*, eds. Davis-Floyd R, Cheyney M, 1–16. Long Grove IL: Waveland Press.

Cooper LA, Roter DL, Carson KA, et al. 2012. "The Associates of Clinicians' Implicit Attitudes about Race with Medical Visit Communication and Patient Ratings of Interpersonal Care." *American Journal of Public Health* 102: 979–987.

Cooper Owens D. 2017. *Medical Bondage: Race, Gender, and the Origins of American Gynecology*. Athens: University of Georgia Press.

Crimmins EM, Hayward MD, Seeman TE. 2004. "Race/Ethnicity, Socioeconomic Status, and Health." In *Critical Perspectives on Racial and Ethnic Differences in Health in Late Life*, eds. Anderson NB, Bulatao RA, Cohen B. Washington DC: National Academies Press, 123–135. Retrieved 12 December 2022 from https://www.ncbi.nlm.nih.gov/books/NBK25526/.

Cuevas AG, O'Brien K, Saha S. 2016. "African American Experiences in Healthcare: 'I Always Feel Like I'm Getting Skipped Over.'" *Healthy Psychology* 35(9): 987–995.

Cullin JM. 2021. "Implicit and Explicit Fat Bias Among Adolescents from Two US Populations Varying by Obesity Prevalence." *Pediatric Obesity* 16: e12747.

Davis DA. 2019. "Obstetric Racism: The Racial Politics of Pregnancy, Labor, and Birthing." *Medical Anthropology* 38(7): 560–573.

Diaz-Tello F. 2016. "Invisible Wounds: Obstetric Violence in the United States." *Reproductive Health Matters* 24(47): 56–64.

Dovidio JF, Kawakami K, Gaertner L. 2002. "Implicit and Explicit Prejudice and Interracial Interaction." *Journal of Personality and Social Psychology* 82: 62–68.

Fryer KE, Vines AI, Stuebe AM. 2020. "A Multisite Examination of Everyday Discrimination and the Prevalence of Spontaneous Preterm Birth in African American and Latina Women in the United States." *American Journal of Perinatology* 37(3): 1340–1350.

Giurgescu C, McFarlin BL, Lomax J, et al. 2011. "Racial Discrimination and the Black-White Gap in Adverse Birth Outcomes: A Review." *Journal of Midwifery and Women's Health* 56: 362–370.

Green AR, Carney DR, Pallin DJ, et al. 2007. "Implicit Bias among Physicians and Its Predictions of Thrombolysis Decisions for Black and White Patients." *Journal of General Internal Medicine* 22: 1231–1238.

Greenwald AG, McGhee DE, Schwartz JLK. 1998. "Measuring Individual Differences in Implicit Cognition: The Implicit Association Test." *Journal of Personality and Social Psychology* 74(6): 1464–1480.

Hagiwara N, Dovidio JF, Eggly S, Penner LA. 2016. "The Effects of Racial Attitudes on Affect and Engagement in Racially Discordant Medical Interactions between Non-Black Physicians and Black Patients." *Group Processes and Intergroup Relations* 19(4): 509–527.

Hall WJ, Chapman MV, Kent ML, et al. 2015. "Implicit Racial/Ethnic Bias among Health Care Professionals and Its Influence on Health Care Outcomes: A Systematic Review." *American Journal of Public Health* 105(12): e60–e76.

Jolly P. 2008. "Diversity of US Medical Students by Parental Income." *AAMC Analysis in Brief* 8(1). Retrieved 15 December 2021 from https://www.aamc.org/download/102338/data/aibvol8no1.pdf.

Le HH. 2017. "The Socioeconomic Diversity Gap in Medical Education." *Academic Medicine* 92(8): 1071.

Liese K, Davis-Floyd R, Stewart K, Cheyney M. 2021. "Obstetric Iatrogenesis: The Spectrum of Unintentional Harm, Disrespect, Violence, and Abuse." *Anthropology & Medicine* 28(2): 1–16.

Maina IW, Belton TD, Ginzberg S, Singh A, Johnson TJ. 2018. "A Decade of Studying Implicit Racial/Ethnic Bias in Healthcare Providers Using the Implicit Association Test." *Social Science and Medicine* 1999: 219–229.

Martin JA, Hamilton BE, Osterman MJK, Driscoll AK. 2019. "Births: Final Data for 2018." *National Vital Statistics Reports* 68(13): 1–37. Hyattsville, MD: National Center for Health Statistics.

Martinez T, Wiersma-Mosley JD, Jozkowski KN, Becnel J. 2018. "'Good Guys Don't Rape': Greek and Non-Greek College Student Perpetrator Rape Myths." *Behavioral Sciences* 8(7): 60.

McGregor DK. 1998. *From Midwives to Medicine: The Birth of American Gynecology.* New Brunswick NJ: Rutgers University Press.

McLemore MR, Altman MR, Cooper N, et al. 2018. "Health Care Experiences of Pregnant, Birthing and Postnatal Women of Color at Risk for Preterm Birth." *Social Science and Medicine* 201: 127–135.

Noël RA. 2018. "Race, Economics, and Social Status." *US Bureau of Labor Statistics: Spotlight on Statistics*. Retrieved 15 December 2021 from https://www.bls.gov/spotlight/2018/race-economics-and-social-status/pdf/race-economics-and-social-status.pdf.

Parker-Benfield GJ. 2000. *The Horrors of the Half-Known Life: Male Attitudes toward Woman and Sexuality in Nineteenth-Century America.* London: Routledge.

Parsons S. 2020. "Addressing Racial Biases in Medicine: A Review of the Literature, Critique, and Recommendations." *International Journal of Health Services* 50(4): 371–386.

Payne DL, Lonsway KA, Fitzgerald LF. 1999. "Rape Myth Acceptance: Exploration of Its Structure and Its Measurement Using the Illinois Rape Myth Acceptance Scale." *Journal of Research in Personality* 33: 27–68.

Prather C, Fuller TR, Jeffries WL, et al. 2018. "Racism, African American Women, and Their Sexual and Reproductive Health: A Review of Historical and Contemporary Evidence and Implications for Health Equity." *Health Equity* 2(1): 249–259.

Rayburn WF, Xierali IM, Castillo-Page L, Nivet MA. 2016. "Racial and Ethnic Differences between Obstetrician-Gynecologists and Other Adult Medical Specialists." *Obstetrics & Gynecology* 127(1): 148–152.

Roberts D. 1998. *Killing the Black Body: Race, Reproduction, and the Meaning of Liberty.* New York: Vintage.

Sacks TK. 2018. "Performing Black Womanhood: A Qualitative Study of Stereotypes and the Healthcare Encounter." *Critical Public Health* 28(1): 59–69.

Saluja B, Bryant Z. 2021. "How Implicit Bias Contributes to Racial Disparities in Maternal Morbidity and Mortality in the United States." *Journal of Women's Health* 30(2): 270–273.

Vedam S, Stoll K, Taiwo TK, et al. 2019. "The Giving Voice to Mothers Study: Inequity and Mistreatment during Pregnancy and Childbirth in the United States." *Reproductive Health* 16(1): 77.

Washington HA. 2006. *Medical Apartheid: The Dark History of Medical Experimentation on Black Americans from Colonial Times to the Present.* New York: Doubleday.

Xu K, Nosek B, Greenwald AG. 2014. "Psychology Data from the Race Implicit Association Test on the Project Implicit Demo Website." *Journal of Open Psychology Data* 2(1): 1–11.

Youngclaus J, Fresne JA. October 2020. "Physician Education Debt and the Cost to Attend Medical School: 2020 Update." Washington DC: AAMC.

CHAPTER 5

Censusing the Quechua

Peruvian *Obstetras* in Light of Historic
Sterilizations, Contemporary Accusations,
and Biopolitical Statecraft Obligations

Rebecca Irons

Introduction: The Demonization of Peruvian *Obstetras*

Despite evidence that a Malthusian government health policy was to blame, individual healthcare providers, and particularly obstetricians, are increasingly being demonized in the ongoing case of Peru's more than 300,000 enforced sterilizations of the 1990s. Even before this blame, obstetricians were already in positions of precarity; the profession is highly gendered, and female *obstetras* (obstetricians) find themselves subjugated to the authority of majority-male gynecologists and surgeons. These *obstetras* are currently fighting a legal battle to maintain their status as fully State-endorsed professionals, and their profession is further under fire for concerns over obstetric violence toward the poorer and Indigenous patients served by the national health service. Literature often suggests that obstetric violence occurs in Peru due to the differential races and classes of university-trained biomedical professionals and their impoverished patients (Guerra-Reyes 2019), but in this chapter, I will refute such generalizations and take a more nuanced approach to the complexities of obstetric violence and the *obstetras* who are accused of perpetuating it.

I will argue that while *obstetras* certainly played significant roles in the condemnable historical sterilizations, even today, the underlying push for "quota-filling" as a condition of employment may encourage similar coercive behaviors that seek to limit poor and Indigenous reproduction via contraception and other methods of family planning. Furthermore, over time *obstetras*' tasks have become increasingly administrative, leading to the suggestion that the role may be a "bullshit job" (Graeber 2018)—one that should be meaningful but is rendered "bullshit" by required state "box-ticking" and "form-filling." I will suggest that a key role of Peruvian *obstetras* is to census and discipline the population as a form of stratified biopolitical statecraft (Bridges 2011a) via administrative tasks and meeting quotas, resulting in dissatisfaction among *obstetras*, patient neglect, and accusations of obstetric violence. Only by exploring this situation from the perspective of the *obstetras* themselves will it be possible to effectively understand how and why structural violence is perpetuated at a local level by those who, under other circumstances, might be victims of structural violence themselves.

Obstetrics in rural Peru is an increasingly precarious position. As a largely female workforce in environments where resources may be scarce and healthcare practitioners often need to live away from their families due to rural health center and hospital isolation, Peruvian *obstetras* face multiple problems. It is not only their working conditions that create tensions, but also the historical context of forced sterilizations within which *obstetras*, gynecologists, and primary care doctors are contemporarily instigated and blamed. In the 1990s, it is estimated that more than 300,000 mostly rural, Indigenous women were sterilized as part of the Fujimori government's national family planning program (*Programa Nacional de Salud Reproductiva y Planificación Familiar*) (PNSRPF). These sterilizations were implemented by State employees such as *obstetras* and doctors working for the Ministry of Health (MINSA), though the details and motivations surrounding these scenarios remain murky. Not all sterilizations were forced, but evidence has emerged that many women were coerced and tricked into accepting the removal of their reproductive capabilities (Rousseau 2009; Ewig 2010). Though there has been an increasing amount of scholarship on the women and communities affected by this important and tragic topic, this chapter will examine the perspective from the opposite side: that of the *obstetras* who participated in the sterilizing and/or who continue to work in the shadow of these memories. I will argue that it is only through careful examination of the realities and precarities of *obstetras* that issues surrounding accusations of obstetric violence in Peru can begin to be addressed, as, again, this group is also implicated and coerced into biopolitical statecraft, which for them is difficult to avoid.

A key issue when addressing biomedical practitioners in rural Peruvian communities is that they are portrayed as "racist" and "regionalist," with the assumption being that their vastly differential status from their patients incites bad behavior such as forced sterilizations, but also general obstetric violence. For example, studying the intercultural birthing policy in the Peruvian highlands and commenting on the inability of MINSA workers to sympathize with the beliefs of the Indigenous Quechua (ethnomedical and otherwise), Lucia Guerra-Reyes (2013:157) concluded: "Health personnel, who are mostly urban professionals, identify as 'white' or 'mestizo' and middle class, and assume that their view of the world is normal, desirable, and correct. This persistent ethnocentric attitude, which is shared by many Peruvians, is replicated at all levels of policy and direct-care in health." This view is also shared by Christina Ewig (2010:6), who describes a Quechua woman's experiences at a health center as she imagines they proceeded:

At the health center, she would face a white or mestizo doctor born and educated on the urban coast who would not comprehend her language or customs. He would likely call her *mamacita* (little mama) rather than by her name. Indigenous health concepts like *pacha* (sickness from the earth) would bewilder him, which in turn would frustrate her.

The fact that most healthcare practitioners lack Quechua language skills was also suggested as a means through which they coerced women into sterilizations during the family planning program (PNSRPF), as they were unable or unwilling to sufficiently explain the procedure or its consequences (Rousseau 2009; Ewig 2010). Therefore, in the literature on healthcare practitioners in Peru, one is faced with what appears to be a definitive racist and classist distinction between *obstetras* and patients. This distinction simplifies the understandings of coercion—*of course* white and mestizo doctors would treat Indigenous patients badly if they have been educated by, and live in, a country with a "persistent ethnocentric attitude" (Guerra-Reyes 2013:157). However, I argue that this view lacks both nuance and sufficient ethnographic data on lived realities and falls into simplistic race/class dichotomies.

Methods

I carried out the research on which this chapter is based around the MINSA healthcare network in the rural Ayacucho province of Vilcashuaman, where the majority of *obstetras* and other healthcare providers not only spoke Quechua but also were Quechua. Having grown up in the surrounding areas, they knew a great deal about ethnomedical health concepts and local customs. During 2018, I lived for a year in the province capital of Vilcashuaman as well as in a smaller village conducting ethnographic fieldwork through participant observation and interviews with Quechua women and healthcare practitioners. I conducted this research as part of my doctoral dissertation project, and sought to investigate the contemporary implementation of the State family planning program in an area previously ravaged by both internal conflict due to Shining Path,[1] as well as the historical sterilization abuses.

Discriminatory Behaviors

With the above-mentioned nuances in mind, the fact that coercive and discriminatory activities still continue may actually seem more significant in the absence of simple binaries with which to analyze those behaviors. Instead, when healthcare practitioners and patients are more similar than the literature would have one believe, a deeper analysis is required to understand discriminatory behaviors, which this chapter addresses. And those behaviors *do* occur.

Khiara Bridges (2011b:38) suggested that such biomedical animosity toward patients of similar backgrounds may be due to practitioners' desires to distance themselves from those patients, as "the staff's animosity . . . is intensified by a recognition of [their] own similarity to the patient's profile and [their] desire to disavow the discursively disparaged patient as an abject version of [themselves]", and that "at least some portion of the hostility . . . demonstrated toward . . . patients can be explained as an attempt to create distance between [themselves and their patients] such that they could not, or no longer, be considered abject forms of [themselves—the practitioners]" (2011b:39). Indeed, in Peru, healthcare workers and other state employees, by virtue of their studies and their differential status, may place themselves "above" those with whom they grew up. Looking at intercultural education, Maria Elena Garcia (2005:118) commented that "even if teachers were from highland towns, their profession placed them in a higher social stratum than the Quechua farmers and herders." Thus, practitioner behaviors may be classist if not racist, or both. These attitudes reflect a common phenomenon in Peru called *choleandao*: when one group of Peruvians looks down on another, who looks down upon another. Walter Pariona Cabrera (2017:41) asserted that in Ayacucho, *choleando* is quite prevalent, and that the healthcare practitioners' attitudes of looking down on their Indigenous patients (who may be similar to them in many ways) is *choleando*. Other Peruvians may look down on those same healthcare workers, and so on.

There are also other factors at work in the ways in which *obstetras* treat patients. Life as an *obstetra* is highly precarious, as the following paragraphs will discuss, and it is important to recognize this precarity when approaching negative behaviors. For example, a change of law was proposed in 2018 that would demote *obstetras* to the category of "non-medical" personnel—a position akin to a "technical" career (e.g., a nurse), that would remove a degree of respect and authority over patients from their jobs. There have been numerous manifestations and marches in protest of this change. However, this situation further underscores both the precariousness in which *obstetras* operate and the belittlement that they receive from the Peruvian government and from other workers within their own healthcare networks.

It is necessary to note here how and why such a legal suggestion could be made, and why Peruvian obstetrics is potentially ambiguous. *Obstetras* are demonstrably *not* the same as midwives in Peru, who are considered "traditional" (there is no official category of "midwife" in the healthcare services), and who themselves have been pushed to the margins due to the increasing biomedicalization of birth in the country. Nor are *obstetras* the same as a North American ob/gyn in terms of their job roles and capabilities. To mark the nuances, I refer to these Peruvian obstetricians using the Spanish term *obstetras*. In Peru, *obstetras* handle all reproductive health issues, including family planning, pregnancy and labor, and cervical cancer screening and consultation, but, unlike obstetricians in other countries, they do not operate. Instead, cesareans and other gynecological surgeries are performed by (mostly male) gynecologists, thereby diminishing the role of the *obstetra*. If the career of the *obstetra* were to be demoted to "non-medical," little would change in terms of their tasks, but they would lose some power of decision-making and respect within the biomedical hierarchy. Therefore, they have been struggling to hold onto their professional categorization.

In addition to these stresses, *obstetras* are constantly aiming to fulfill targets, or *metas* (goals), set forth by their employers—an activity that results in stressful working situations, which, at the same time, may incite coercive behaviors by the *obstetras*, for which they are later personally blamed. Thus, I argue that it is not possible to understand the treatment of Quechua women in Peruvian healthcare networks without also addressing the situation of the *obstetras* who serve them.

Contemporary Quota-Filling and Historical Sterilization Accusations

> "We belong to a network that give us *metas* [goals] to reach every year. Like, we must cover 200 couples each per year [with family planning]. But you can't obligate—no, no, no."
> —*Obstetra*, Vilcashuaman

Obstetras and gynecologists are being blamed for the forced sterilizations, and furthermore, these accusations are increasingly gunning for individual blood rather than collective punishment. In Vilcashuaman, specific names of those who performed the sterilizations have been identified by patients, and therefore this mounting tension may directly affect those *obstetras* in Vilcashuaman who were working at the time. Importantly, *obstetras* are not actually licensed to perform tubal ligation sterilizations. However, they have been directly mentioned in sterilization testimonies given to me, and *obstetras* whom I interviewed also spoke about "sterilizing" women. This may mean that they either illegally performed the sterilizations themselves, or accompanied and assisted the doctors and/or gynecologists who were qualified to do so. Either event would render them culpable, although to varying degrees of legality and intent. Therefore, when the literature speaks of "doctors" sterilizing women in regard to *obstetras*, they were arguably either acting in the role of doctor or directly supporting a doctor by rounding up and coercing patients and/or assisting the actual surgery. As *obstetras* admit to having quotas, it can be concluded that, at the very least, they acted as the initial vehicle through which women were brought into the clinics for sterilization. Although there are those who argue that the Fujimori government is the culpable party because it obligated gynecologists to sterilize certain numbers of people through enforced quotas, or *metas* (Ewig 2010; Rousseau 2007), the condemnation of individual *obstetras* and gynecologists as acting alone operates as a counter to this idea.

Gonzalo Gianella (2014) claimed that, owing to the mounting evidence released against the *Colegio Medico de Peru* (Peruvian Medical College), its members felt obliged to create their "own version of the story" (2014:80). This story, Gianella suggested, sought to portray biomedical staff as victims of a perverse system, just as were the women whom they were sterilizing (2014:81), and blamed the structure of the Peruvian healthcare system, as opposed to individual will, to sterilize without consent. However, Gianella (2014:84) concluded that if this were really the case, MINSA would be apologizing for the past, when it has not. He went on to note that, as a doctor himself, he has never known a surgeon who did not enjoy his own authority (2014:88). Gianella also noted that if there had been a lack of medical will to do so, then thousands of sterilizations would not have occurred, and that no one resisted (2014:89)—an observation that Jorge A. Villegas (2017:109) also made—and that Peruvian doctors have blamed other actors in society (e.g., MINSA or the government) for their own actions (2014:86–87). Finally, Gianella (2014:89) stated that "the Peruvian doctors who sterilized thousands of women . . . did it convinced that they were doing what was medically correct."

As previously noted, healthcare practitioners, and particularly female *obstetras*, are already in precarious situations in Vilcashuaman, and were somewhat disempowered during the family planning program (PNSRPF; *Programa Nacional de Salud Reproductiva y Planificación Familiar*) regarding autonomy in the clinic. They argued that they were responding to the demands of the job to save their own livelihoods. This argument is not necessarily enough to exonerate these *obstetras* from perpetrating serious obstetric violence, if that is indeed the case, but it is also necessary to hear their voices to better understand their motivations for doing so.

Perhaps understandably, *obstetras* shied away from being interviewed about the PNSRPF. It is not necessarily that these *obstetras* feel guilty or deny that the sterilizations happened. Many practitioners maintain that women were not *forced* but *convinced*, and that *they were obliged* to reach certain goals as biomedical professionals, or they might lose their jobs. One *obstetra* put a figure to this situation: "They told us that we had to convince five women a month to have the *ligadura*." Another elaborated further on her experiences of working during this period:

> Women who had up to three children were ok [to sterilize], but less than that, one or two, no. In the rural places it was more—those who worked in that time had a kind of contract where *si o si* (yes or yes)—you had to capture (*captar*) people. If you didn't capture enough women, then you would lose your contract, so the staff, for fear of losing their jobs, had to complete their contracts however they could, even using force (*a la fuerza*). I didn't see any violence—the idea was to convince (*convencer*) the patients, although the reality I saw might have been different from what others saw—I have colleagues that *si o si* had to take people with violence . . . We had to work 12 hours a day, so we had to do more extra-curricular activities . . . go to the communities . . . it was like that.

The "capture" of patients refers to the targets given to practitioners. Stéphanie Rousseau (2007:108) wrote that "the government's prioritization of tubal ligation was . . . reflected in target quotas and incentives offered to medical personnel . . . quotas were pursued, notably, by holding 'tubal ligation and vasectomy festivals' organized by MINSA staff in various poor regions of Peru." Ewig (2010:152) also concurred with the notion that "If quotas for sterilizations were not met, then within this labor structure, professionals risked losing their jobs." However, because of these pressures, it was claimed that the workers "overstepped the norms in order to fulfil a quota and touched people who should not have been touched" (2010:152).

Although practitioners in Vilcashuaman continue to express innocence and to claim that they were "only following orders" when sterilizing, it is worth mentioning that the files containing medical information about the known sterilization victims had "gone missing" from the health posts when I tried to locate them. It should also be noted that this was a fact that not one healthcare worker tried to conceal from me, so the absent files do not necessarily express guilt, but may highlight the unease produced in *obstetras* when they are singled out for "justice." It is also worth reiterating that in Vilcashuaman, it is known who specifically participated in the sterilizations. Rural healthcare networks are small, and, again, *obstetras* and other healthcare practitioners are recognizable. Therefore, the threat of denunciation constantly lingers over those who performed the sterilizations. Indeed, *obstetras* are fearful of being denounced by patients, not only for past sterilizations, but also for contemporary maltreatment. For example, one *obstetra* told me that it was always important to ensure that the forms (described below) were filled out correctly, and that the patient had given their fingerprints as consent; otherwise, the patients would *denunciar* (denounce) them.

Although I never actually heard of a case where a patient had successfully taken any healthcare provider to court or "denounced" them, the increasing focus on individualized guilt for their sterilizations may heighten *obstetras'* awareness of this possibility. *Obstetras* often fretted over this. For example, when one *obstetra* was discussing the day-to-day realities of her work, she said:

> *Obstetra*: In reality it's difficult . . . it becomes difficult because of legal things (*se hace difícil por las cosas legales*).
>
> *Rebecca*: What do you mean by *cosas legales*?
>
> *Obstetra*: The patients can denounce you for everything, they want to denounce you (*te quieren denunciar*). It's not easy working here for sure because of this.

She was not alone in her concern about being denounced. Another *obstetra* said that her work was difficult because her patients would often neglect their contraceptive method, or the method would inexplicably fail, and she would be blamed for their unwanted pregnancy: "If she becomes pregnant, it's you who she will denounce, and why? Because now she has four children, and who is at fault? Because sometimes we say that a method is *seguro* (safe), but instead we should say that it is 'highly effective.'"

The fact that *obstetras* showed concern over a patient taking legal action underscores one important thing—that those patients are not entirely without agency in their interactions with healthcare workers. Although it may prove legally complicated and expensive should a patient wish to officially report malpractice on the part of an *obstetra*, the fact that the threat of this possibility is felt in the health posts suggests that Quechua patients may have a degree of agency and power within this situation, perhaps more than they are aware of. However, Quechua women are also wary of being denounced by official workers in turn. As one woman suggested to me, people in her village were previously asked to sign paperwork that was used "to denounce us" (though it was unclear what for); hence she no longer wanted to sign anything official nor to respond to questions.

Denouncement can be a weapon of agency on both sides; thus both sides are suspicious of it, perhaps underscoring the shared cultural approach to certain State mechanisms by Indigenous *obstetras* and their patients. Yet despite these concerns over potential legal problems with patients, *obstetras* did not necessarily cease certain behaviors. In all this, of vital importance and contemporary concern is the subject of quotas, or *metas* (goals). This subsection of this chapter opens with a quote from the head *obstetra* at the healthcare center in the village. She admits that goals are given by "the network"—the MINSA network—which decides how many people healthcare workers need to "capture," similarly to the Fujimori quotas. But this is not a quote from 20 years ago, as may be inferred; instead, it is happening right now.

Obstetras face mounting blame for the sterilizations they performed, or helped to perform, whereas they claim that they were responding to government-set quotas. However, *obstetras* must fulfill *metas* or risk loss of work. Sterilization as a specific target has long been off the table, an *obstetra* argued—yet in a bid to fulfill their mandated goals, coercion may still occur in regard to other contraceptive methods (although she insisted that they could not obligate people). In fact, *obstetras* are somewhat hushed about these contemporary targets, as they are aware of the implications. One *obstetra* directly (and misleadingly) told me, "We don't have targets because then we'd have to obligate, like in the time of Fujimori." Her superiors said otherwise. Furthermore, the achievement of *metas* is also still implicated in *obstetras*' job security, as evidenced by the frequent evaluations.

Evaluations, Paperwork, and Precarity

Unless an *obstetra* has earned a "named" position after years of service, she will need to undergo an evaluation at the end of every contract period. To be "named," or *nombrada*, grants a worker special privileges and permissions not available to those under contract, and is usually granted after a minimum of ten years of service within one healthcare institution (Ewig 2010:105). Without this status, whether or not an *obstetra* will have her contract extended or terminated will depend on the positivity of this evaluation.

To pass the evaluation, *obstetras* need to prove that they are reaching the *metas* assigned to them for "capturing" women for prenatal care or contraception. This proof is shown through documentation of work completed and lists of patient records that show how many people have been attended by each practitioner. In a rural network such as Vilcash-uaman with little technology, this is all done by hand, leading to an excess of paperwork and administration due to the evaluations that non-named workers (who are the majority) must undergo every three to six months, depending on their particular contract. No paper trail, no proof; no proof, no positive evaluation; no evaluation, no contract renewal.

During fieldwork one day, I found an *obstetra* in her consultation room sitting behind a stack of papers and forms when I came to interview her. Her contract was coming to an end, and with the evaluation looming, she was hurriedly trying to complete the necessary forms to prove that she had reached her *metas* and should be kept on as an employee. Stressed by her imminent professional "Judgment Day," she was keen to offload about the evaluation and contracts:

> *Obstetra*: Look, when you have this kind of contract [short term, renewable] it's not that stable, in any moment they can tell you that you have to go and look for another job . . . if they want to put someone else . . . it's not stable. It's stressful. What papers you might have to prepare, maybe you need to study a bit more, so you are ready for the evaluation. If you don't pass it, then *hasta aquí chau* (until here, then goodbye). The modality of work is like that: they contract you, they evaluate you, then they contract you . . .

Rebecca: What are the duties that you must fulfill to pass the evaluation and be contracted again?

Obstetra: It's according to your profile. Yes, you have to *captar* pregnant women [*gestantes*], yes, you have to *captar* women for *métodos* [contraceptive methods]. If you achieve this according to your profile, then there's no problem . . . In the case that you don't fulfill your profile, then yes, the superiors have the obligation not to contract you again.

Rebecca: Do they give different "profiles" to different workers depending on their experience or abilities?

Obstetra: It depends; it's personal. If you are doing well, then they will renew your contract.

If, as this *obstetra* states, she and other healthcare workers are still at risk of job loss lest they fail to fulfill certain *meta*s outlined in their contracts, then, arguably, those same incentives that resulted in past coercive sterilizations continue to exist in some healthcare networks. It is not hard to conclude that if an *obstetra* is given a goal of reaching say, 200 people per year for family planning, and her job depends on successfully fulfilling that *meta*, then she may do so by whatever means possible—including coercion.[2] However, if such activities continue to exist as they did under the Fujimori presidency, it should be questioned whether or not coercive behaviors and accusations of obstetric violence occur due to racism and discrimination, as suggested by Ewig (2010) and Guerra-Reyes (2013); or due to power-mad authority abuse and self-righteousness, as suggested by Gianella (2017:88); or if in fact they may be due to institutional and structural conditions that *obligate obstetras* to pursue certain activities and behaviors on behalf of the State in order to keep their jobs. Of course, it is tempting to suggest that they should "just say no." However, realistically, losing one's employment is unlikely to be a viable option for these *obstetras*, who also need to survive financially.

A further problem with this kind of system is that so concerned are *obstetras* to produce a positive evaluation that they necessarily concentrate a large part of their working time attending to the accompanying paperwork to prove that they have performed successfully. To complete an evaluation, *obstetras* need to not only provide evidence of patient records through the FUA and HIS (discussed below) but also to complete large quantities of other documentation to prove that they have been working hard (such as, for examples, lists of houses visited, regardless of patient attendance once there, and records of additional training and professional development). Though there may be some use to forms that collect patient data, as will be later argued, much of the paperwork that goes toward the evaluation cannot necessarily be considered as such. Impossible to overstate is the sheer volume of the working day, during which *obstetras* and other practitioners can be observed completing paperwork and forms at every level of the healthcare network. *Obstetras* will fill forms during lunch breaks, during consultations, and even on days off, for if the forms are incomplete, the employee faces penalties. Indeed, paperwork administration is not confined to MINSA, but is a feature of government offices across Peru. As Joaquín Yrivarren Espinoza (2011:22) suggested in his study of a Lima municipality's transition to an electronic system, for most public service workers, "paper is king" (*papelito manda*). Many sectors of the government, especially in rural areas, lack the resources to move to an electronic system, and all "paperwork" in the Vilcashuaman MINSA network is just that—written on paper.

This heavy reliance on paperwork also produces another effect: it turns the practitioners into administrators. There are obvious negative effects of this transformation—more time spent filling forms and filing them away means less time with patients. It also takes a toll on the practitioners themselves. Everyone always complained about the amount of paperwork required of them, and I can attest that it is genuinely excessive.

Obstetra evaluation paperwork aside, the principal forms that must be completed for each patient are the FUA (*formato único de atención/* care records form) and the HIS (*historia/*patient history) along with other specific forms for the patient's medical concerns (e.g., family planning record, pregnancy record, etc.), as well as the medication(s) and contraceptive methods a patient has been prescribed or has discussed. These forms are then filed in a paper folder stored within the patient's corresponding healthcare center. When patients come for an appointment, they must fetch their corresponding folder from the records room, and the *obstetra* will return it once the new paperwork is filed. The following section addresses the political function of these specific forms themselves; however, for now, it is instructive to examine how the workers relate to these forms and to paperwork more generally.

It may be telling that those who are undertaking their mandatory year of rural service (SERUM), the *serumistas*, who are new to the MINSA system, make jokes about the patient forms, both verbally and in the form of shared memes. For example, one meme shows a shocked "Lisa Simpson" staring down at an FUA and reads: "My face the first time that I saw the FUA and HIS [forms]." The second shows a cross-armed, grumpy "Pingu the Penguin" and reads, "I want to fulfil my *meta*, but I don't like to fill out FUA or HIS." Daniel Miller and colleagues (2016:172) argue that memes are a way to reinforce norms; in this case, the begrudging acceptance of certain paperwork to reach one's goal (and the importance of fulfilling that goal) through humor: "Memes circulate as a mode of moralizing and humor; as such they are a way of reinforcing social norms . . . there seems to be a case for regarding memes more generally as a kind of 'internet police,' attempting to assert moral control through social media." Thus, the sharing of discontent with MINSA paperwork through memes may be part of the process by which *serumistas* come to understand the gap between their studies at university and their actual roles within the healthcare network—fewer patients and less hands-on health care, more forms and tedium. However, *serumistas* are new to their roles, and after years of such tasks, one's humor may change. *Obstetras* would often lament about how frustrated they felt with the situation. An *obstetra* sighed, "Look, it's all paperwork. *Todo papeleo*."

On this subject, David Graeber (2018:9–10) discusses the rise of unsatisfactory work through the "phenomenon of bullshit jobs"; work which he defines as: "a form of paid employment that is so completely pointless . . . that the employee cannot justify its existence even though, as part of the conditions of employment, the employee feels obliged to pretend that this is not the case." Neither Graeber nor I would ever suggest that the work of *obstetras* and other healthcare workers is in any way pointless (for example, Graeber [2018: xix] mentions nursing as the opposite of "bullshit"). However, the rise of the administrative sector, which results in reams and reams of paperwork destined for nowhere *is* highlighted as "bullshit" by Graeber (2018: xv).

Of course, not all forms are useless, as the following section will discuss; however, here I refer principally to those forms that justify an *obstetra*'s evaluation (as opposed to the FUA and HIS), and that must be completed over and over as every new evaluation cycle begins. As such, a job that is vital in many aspects, yet reduces itself to mindlessness through State-mandated necessity, could be seen as "partly bullshit" (Graeber 2018:24). What should be an active, engaging job such as obstetrics is arguably becoming pointless to an extent in the eyes of *obstetras* and other practitioners due to the endless march of paperwork and form-filling (and lack of patient interaction). Furthermore, the destination of these forms is likely at the bottom of a cabinet or a dank records room, alongside other forms like the contract evaluation records, which may never even be properly reviewed due to the volume and frequency with which all un-named staff submit them. The tasks of filling out the FUA and HIS forms are specifically what Graeber (2018:46) calls "box-ticking," which is often a form of government, and functions to "allow an organization to be able to claim it is doing something that, in fact, it is not doing" (2018:45) (e.g., to satisfy MINSA *metas*). The effect that this "box-ticking" has on a person is far more serious than idle boredom, Graeber argues, and can be "soul destroying" (2018:133). Humans, he suggests, are wired to produce a cause and an effect (2018:113), the lack of which can result in stress (2018:117) and physical illness (2018:119). Furthermore, the very act of forced pretense—of pretending that one is undertaking something meaningful while realizing that this is untrue— can be particularly damaging. *Obstetras* do realize that the paperwork is stopping them from spending any real time with patients but are forced to do it anyway for their evaluations. Graeber (2018:113–134) muses:

> It is hard to imagine anything more soul destroying than . . . being forced to commit acts of arbitrary bureaucratic cruelty against one's will. To become the face of the machine that one despises. To become a monster. It has not escaped my notice that the most frightening monsters in popular fiction do not simply threaten to rend or torture or kill you but to turn you into a monster yourself: think here of vampires, zombies, werewolves. They terrify because they menace not just your body but also your soul.

Following on from Graeber's rather haunting premonition, if *obstetras'* jobs are becoming partly bullshit through the perpetuation of the *administerization* of biomedical care, nevertheless they must continue to do so in order to satisfy the evaluations that will ensure the continuation of their employment—the evaluations that are based upon the target-reaching that has historically led to mass sterilizations and subsequent blame. Thus, how can *obstetras* be expected to offer optimum care to their patients when they can barely find time to be with them, and the system that measures their success is geared toward reproductive coercion? When addressing obstetric violence, this situation clearly needs to be taken into consideration, and the literature has yet to do so

Although healthcare networks are set up to provide biomedical care, the aforementioned situation suggests that there may be other motives; it seems clear that paperwork and form-filling data collection are being prioritized over patient primary care. Thus, there may be an impetus and a motive for the patient forms beyond optimum care provision. It has been suggested that the very nature of paper-based forms and medical reporting may have implications for the ways in which the healthcare system and employee relations (both with patients and with each other) are constructed through the act of writing, which would be lost in an electronic system, thus supporting the continuation of paperwork. Marc Berg (1996) argued that the patient record itself can be taken as a "Latourian force" that transforms the social interactions around it (1996:501) and renders the patients "manageable" (1996:507)—an important point to which I return in the following section. Significantly, the use of paper administration made the previously mentioned disappearance of sterilization records possible, thereby directly mediating relationships not only of provider-patient interaction, but potentially also of justice. As Yrivarren Espinoza (2011:22) stated, "For many Peruvians, to be 'papered' (*empapelado*) means to be submitted to an unjust power." Indeed, this issue of paperwork tying one to a power system is not inconsequential; it does exactly that, through the census.

Data, Census, and Biopolitical Statecraft

As noted in the Series Overview in Volume I of this three-volume series (Davis-Floyd and Premkumar 2023a, 2023b, 2023c, 2023d), "'biopolitics' refers to a way of regulating populations through 'biopower'—the application and impacts of political power on human biology in all aspects of human life" (Davis-Floyd and Premkumar 2023b:xiv). The paperwork that *obstetras* and other healthcare workers must complete not only contributes to suboptimal patient care, but is also intimately related to the State and its power. Gathering and recording data on patients tells MINSA a great deal about the population with whom the contracted workers are dealing—information that is very important for the exercise of State biopower—though indeed it is worth noting here that this information-gathering is only useful where specific kinds of data are collected through an FUA or HIS. Taken as such, the focus and importance placed upon data-gathering and record-keeping through staff incentives (i.e., "complete the tasks or lose your job") becomes unpacked. Indeed, *metas* may be about encouraging contraception coverage by any means to control the fertility of a population, but they also ensure that healthcare workers collect information from as many patients as they possibly can to achieve their *metas*/work targets. Thus, in this section I argue that the FUAs and the HISs are more than just paperwork; *they are also agents of power.*

Berg (1996:513) suggested that "the medical record is one of the ways power differences are materially constituted," as "the reality of a patient's body is assessed and transformed through layers of paperwork" (1996:511). Furthermore, Berg (1996:501) wrote that the medical record is a "force" in and of itself, *mediating* the relations that act and work through it . . . social interaction is *transformed through* it" (italics in original). The information recorded on these seemingly innocent sheets of paper does not and cannot reflect "reality" or "the truth," as these are highly subjective. The papers thus are records made by individual actors to interact with other actors; their contents and consequential calls-to-action dictate the social interactions (perpetuated by the papers) that occur during the evaluations. In Berg's discussion, such interactions take place among those within the hospital network. Yet the relationships that are mediated by the medical forms may be much larger than that. Such relationships may occur with patients, other practitioners, the State, and on to the global health communities with a vested interest in the national government, such as USAID in the case of Peru—if we consider the destinies of health statistics and their influences on donor programs, for example—and on it goes. It thus further follows that medical records such as the FUA and the HIS should be understood as actors within a human-nonhuman relationship, and should be treated as equal agents of power.

From this perspective, we can see that the information on the MINSA forms does not just record a patient's "reality," but actively incites a transformation in that reality. Simply put, the data collected on the forms—data about children, fertility, contraceptives etc.—is fed back to the State (or at least has the *possibility* to be so), which can then take steps toward its own goals for the population based upon this information—which can be seen as biopolitics. On this subject, Michel Foucault ([1978] 1990:25) stated that governments perceive that they are "not simply dealing with subjects or even with a 'people,' but with a 'population' with its specific phenomena"—a population whose reproduction becomes a "thing one administered" ([1978] 1990:24). Ways to achieve this "administration" include "analysis, stocktaking, classification, and . . . quantitative . . . studies" ([1978] 1990:24), all of which culminate in the census—the ultimate way to analyze and take stock of a group of people (or a nation). To expand, Dianna Taylor (2011:46) writes:

> Biopower administers life rather than threatening to take it away. In order to administer life, it is important for the [national government] to obtain forecasts and statistical estimates covering such demographic factors as fertility, natality . . . for this reason, an important moment in the history of biopower is the development of the modern census.

The "administration of life" is possible through governmentality, and James Scott (1999) suggested that the State needs to collect comprehensive data on its citizens to achieve the "legibility" to govern effectively. The census—an "instrument of statecraft" (1999: 343)—is the tool used to collect this data. Scott (1999:77) outlined the aim and scope of the census thusly:

> State simplifications such as maps, censuses, cadastral [surveying] lists, and standard units of measurement represent techniques for grasping a large and complex reality; in order for officials to be able to comprehend aspects of the ensemble, that complex reality must be reduced to schematic categories.

It is important to note that in Peru, the 2017 State census re-introduced ethnic categories, including Indigenous self-identification, and that this re-introduction was analyzed as highlighting the Peruvian government's re-emerging interest in identifying these communities within the country (Chirapaq 2017). Thus, it follows that the FUA, HIS, and other forms of data collection undertaken in MINSA are also forms of census-taking that may eventually contribute to the whole State snapshot of population demographics.

In the case of the medical records, the term "census" can be applied if one considers the motivation and execution of the modern census and notes the same manner of reductionist statistical collection in the FUA and HIS. However, if the national census can identify the ethnicities of communities in the county, then the health census can identify bio-elements of the people within those ethnic categories and "report back" to the central government statistics and population demographic databases. The work of MINSA can help to flesh out the realities of the population's health to make them "legible" (Scott 1999). Yet this work is arguably not only about understanding these realities. The health data gathered can also help the State to "administer life" (Foucault [1978] 1990) for these groups. For example, *obstetras* are careful to ask questions about a patient's fertility, infant mortality, use of contraception and reasons for discontinued use, number of sexual partners, and so forth—all of which is written down in the medical record. Combined with the national census information on ethnicity, one would now be able to infer the relationship between, say, Quechua women's fertility compared to the also Indigenous Aymara of Peru, and therefore create more meticulously targeted healthcare programs based upon this new information, for better or for worse.

It is important to note that the gathering and tabulation of statistical data about a "population" is a constructive activity in and of itself. As Khiara Bridges (2011b:148) argued: "The measurement and quantification of population does not occur after the population has been constructed; rather, population is constructed simultaneously with its measurement and quantification." Ian Hacking (1990:3) calls this population construction "making up people." To count people and their characteristics, it must first be decided which categories will be presented for them to be placed into. For example, Indigenous/ethnic categories must be reduced into quantifiable categories, thereby producing those ethnic categories through the act of the national census's insistence on citizens self-selecting only one such category, when they might actually also belong to another, or to several.

In terms of the census information that the *obstetras* collect, this categorization and quantification may be even more ambiguous. For example, listing a contraceptive for the FUA may be made more difficult if the woman did not consent to past contraceptives that she has had, or if she and her sexual partner(s) use natural or traditional methods (such as the rhythm method or withdrawal) that do not feature as an acceptable biomedical census category. One risks being a non-user statistic through the necessary rigidity of quantitative State data collection. The census forces people to put a number on things that may be too complicated to quantify, thus inventing the categories "in which people could conveniently fall in order to be counted" (Hacking 1990:3). This not simply counting, either. As Hacking argued, statistical inference and the census are based upon an idea that through classification, "one can improve-control a deviant subpopulation" (1990:3) The forms of data collection that make up *obstetras'* days, then, are arguably themselves agents of State biopolitics. In light of the recent national census's focus on ethnic, particularly Indigenous, categorizations, the mass collection of family planning and contraception use data and statistics should not be brushed off as "business as usual." The Peruvian state seemingly wants to know the ethnic and bio-realities of the Quechua (and other) population(s), and the already-stretched and demonized *obstetras* are apparently charged with this task.

Conclusion: The Limited Agency of *Obstetras*

As I have shown, life as an *obstetra* in a rural Peruvian health network is precarious, and is complicated by significant expectations of goal-fulfilling, census-taking, and form-filling to keep one's job. All such acts may indeed contribute toward the realization of questionable outcomes, as with the past forced sterilizations of Indigenous women. However, in this chapter, I have attempted to underscore the limited agency held by *obstetras* in the face of such scenarios, and have discussed the ways in which their lived realities are imbued with bureaucratic stresses that detract from providing optimal services to Quechua patients. Thus I argue that, particularly when addressing sterilizations but also when discussing contemporary issues in rural Peruvian reproductive care, it is important to take note of the ways in which healthcare providers fit into the wider State system. Under other circumstances, many *obstetras* in Vilcashuaman may also be considered Indigenous women for whom protections could be sought, and it is important to extend certain considerations, such as their positionality and working conditions, to them when they are employed by, and subsumed under, the State apparatus. Medical anthropologist Paul Farmer once advised that "You can't sympathize with the staff too much, or you risk not sympathizing with the patients" (quoted in Kidder 2009:25); this chapter has been an attempt to refute such a statement. Instead, I argue that to sympathize with and understand the experiences of care receivers, we need to also understand and sympathize with the care providers.

Rebecca Irons is a medical anthropologist at University College London (UCL), where she is based in the Institute for Global Health. She holds a PhD in Medical Anthropology (UCL), Master of Research (UCL), and an MA in Development (University of Sussex). Her research interests include reproductive and sexual health, family planning and kinship, race and ethnicity, coloniality, and migration. She has worked extensively in Peru on projects addressing social determinants of health, including with Quechua Indigenous communities on reproduction and State health care, and more recently, on Venezuelan migration and HIV/AIDS.

Notes

1. Shining Path was a Peruvian Maoist revolutionary movement founded in Ayacucho in 1970 and led by Abimael Guzmán until his capture and imprisonment in 1992.
2. It is possible that *obstetras* falsify information in order to reach *metas*. As Cal Biruk suggests in an ethnography of African healthcare system staff "inventing" information that goes toward statistics: "Cooking data refers to fabricating, falsifying, or fudging the information one is meant to collect from survey respondents in a standardized and accurate manner" (2018:3). However, in the absence of any evidence to suggest this possibility, it cannot be included as an argument in this present chapter.

References

Berg M. 1996. "Practices of Reading and Writing: The Constitutive Role of the Patient Record in Medical Work." *Sociology of Health & Illness* 18(4): 499–524.

Biruk C. 2018. *Cooking Data: Culture and Politics in an African Research World.* Durham NC: Duke University Press

Bridges K. 2011a. "Pregnancy, Medicaid, State Regulation, and Legal Subjection." *Journal of Poverty* 16(3): 323–352.

———. 2011b. *Reproducing Race: An Ethnography of Pregnancy as a Site of Racialization.* Berkeley: University of California Press.

Cabrera WP. 2017. *Hampiq: Salud y Enfermedad en Ayacucho* [Doctor: Health and Disease in Ayacucho]. Ayachucho, Peru: Universidad San Cristobol de Huamanga.

Chirapaq. 2017. *Es Útil Ser Indigena? Identidad, Censos y Politicas Publicas* [Is It Useful to Be Indigenous? Identity, Censuses and Public Policies]. Lima, Peru: Chirapaq.

Davis-Floyd R, Premkumar A, eds. 2023a. *Obstetricians Speak: On Training, Practice, Fear, and Transformation.* New York: Berghahn Books.

———. 2023b. "The Anthropology of Obstetrics and Obstetricians: The Practice, Maintenance, and Reproduction of a Biomedical Profession." In *Obstetricians Speak: On Training, Practice, Fear, and Transformation,* eds. Davis-Floyd R, Premkumar A, Series Overview. New York: Berghahn Books.

———. 2023c. *Cognition, Risk, and Responsibility in Obstetrics: Anthropological Analyses and Critiques of Obstetricians' Practices.* New York: Berghahn Books.

———. 2023d. *Obstetric Violence and Systemic Disparities: Can Obstetrics Be Humanized and Decolonized?* New York: Berghahn Books.

Ewig C. 2010. *Second-Wave Neoliberalism: Gender, Race, and Health Sector Reform in Peru.* Pittsburgh: Pennsylvania State Press.

Foucault M. (1978) 1990. *The History of Sexuality: The Will to Knowledge,* Vol. 1 London: Penguin.

Garcia, M.E. 2005. *Making Indigenous Citizens: Identities, Education and Multicultural Development in Peru.* Stanford CA: Stanford University Press.

Graeber D. 2018. *Bullshit Jobs: A Theory.* London: Allen Lane.

Gianella G. 2014. "Los Medicos Peruanos y Las Esterilizaciones Forzadas: La Historia Aun No Termina" [Peruvian Doctors and Forced Sterilizations: The Story Is Not Over Yet]. In *Memorias Del Caso Peruano De Esterilización Forzada,* ed. Ballón A, 73–92. Lima, Peru: Biblioteca Nacional del Perú.

Guerra-Reyes L. 2013. *Changing Birth in the Andes: Safe Motherhood, Culture and Policy in Peru.* Ph.D. dissertation. Pittsburgh PA: University of Pittsburgh.

———. 2019. "Numbers that Matter: Right to Health and Peruvian Maternal Strategies." *Medical Anthropology* 38(6): 478–492.

Hacking, I. 1990. *The Taming of Chance.* Cambridge: Cambridge University Press.

Kidder T. 2009. *Mountains Beyond Mountains: One Doctor's Quest to Heal the World.* New York: Profile.

Miller D, Costa E, Haynes N, et al. 2016. *How the World Changed Social Media.* London: UCL Press.

Rousseau S. 2007. "The Politics of Reproductive Health in Peru: Gender and Social Policy in the Global South." Social Politics 14(1): 93–125.

———. 2009. *Women's Citizenship in Peru: The Paradoxes of Neopopulism in Latin America*. London: Palgrave Macmillan.

Scott J. 1999. *Seeing Like a State: How Certain Schemes to Improve the Human Condition Have Failed*. New Haven CT: Yale University Press.

Taylor C. 2011. "Biopower." In *Foucault: Key Concepts*, ed. Taylor D, 41–54. Durham NC: Acumen.

Villegas JA. 2017. "Commentary: Perception and Performance in Effective Policing." *Public Administration Review* 77(2): 240–241.

Yrivarren Espinoza J. 2011. *Gobierno Electrónico: Análisis de los Conceptos de Tecnología, Comodidad Y Democracia* [Electronic Government: Analysis of the Concepts of Technology, Comfort and Democracy]. Lima, Peru: Universidad Peruana de Ciencias Aplicadas.

PART 2

Decolonizing and Humanizing Obstetric Training and Practice?

Obstetricians, Midwives, and Their Battles against "The System"

CHAPTER 6

Decolonizing Biomedical Education in the UK

Amali U. Lokugamage, Tharanika Ahillan, and S.D.C. Pathberiya

Introduction

In the wake of the Black Lives Matter movement, another movement to "decolonize" traditional university biomedical curricula has gathered momentum. Its aims are to dismantle the lingering colonial biases of traditional, Eurocentric, white, male-oriented curricula to provide a more inclusive education. This decolonization movement aims to create curricula that equip students with the critical tools to question historical power imbalances to shift and co-produce curricula that are fair and just regarding race, ethnicity, nationality, class, gender, sexual orientation, and disability.

According to Sarah Wong, Faye Gishen, and Amali Lokugamage (2021), the term "decolonizing" refers broadly to a movement that:

1. Recognizes how forces of colonialism, empire, and discrimination have shaped the systems of the societies in which we live our day-to-day lives; and
2. Offers alternative ways of thinking about the world, re-centering perspectives of populations that have been historically oppressed and marginalized by these forces.

Higher educational curricula in the spheres of the arts, humanities, and social sciences have led the "decolonizing the curriculum" movement. This has been seen in the University College London (UCL) 2015 initiative entitled *Why is My Curriculum White?*; in Priyamvada Gopal's (2017) (University of Cambridge) provocative article, "Yes, We Must Decolonise: Our Teaching Has to Go Beyond Elite White Men"; James Muldoon's (2019) article "Academics: It's Time to Get Behind Decolonising the Curriculum"; and the School of Oriental and African Studies (SOAS) University of London blog "Decolonizing the Curriculum: What's All The Fuss About?" (Sabaratnam 2017).

Biomedical schools have been historically slower to embrace a decolonizing approach, but there has been a rapid recent effort in the UK to catch up. Although equality and diversity policies have had roles in alleviating healthcare inequalities at both population and individual levels, it could be argued that this is tokenistic until a fully decolonial approach is adopted. A decolonial perspective reveals the structural biases that a purely inclusive policy cannot not reveal, as we will further discuss later on in this chapter.

In recent years, biomedical educators have been recognizing that the biomedical hierarchy of knowledge is not immune to the deep entrenchment of colonial historical bias. The efforts toward inclusivity being made by academic Humanities and Social Science departments find their parallels in biomedical discussions on how more inclusive curricula can improve disease diagnosis and treatment, patient management, professionalism, and quality of care. Speaking from a *planetary health* education curriculum perspective, Sara Stone, Samuel Myers, and Christopher Golden (2018:193) state:

> Understanding the differences between equality and equity in theory and practice, and concepts of marginalisation, vulnerability, resilience, and who benefits and is harmed in a given scenario, is a core objective of planetary health teaching. Since the effects of environmental change on human health are heterogeneous and are mediated by factors such as geographical scale, temporal scale, socioeconomic factors, and political and cultural context, students should think critically about whose health is at stake and how it is measured.

As a result, more recently, biomedical educators have started to think of how a process of decolonization could produce doctors who can meet the complex needs of a diverse population, while recognizing the colonial influences that created the origins of biomedicine. The influence of biomedical education in propagating healthcare inequalities in the post-colonial hierarchy, in which marginalized groups have poorer healthcare outcomes than patients who are white, male, high social class, and heterosexual, is being realized. In this chapter, we look at the professional and legal impetus to decolonize biomedical curricula and at how elements of decolonization can be applied to contemporary biomedical curricula.

This chapter is based on an article published in the *Journal of Medical Ethics* (Lokugamage, Ahillan, and Pathberiya 2020a; used with permission), which we have revised and updated, and is centered around biomedical education in the UK, influenced by the Commonwealth origins of the three British authors. (We have not refocused this chapter to deal only with obstetric education, as its purpose is broader, yet its general points can be extrapolated to the education of obstetricians and other maternity care providers.) Furthermore, in taking a decolonial perspective, we acknowledge the caveat that across the colonized world, there are differences in law, histories of oppression, and healthcare infrastructures, yet we authors are only capable of commenting with expertise on the UK situation. We advise readers outside the UK to extract from this chapter the subject matter that is relevant to their unique geographical situation, colonial history, law, infrastructure, and resources.

The Colonial Backdrop of Dehumanized Care

Decolonizing the history of biomedicine promotes awareness and questions the traditional narratives and power imbalances to disrupt the prejudiced legacy of the colonization of biomedicine; these prejudices are not limited to racism, but also include classism, sexism, ableism, xenophobia, and gender discrimination (Wong et al. 2021). Re-framing, re-orienting, and reforming the profession require the reassessment of past biomedical colonial legacies.

According to Lindsay Porter (2018), a cultural historian, the 18th-century European "Enlightenment" and the subsequent professionalism of biomedical practice encouraged a sphere of scientific inquiry that compromised on empathy to prioritize experimentation and to further scientific advancement. Practitioners were encouraged to perceive the patient as an object first and a human second. Over the course of centuries, this ideology emboldened European male practitioners and molded a patriarchal biomedical system, and a state of biomedical cultural arrogance was allowed to grow. In the process of establishing biomedical criteria in which reason was favored over "superstition," power hierarchies became ingrained, and other types of healing were denigrated and ostracized. Diversity in types of practitioners, such as midwives and folk healers and schools of thought such as Indigenous healing systems in the colonies, were excluded or oppressed. *Medical pluralism* was squeezed out of the growing biomedical power hierarchy.

It is argued that the story of Dr. Marion Sims (named the "father of gynecology" due to his development of the Sims speculum and of surgical techniques for the repair of vesico-vaginal fistulas in the United States) should be included in biomedical curricula. It is well known that Sims's motivation followed the 18th-century "Enlightenment's" aspect of dehumanization (White 2020): he repaired fistulae in Black women slaves both to perfect his techniques and to facilitate their return to the workforce, rather than to heal them. What is perhaps more incomprehensible and alarming is that the fistulas in these women were a result of disregarding Indigenous practices of midwifery in favor of acquiring the skills of forceps delivery by obstetricians. The Black women slaves who were experimented on to improve surgical techniques did not give their consent to this experimentation, nor were they given any sort of analgesia. Indeed, this latter fact may have some relation to the well-documented racial bias in pain management, in which false beliefs are held about biological differences between Black and white people that shape the ways in which pain assessment and treatment recommendations are perceived (Hoffman et al. 2016). Following protests regarding their treatment, Sims's statue in Central Park, New York, was relocated, and the names of three of these women—Anarcha, Betsy, and Lucy—have now found equal fame from a human rights perspective (Brown 2017). In the UK, there have been calls to the Royal College of Obstetricians and Gynaecologists to also honor these slaves, as the knowledge in the UK curriculum about fistulae stems from Sims's work on their bodies (Downes 2020).

Likewise, proponents of decolonization argue that the story of the Tuskegee syphilis experiments in the United States (Centers for Disease Control and Prevention 1929–1972), in which 600 Black men were recruited to eugenics experiments to follow the natural course of untreated syphilis, should be taught within the ethics and law syllabi of biomedical schools. These men were intentionally denied treatment within a background of dishonesty, whereby they were misled with "special free treatment" and enrolled without informed consent. (The US government has since formally apologized and has compensated the families.) Proponents of decolonization argue that this study, often compared to the horrific Nazi experiments, should be taught as a prime example of what happens when, for powerless subjects, the State's coercive power, racism, and biomedical research ignore ethical considerations (Reverby 2001). The discussion of such stories to contextualize them within the history of biomedical colonization, and to explore the dominant ideologies that have been assimilated into modern biomedical education, can provide meaningful professional development for biomedical practitioners.

The propensity of Euro-American healthcare systems and institutions to label themselves as "rational," "modern," and "objective" seeks to absolve their practitioners of their roles in perpetuating the systemic marginalization of minority populations. This consequently exacerbates healthcare inequalities in minority ethnic populations, among other groups that traditionally have been sidelined based on disability, sexual orientation, or gender identity (Wong et al. 2021). For instance, there are higher rates of maternal mortality among ethnic minority women as compared to white women in the UK and the US, and there is evidence that Black women in these countries are less likely to receive epidural analgesia during labor and delivery, despite reporting similar or even higher levels of pain than white women during childbirth (Wong et al. 2021).

Lack of knowledge about services, structural barriers, and wider Western beliefs, such as autonomy in decision-making and the appropriateness—or lack thereof—of biomedical control over birthing and dying often do not universally reflect the views of different cultures and can violate a patient's sense of family, beliefs, and identity. Thus, there is a prerequisite for dismantling the existing power hierarchies. The process of dissipating cultural arrogance in favor of *cultural humility* (see Table 6.1) as part of decolonization entails disrupting elements of the hidden biomedical curriculum, in which the legacies of colonial norms operate as unconscious bias in practitioners' professional behaviors. To an equal degree, *Cultural Safety* exposes implicit and structural biases, offering a way of achieving social justice and ensuring that the pillar of non-maleficence is upheld (Lokugamage et al. 2021).

A body of work undertaken by Indigenous Māori nurse and educator Irihapiti Ramsden in New Zealand led to her realization that student and graduate midwives and nurses could not connect the impacts of colonization to ill health and disparities for Māori. Ramsden (2002) recognized that midwifery and nursing education needed to incorporate the concept of *Cultural Safety*—which, as she and the Māori insist, should always be capitalized; not to do so is considered a subtle insult to the Māori and to others who are also promoting this concept. It is vital to distinguish *Cultural Safety* from *cultural competence* (see Table 6.1). "Cultural Safety" acknowledges the inherent power imbalances between clinician and patient, requiring practitioners to use critical self-reflection on their own beliefs, values, biases and assumptions, but *cultural compe-*

Table 6.1. Useful Definitions © Amali U. Lokugamage, Tharanika Ahillan, and S.D.C. Pathberiya.

UNCONSCIOUS BIAS refers to a bias that we are unaware of and that happens outside of our control. It is a bias that is triggered automatically by our brain making quick judgments and assessments of people and situations, influenced by our background, cultural environment, and personal experiences (Equality Challenge Unit 2013).
CULTURAL COMPETENCE: A broad concept with various definitions based on a number of frameworks: • Originally defined by Terry Cross and colleagues (1989:13) as: "A set of congruent behaviours, attitudes, and policies that come together in a system, agency, or among professionals to work effectively in cross cultural situations." • Limited by focusing on mastery of knowledge, skills, and attitudes by inferring a static outcome that can be checked off some list. • Relies on recognition of social and cultural influences and on creating interventions that take these into account. • Has the potential to confuse practitioners with complex jargon. Multiple terms are often used interchangeably: cultural awareness; cultural sensitivity; cultural security (Lokugamage et al. 2021).
CULTURAL HUMILITY emphasizes openness, self-awareness, egolessness, supportive interactions, self-reflection and critique, and respect for other cultures and their beliefs and customs. Its antecedents and prerequisites are biomedical treatments that ignore cultural diversity and reflect power imbalances; such treatments still characterize much of biomedical practice. Its consequences are mutual empowerment, partnerships, respect, optimal care, and lifelong learning. With a firm understanding of the term, individuals and communities will be better equipped to understand and accomplish an inclusive environment with mutual benefit and optimal care (Foronda et al. 2016).
CULTURAL SAFETY • Requires practitioners to use critical self-reflection on their privileges, biases, assumptions, stereotypes, and power imbalances. • Recognizes that sociocultural differences manifest, in part, as power imbalances among different ethnicities. • Recognizes the dynamics of institutional racism: that cultural differences, while centrally important to many Indigenous peoples and other ethnic minorities, are not recognized as "ordinary" by institutions and therefore are often not properly provided for. • Recognizes that it is not just that services need to be culturally appropriate; but also, if services are delivered inadequately, then the delivery method of those services can become a negative determinant of health outcomes. • Requires care to be determined by the recipients of care in ways that make them feel safe, both culturally and individually (Lokugamage et al. 2021).

tence does not include this important reflexivity on power (Lokugamage et al. 2021). By directly tackling the history of biomedicine through the lens of decolonization within the course syllabi of ethics and law and of anthropology or global health frameworks, biomedical educators can critically evaluate the evolution of patient-centered care and can reflect on why and how the profession chooses to commemorate knowledge, and on who decides to commemorate what knowledge. Educators can then contextualize the legal advancements of human rights in health care.

Professional and Legal Incentives to Decolonize the Medical Curriculum

Professional Incentives

The case for decolonizing biomedical curricula stems from a social justice perspective on the persistent legacies of colonialism, which result in power imbalances and healthcare inequities (Gishen and Lokugamage 2018). By flattening entrenched colonial era power hierarchies, we can ensure that healthcare policies, education, and research are informed by the perspectives of the communities they affect (Lokugamage et al. 2021). Decolonizing biomedical curricula could also equip future doctors with the professional and cultural literacy and confidence that are needed to deal with the complexities and uncertainties of growing grassroots decoloniality activism by patients, academics, and the public. This debate has started difficult conversations that we will describe below.

White fragility is the refutation of the existence of structural racism, as described in the best-selling book *White Fragility: Why It's So Hard for White People to Talk about Racism* (DiAngelo 2019). Defensive responses and swift negation of results related to decolonization and the challenge of the epistemic status quo from doctors who have "white coat privilege" (Lokugamage, Ahillan, and Pathberiya 2020a, 2020b) can be regarded as demonstrations of *privilege fragility*—a term that we have coined for this chapter. "Privilege fragility" is at odds with the embodiment of the diversity and equality agenda within professional behaviors, such as through "cultural humility" (as described in Table 6.1) for the purposes of neutralizing power imbalances in education and health care.

Diversity-related teaching has been shown to increase the confidence of medical students in handling communication barriers in clinical practice with the potential for reducing prejudices and negative stereotyping behaviors, which are well-documented as deterring patients from minority and marginalized groups from seeking biomedical care (Wong et al. 2021). By rewriting the discourses around what should be included and excluded in biomedical curricula, biomedical educators can contribute toward the dismantling of existing power structures and norms.

Within the makeup of the biomedical profession itself, "decolonizing" has been identified as important for ethnic minority students—a population that has experienced an attainment gap, lower feelings of belonging, and perceptions of being less welcome into the profession than their white counterparts (E. Charles 2019; Mbaki and Todorova 2020). These "prejudices are not limited to racism but also [to] classism, sexism, ableism, xenophobia, and gender discrimination" (Lokugamage et al. 2021). Decolonizing and diversifying biomedical curricula can provide important steps toward improving the experience and sense of belonging of minority students to create a population of biomedical doctors that reflects the patient population it serves.

The General Medical Council (GMC), which is the regulatory body for biomedical doctors in the UK, has official guidance regarding the importance of supporting doctors to serve a diverse population with awareness of equality and human rights (GMC 2018a, 2018b). However, the GMC has yet to attempt a decolonial analysis of its historic institution and has been criticized for institutional racism (Bamrah et al. 2021).

Legal Incentives

The legal incentives for promoting the decolonization of biomedical curricula are inextricably tied up with the relevant laws in statute, case law, and international legal instruments. Internationally, the European Convention on Human Rights (Council of Europe 1950) has a number of provisions that protect an individual's rights in a healthcare setting. Articles 2, 3, 8, 12, and 14 allow patients to "make choices in line with their own opinions and values—even if those choices seem irrational, ill-advised or rash to others" (ECHR-CEDH 2021: 86). Article 9 goes further, stipulating that the rights to freedom of thought, conscience, and religion are also pivotal, in that some forms of treatment, from the perspectives of the patients, may also have significant spiritual/religious components. (These include the many international cases relating to Jehovah's Witnesses refusing blood transfusions ([ECHR 2010]). Restricting Indigenous modalities of treatment, which often have religious/spiritual elements, may thus breach the patient's Article 9 rights.

Montgomery v Lanarkshire Health Board (2015) is an important legal case in the UK that is significant from a global perspective as it signals a legal decolonial shift to challenge centuries of biomedical paternalism. The UK Supreme Court in *Montgomery* stated that a "patient is entitled to take into account her own values, her own assessment of the comparative merits" on whether or not she decides to expose herself to a risk regarding her care. Further, the "relative importance attached by patients to quality as against length of life, or to physical appearance or bodily integrity as against the relief of pain, will vary from one patient to another," because many reasons "may affect their attitude towards a proposed form of treatment and the reasonable alternatives. The doctor cannot form an objective, 'medical' view of these matters, and is therefore not in a position to take the 'right' decision as a matter of clinical judgment" (*Montgomery v Lanarkshire Health Board* [2015] UKSC 11, 2015:46). A possible explanation for why biomedical physicians are unable to attach a similar level of significance as patients do to issues of relevance to doctors may be that these sorts of decision-making do not fit within doctors' paradigms of biomedicine or health care. (For descriptions of such paradigms, see Pathberiya 2016; Davis-Floyd 2018, 2022; and the Introduction to this present volume). Furthermore, *Outcomes for Graduates 2018* specifies that graduates "must demonstrate knowledge of the principles of the legal framework" as well as "the importance of the links between pathophysiological, psychological, spiritual, religious, social and cultural factors for each individual" (GMC 2018b:10,16).

Doctors need to be able to act in a person-centered manner. In diverse populations, this entails being culturally safe by exercising cultural humility (Table 6.1); without these, their actions may fall short of required standards of duty of care, and thus become open to litigation. Therefore, as Lord Kerr and Lord Reed in the UK Supreme Court put it, it is "necessary to impose legal obligations, so that even those doctors who have less skill or inclination for communication, or who are more hurried, are obliged to pause and engage in the discussion which the law requires" (*Montgomery v Lanarkshire Health Board* [2015] UKSC 11, 2015:93).

Decolonization and Biomedical Education

Within the UK, public engagement events were held from 2017 to 2019, inspiring an ideology of decolonization in biomedical education, and through which we formed our preliminary thoughts for this chapter. For instance, in 2017, the UCL Medical School (2017) held a public engagement event titled "Practically Creating an Inclusive Curriculum," the feedback from which in turn inspired a second event in 2018 named "Decolonising the Medical Curriculum" (UCL 2018). The latter event focused on the following six major topics on which this chapter is based:

- decolonizing the body;
- decolonizing biomedical curricula;
- decolonizing learner experiences;
- decolonizing educational spaces;
- decolonizing professional behaviors;
- decolonizing ideas of healing.

In 2018, the Wellcome Collection held an exhibition titled *Ayurvedic Man: Encounters with Indian Medicine*, which was accompanied by an associated "Decolonizing Health" symposium. The exhibition explored Ayurvedic medicine in South Asia, interrogating how medicine is transformed by biomedical and cultural exchanges and surveying the impacts of colonialism on medical heritage. As the Wellcome explained:

> We are at a time of growing popularity of pluralistic approaches to health; societies around the world are at increasing risk of losing natural resources, medicinal plants, and traditional knowledge. Ayurvedic Man highlighted the delicate balance between sharing and protecting heritage, cultural resources, and environmental biodiversity. (Wellcome Collection 2017)

Building on this exhibition, in September 2019, a series of high-profile events were held in London that promoted key messages about sustainability, climate change, Indigenous land rights, Indigenous ideas of healing, and collective sharing of Indigenous knowledge: the "Flourishing Diversity Series" (UCL Anthropology Department 2019; BBC World Service 2019; Pyānko, Benki, and Haynes 2019). Following our active listening to the above events, we have refined concept areas specific to the concept of healing in the individual and in the population. These may have been omitted from conventional top-down organizational equality and diversity policy in the context of biomedical education. We argue that the emerging grassroots interest in decolonization is a liminal space for biomedical educational transformation.

Medical Pluralism

The Tensions between Biomedical and Traditional Healing Systems

In the East (India, Sri Lanka, China, etc.), overcoming illness through Indigenous medicines (e.g., Ayurveda, Traditional Chinese Medicine,

Unani-Tibbi [Arabic or Islamic traditional medicine], etc.) can be viewed, on a superficial level, as symptom relief/cure, but their philosophies have a deeper endpoint of paving the road to "enlightenment" of mind, body, and spirit by attempting to create ecological balance by working with nature. In the West, the 18th-century "Enlightenment" refers to the overturning of "superstition" with science and logic; in European colonies, this contributed to the suppression and oppression of Indigenous medicines in favor of Western healthcare practices. Eastern practices, such those mentioned above and other Indigenous healing systems, were regarded through the skeptical lens of a Western biomedical perspective, and their efficacy was rejected. Indeed, as Atwood Gaines and Robbie Davis-Floyd (2003:96) stated: "Like science, Western medicine was assumed to be acultural—beyond the influence of culture—while all other medical systems were assumed to be so culturally biased that they had little or no scientific relevance."

Colonialism led to Europeans establishing their own biological, structural, and cultural superiority and their own biomedical system as the only legitimate medical knowledge base in the countries they colonized (Quijano 2007). Thus the unique context of the decolonization of healing practices depends not only on dismantling colonial epistemologies and aspects of patriarchal institutions but also on simultaneously re-centering the displaced Indigeneity. Indigenous/traditional ideas of healing involve mind, body, spirit, and society. These treatments are nuanced and individualized. (See Davis-Floyd 2018, 2022 and the Introduction to this volume for a description of "the holistic model of birth and health care" as encompassing body, mind, spirit, and energy, as many Indigenous healing systems do.) Despite colonial efforts to stamp them out or discredit them, today diverse healing traditions are now labelled "alternative" or "complementary" to biomedicine (Wong et al. 2021) and are thriving in many countries. Yet their jarring juxtaposition against "Western medicine," which is referred to as "modern" or "evidence-based," is in part due to the fact that the outcomes of such healing systems are difficult, and sometimes impossible, to capture with standard biostatistical methods and "one-size-fits-all" study designs, which prefer to look at one primary endpoint. Hence, it is challenging to develop an evidence base for such healing systems according to Western criteria (see Johnson 1997). However, as conversations relating to decolonization in health care circulate and contribute to ongoing health activism, it will be interesting to see what will unfold and what patients will want from their healthcare systems.

The decolonizing agenda to "re-center" displaced Indigenous healing systems will be challenging for those in biomedicine due to the paucity of epidemiological evidence. To address this issue, equality and diversity training within education call for an anthropological component that includes the concept of cultural humility (Table 6.1); in this case, that is the awareness that Western biomedicine is just one of many global healing systems. Such awareness could throw light on unconscious biomedical biases. Often these unconscious biases stem from the assumed superiority of Western biomedicine, which is presumably grounded in "evidence-based" research. However, reviews of the evidence base of biomedical guidelines, such as that of James Wright, say that "Practice guidelines by specialist societies are surprisingly deficient," indicating that only a minority of medical guidelines are based on Grade A evidence, and suggesting that the majority of biomedical practices are not based on evidence or are based on lesser grades of evidence (Wright 2007; Lee and Vielemeyer 2011). Indeed, analyses of evidence levels in the guidelines for obstetrics and gynecology produced by the Royal College of Obstetricians and Gynaecologists (UK) (Prusova et al. 2014) and the Society of Obstetricians and Gynaecologists of Canada (Ghui et al. 2016) have found patterns of predominantly low grades of evidence for the majority of perinatal biomedical procedures (see also Enkin et al. 2000 and Davis-Floyd 2022 for descriptions and analyses of those low grades of evidence).

Further, the prioritization of quantitative over qualitative data arguably reflects a fixed preconception in clinical research about what constitutes good treatment outcomes; such fixation based on a privileged hierarchy has affected current study designs of "alternative medicines." For example, randomized controlled trials around medical acupuncture have encountered challenges in finding an adequate placebo control, and patients' experiences of care as qualitative outcomes are devalued by the power hierarchies of "evidence-based" biomedicine (Wong et al. 2021). Again, as overarching analyses of evidence-based guidelines are revealing low levels of high-quality evidence in specialty guidelines, biomedicine may be more belief- and tradition-based than is generally presumed, as explored in Cathy Charles, Amiram Gafni, and Emily Freeman's (2011) article "The Evidence-Based Medicine Model of Clinical Practice: Scientific Teaching or Belief-Based Preaching?" Given that both Western and Indigenous healing systems have deficits of high-quality scientific evidence, we suggest looking beyond Western versus traditional antagonisms to explore opportunities for synergy and co-delivery in medically pluralistic, person-centered approaches to health care (for examples, please see Ali and Davis-Floyd 2022).

Transgenerational Traumas and Indigenous Ideas of Healing

Demographic studies show ethnic differences in the diagnoses of psychiatric diseases (Coleman et al. 2016). Attention also needs to be paid to research on intergenerational traumas originating from the legacies of slavery and the subjugation of Indigenous ways of life (Chavez-Dueñas et al. 2019). Decoloniality scholars have proposed that those affected should be approached with respect for the Indigenous systems of beliefs and healing systems of their ancestors and by making available standard psychological therapies. Social science and humanities publications, such as Aníbal Quijano's (2007) "Coloniality and Modernity/Rationality"; Renee Linklater's (2014) *Decolonizing Trauma Work: Indigenous Stories and Strategies*; Stephanie Davis's (2017) PhD dissertation *Being a Queer and/or Trans Person of Colour in the UK: Psychology, Intersectionality and Subjectivity*; and Jonathan Fay's (2018) "Decolonizing Mental Health One Prejudice at a Time: Psychological, Sociological, Ecological and Cultural Considerations," have highlighted the inadequacies of current psychological and psychiatric practices in dealing with such intergenerational traumas.

The Office of Hawaiian Affairs has backed a Bill promoting Native Hawaiian concepts of wellbeing, culturally grounded healthcare methodologies, and traditional healing and health practices (State of Hawaii 2019). This was a governmental response to findings that the colonized style of Western health care did not meet the mental health needs of Indigenous people in Hawaii. The white paper to the Bill says that the "health programs and services that are aligned with Native Hawaiian cultural identity, values and beliefs can significantly increase the number of Native Hawaiians who utilize mental health services" (The Office of Hawaiian Affairs 2018:1).

Underlying relevant factors may be the stigmas attached to psychiatric disorders, which are seen differently from Indigenous treatment perspectives. For instance, psychiatric conditions may be seen as invasions of an external entity that can be remedied through rituals or as symptoms of disharmony in the community as opposed to in the individual; such views are common in Indigenous communities. Another perspective might be that psychological conditions are a result of Westernization and the biomedical labelling of such conditions. It is probably for all the reasons listed above that the *Diagnostic and Statistical Manual of Mental Disorders* DSM-5 (American Psychiatric Association 2013) incorporates greater cultural sensitivity in its latest update. The article by Alannah Earl Young and Denise Nadeau (2005) on "Decolonizing the

Body: Restoring Sacred Vitality," which describes these authors' experiences of setting up a program in Canada to help native women who have suffered sexual, racial, and colonial violence makes a valuable contribution to this area.

Molecular medicine has also started to accrue epigenetic evidence (Youssef et al. 2018) that suggests the transgenerational transmission of DNA methylation changes from parents to children derived from the experiences of traumas. Similarly, specific to the field of obstetrics and gynecology, the negative impacts of postpartum PTSD (Post-Traumatic Stress Disorder) could extend beyond the mother, impacting child development and demonstrating a transfer of trauma-related consequences from the mother to her child (Horsch and Stuijfzand 2019). It follows that there could be cross-linkages between biomedicine and the humanities to act synergistically to explore new conversations on intergenerational traumas and their treatments. We introduce these ideas into this chapter within the context of decolonizing biomedical education and propose inclusion of this aspect of *cultural psychiatry* (Kleinman 1987) within relevant course syllabi to include the intersections between mental health and social determinants of health.

Effective educational vehicles for creating professional awareness in future doctors regarding cultural sensitivity around Indigenous systems of healing would be for biomedical curricula to continually evolve teaching materials based on decolonial aspects of medical anthropology, Cultural Safety, and patient experiences. One instance of this evolution is the UCL Medical School curriculum, which gives students the opportunity to take a special study component—an anthropological project looking at mental health from Indigenous perspectives in a mini-course on "Culture, Ethics, and Religion in the Clinical Encounter." This course explores some of the complexities of clinical practice with culturally diverse patients.

Elements of Decolonized Biomedical Curricula

It is invariably difficult to define the areas that should be included regarding decolonization within biomedical curricula. However, in addition to the areas discussed above, the following areas have been highlighted as important by the public who attended the aforementioned decolonizing public engagement events. Due to the nature of such events, the public's contribution, identified through active listening, at times does not emerge in a logical and structured way. However, Wong, Gishen, and Lokugamage (2021) have framed the dominant themes that emerged within three scaffolding concepts of decolonizing biomedical curricula: epistemic pluralism, Cultural Safety, and critical consciousness.

Epistemic pluralism generally refers to the use of more than one perspective or approach to dealing with a knowledge-related problem. In application to biomedical education, a medically plural curriculum should accept that a healthcare system, much like culture, does not exist as a discrete and immutable entity, and has been shaped by a long history of interactions with other traditions within an interconnected global landscape (Wong et al. 2021).

Critical consciousness, developed and popularized by the Brazilian educator Paulo Freire (1973), integrates critical theory, pedagogy, and social justice within a three-component formulation:

1. Critical social analysis and reflection;
2. Political efficacy—the perceived ability to enact political change; and
3. Participation in civic and political action.

Thus, equipping clinicians to integrate knowledge of the origins of these structures, along with their agency to effect changes within their respective healthcare systems, are crucial components of the arduous task of dismantling barriers to healthcare justice (Freire 1973). Further, these identify the public's contribution via a lens through which colonial era power imbalances in biomedical education can be evaluated within epistemology, diversity teaching, and curricular scope (see Figure 6.1).

Decolonizing Global Health and Research

At the Wellcome "Decolonizing Health" symposium described above, Branwyn Poleykett, anthropologist and postdoctoral research associate at the University of Cambridge, pointed out that decoloniality is rising as a challenge to the conventional—and highly biased—biomedical view of global health and to biomedical research funding. She referred to Richard Smith (who served as the editor of the *British Medical Journal* [BMJ] from 1991 until 2004), who said in his BMJ blog (Smith 2013) that there was a popular way of talking about developments in global health circles—namely that the "Global Health 3.0" model was being upgraded to the more decolonized "Global Health 4.0" model. But Poleykett reasoned that there are decolonizing arguments saying that if we are to use a "computer upgrade" type of terminology for global health development, then it should be acknowledged that Global Health "1.0" was colonialism, and that Global Health "2.0" was post-colonial inter-

Shifting from a Colonial to a Decolonial Lens in Biomedical Curricula

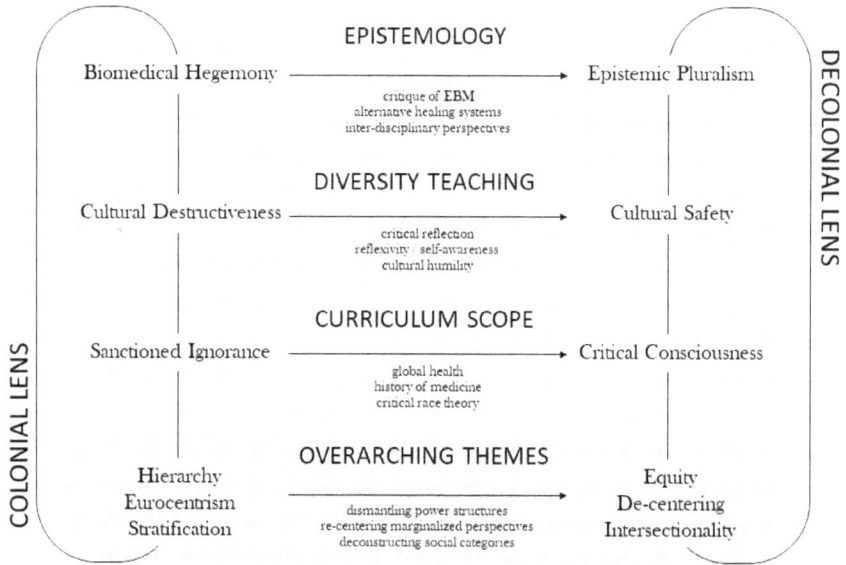

EPISTEMOLOGY

Biomedical Hegemony ⎯⎯⎯⎯⎯⎯⎯⎯→ Epistemic Pluralism

critique of EBM
alternative healing systems
inter-disciplinary perspectives

DIVERSITY TEACHING

Cultural Destructiveness ⎯⎯⎯⎯⎯⎯⎯→ Cultural Safety

critical reflection
reflexivity / self-awareness
cultural humility

CURRICULUM SCOPE

Sanctioned Ignorance ⎯⎯⎯⎯⎯⎯⎯⎯→ Critical Consciousness

global health
history of medicine
critical race theory

OVERARCHING THEMES

Hierarchy   Equity
Eurocentrism ⎯⎯⎯⎯⎯⎯⎯→ De-centering
Stratification   Intersectionality

dismantling power structures
re-centering marginalized perspectives
deconstructing social categories

COLONIAL LENS

DECOLONIAL LENS

Figure 6.1. Shifting from a Colonial to a Decolonial Lens in Biomedical Education. © Amali U. Lokugamage, Tharanika Ahillan, and S.D.C. Pathberiya.[1]

national health. The Global Health 2.0 model had contained many unresolved aspects of discrimination, inequality, and power imbalances between and among former colonizing nations and those colonized. From Poleykett's anthropological viewpoint, the legacies of models 1.0 and 2.0 are still eroding and undermining the ideologies of Global Health 3.0 and the aspirations of version 4.0. Thus, Global Health 3.0 is still riddled with the legacies of colonization and is not a completely virtuous crusade for healthcare improvements. Hence, this complexity needs to be incorporated from a decoloniality perspective into biomedical syllabi on global health education.

Also circling back to the arguments of global health and the power imbalances of the *able* and the *disabled*, Helen Meekosha's (2011) article on "Decolonizing Disability: Thinking and Acting Globally" highlights the lack of a global health focus on the challenges that impaired people face from a multiplicity of phenomena, including war and civil strife, the growth of the arms trade, the export of pollution to "pollution havens," and the emergence of sweatshops. As highlighted by Mark Skopec, Molly Fyfe, Hamdi Issa, and colleagues (2021), just as diversity and the inclusion of marginalized groups are important, so too is the inclusion of marginalized epistemologies and knowledges.

Research methodologies are often accused of being dominated by Western perspectives of looking at the individual body in isolation from other elements such as mind, spirit, and/or nature, contradicting the ways that other cultures have of conceiving knowledge, which in turn distorts the outcomes of the research, as well as research being dictated by funders' objectives that may not have direct public health benefits (Centre for Education Studies 2018). Attention has been drawn to global geographic disparities in knowledge production, as seen in Raj Kumar Pan, Kimmo Kaski, and Santo Fortunato's (2012) global map within their publication "World Citation and Collaboration Networks: Uncovering the Role of Geography in Science," in which authors from the Global South are grossly underrepresented. Indeed, evidence from Skopec, Fyfe, Issa, and colleagues (2021) highlights that 97.8% of first authors in one reading list analysis on STEMM (science, technology, engineering, math, and medicine) subjects were affiliated with institutions based in high-income countries. Further evidence from one systematic review (Skopec, Fyfe, et al. 2021) demonstrated that two of the three included studies identified that geographic bias in some form was impacting peer review. Likewise, an event held at the SOAS University of London, UK, in 2019, titled "Applying a Decolonial Lens to Research Structures, Norms and Practices in Higher Education Institutions" drew further attention to how global research has been influenced by colonial legacies that affect the knowledge imparted in biomedical education. Attention was drawn to geographic biases in research outputs, whereby the institutions of the Global North dominate the evolution of global knowledges. Conversations explored how funders could mitigate these geographical biases through active partnership with research bodies of the nations of the Global South and also through active listening to the voices of Indigenous peoples.

This lack of research and knowledge production from lower- and middle-income countries (LMICs) is systemic, resulting from a "colonial matrix of power" that engenders a lack of resources and upholds the Western "modern" constructions of knowledge and power, stacking the odds in favor of researchers in the Global North (Skopec, Fyfe et al. 2021). This hegemony in the higher education setting needs to be challenged, and it must be ensured that knowledge created in LMICs is considered to be equal to knowledge and research originating from higher-income countries (HICs) (Skopec, Fyfe et al. 2021). Consequently, funders of global health research should actively engage in decolonization to deal with this complex arena, which is brimming with the power imbalances inherent between the research centers of the Global North and those of the Global South, not least of which is having to write academic articles in English when it is not the researcher's native language. On decolonizing global health, Amali Lokugamage, Sarah Wong, Nathan Robinson, and Sithira Pathberiya (2021:969) noted that "By being honest about the difficulty of engaging with decolonial perspectives—and the psychological inertia that precedes the cognitively taxing task of undoing one's deeply ingrained narratives about the world"—then transformational learning can occur.

The Imperial College London is one example of an institution leading the way in examining these biases in their educational development units. Their work, described on the website "Examining Geographic Bias in our Curricula" and by Skopec, Fyfe, and colleagues (2021), chronicles faculty workshops in which students and staff are invited to explore these biases and to stimulate debates and reflections around the sources of course readings and the barriers to the inclusion of literature from scholars in the Global South (Imperial College London 2021).

Ecology and Public Health

The terminology around ecology and human health is developing, and is discussed by Chris Buse and colleagues (2018) in the article "Public Health Guide to Field Developments Linking Ecosystems, Environments and Health in the Anthropocene." The *Anthropocene* is defined as the new geological epoch of humanity's own making, based on evidence of damaging human influence on the biosphere. This article describes seven emerging fields: occupational and environmental health; the political ecology of health; environmental justice; ecohealth; One Health; ecological public health; and planetary health (Buse et al. 2018). "Planetary health" (Horton and Lo 2015) is the most recent development in this area, and it is significant that *The Lancet* has a stand-alone journal dedicated to the topic, titled *The Lancet Planetary Health*. This shines the light of importance on the public events such as the aforementioned UCL "Flourishing Diversity Series," in which displaced Indigenous ideas were re-centered and foregrounded to highlight the importance of human health within planetary ecology.

In her article on "How Decolonizing Health Could Save the Planet," Rebekah Jaung (2019) states:

> Indigenous people have always had ecological perspectives on health, which have only recently entered "mainstream" health discourse. The

scope now is planetary health—approaches which benefit all people and the natural environment. Ideas we have learned from Indigenous people include seeing climate breakdown as a symptom of non-reciprocal and exploitative relationships with land and acknowledging that such a relationship exists. Ways of honouring the land will not only restore it, [they] will lead to good health for the people who live on it. This is not just a nice sentiment but the approach on which cutting edge thinking on global climate action is structured.

Presently, there is a rising social tide of interest in climate change and health, as popularized by the extinction protests seen in major cities and by activists such as Greta Thunberg (see below). These issues are likely to challenge the present and future generations of doctors. It is therefore important to incorporate non-biased critical thinking about these issues on global health and ecological public health, and to raise awareness of the emerging field of *planetary health* within biomedical education curricula (Asakura et al. 2015).

Cultural Appropriation

"Cultural appropriation" occurs when members of one culture (usually a historically dominant culture) adopt or misappropriate elements of another culture (usually a historically disadvantaged culture). In the context of health care, many biomedical therapeutic discoveries have an Indigenous knowledge basis (Maridass and De Britto 2008; Jones 2011). In "Origins of Plant Derived Medicines," Muthia Maridass and A. John De Britto (2008:374) noted that the discovery of many new medicines is credited to traditional approaches, which were based on "trial and error over many years in different cultures and [different] systems of medicine." They go on to say that natural products have been the sources of multiple pharmaceutical drugs such as quinine, morphine, paclitaxel, camptothecin, etoposide, mevastatin, and artemisinin, among many others (2008:374). Similar accusations of cultural appropriation are also seen in respect to meditation, acupuncture, yoga, and other Indigenous modalities of treatment that are used and re-branded in the West (Gandhi and Wolff 2017; Surmitis, Fox, and Gutierrez 2018). The fact that this information is not conveyed in biomedical education exemplifies an aspect of biomedical cultural appropriation that involves Indigenous cultural knowledges not being acknowledged, respected, or learned by this historically dominant group.

Within maternity care, there are ongoing unresolved areas of conflict and debate about the cultural appropriation by Western midwives and doulas of Mexican *rebozo* (shawl) techniques for pregnancy yoga, for turning babies in utero into optimal uterine positions, for facilitating labor, or as methods of baby-wearing, among other maternity-related uses (Foster-Scales 2017; Stub 2017; Baitmangalkar 2021). To avoid cultural appropriation, these techniques or systems should be used/delivered with due respect (epistemological and economic) to the Indigenous or traditional knowledge sources and experts. There are no ready-made solutions to redressing cultural appropriation, and there is no consensus on how best to do so; we are merely highlighting that these are areas of ongoing decolonizing tensions.

Intersectionality

"Intersectionality" is a term used to describe the multiple interlocking, simultaneous oppressions involving race, class, gender, sexuality, and disability. This term was originally coined by Kimberlé Crenshaw (Columbia Law School 2017), a Black US feminist, in describing the experiences of Women of Color. Social activism has highlighted the health inequalities and higher mortality rates for Black women, who are disadvantaged by both their race and their gender. These health disparities are noted in both the UK and the US in routine national datasets (Krieger et al. 2014; McCarthy, Yang, and Armstrong 2015; Nair, Knight, and Kurinczuk 2016; Knight et al. 2018). Indeed, a report from MBRRACE-UK states that "it is striking . . . we seem to be making little impact. Research is urgently needed to understand why Black women are five times more likely and Asian women twice as likely to die during pregnancy and childbirth compared to white women" in the UK (Knight et al. 2018:i).

We recommend that biomedical curricula should utilize the term "intersectionality" as part of the social determinants of health, and to teach cultural competence in ways that integrate self, social, and global awareness, as demonstrated at Columbia University in New York as described by Linda Cushman and colleagues (2015). These authors recognized the associations between power, privilege, and intersectional identities, which often go unrecognized and unacknowledged by the individuals and groups that hold such power and privilege, and ultimately can affect professional behaviors toward patients and the public. Using the voices of marginalized individuals or groups to explain their intersectional experiences within teaching sessions would fit in with the concept of *social accountability* as defined by the World Health Organization's report, which states that there is an "obligation for medical schools to direct their education, research and service activities towards addressing the priority health concerns of the community, region and/or nation they have a mandate to serve" (Beolen and Heck 1995:3). In this way, marginalized groups experiencing simultaneous oppressions can act as patient educators and become future changemakers in finding decolonizing solutions for health inequalities (Towle et al. 2010; Lokugamage and Pathberiya 2017).

Decolonizing Symptoms, Signs, and Investigations

Decolonizing disease diagnoses requires an awareness of studies that have shown ethnic differences in chemistry, fertility, endocrine, cancer, and hematological markers, as well as in vitamins and carotenoids in children, adolescents, and adults. These variations in markers are extensively discussed by Houman Tahmasebi and colleagues (2018), who provide a useful Table on the available evidence for ethnic differences in biomarker levels. It follows that if white European biochemical normal values are used by laboratories and clinicians with diverse populations, then Black, Asian, and other ethnic minority populations are likely to be placed at an increased risk of misdiagnosis. This in turn results in ethnic minority patients either being treated for conditions they don't have or not receiving appropriate treatment in a timely manner. For instance, if biomedical students and doctors are not trained in skin issue diagnosis for darker skin tones, then delays in diagnoses or misdiagnoses in detecting conditions such as skin cancer (Hu 2011) or cyanosis (blueness or lividness of the skin, as from imperfectly oxygenated blood, or a pooling of blood due to congestion of blood vessels) become more likely. Indeed, the lack of teaching on the appearance of cyanosis in darker skin tones in Global North biomedical schools could feasibly contribute to ethnic minority patients' intersectional excess of mortality.

Efforts to address this issue in biomedical education have come into mainstream ideation, with one initiative titled "Mind the Gap"—a clinical handbook of signs and symptoms in Black and Brown skin that highlights the lack of diversity in biomedical literature and education (Mukwende, Tamony, and Turner 2020). Furthermore, the scientific validity of social racial constructs has been disputed by findings in genome science and physical anthropology, leading to calls to deconstruct the notion of "race" in biomedical curricula. According to Sarah Wong and Amali Lokugamage (2021):

> The lack of substantiation for a biological basis for race has not deterred its inclusion in medical discourse, whether as a variable in clinical algorithms or a risk factor for an array of conditions. Aside

from its role in confounding the association between discrete genetic markers and specific medical conditions, the racialization of medicine distracts from the structural determinants of health that produce health inequalities. If medical students are not exposed to critical perspectives around race and ethnicity, the danger is that medical schools will serve to reinforce the false (and generally racist) notion that these are inviolable categories that exist in nature.

We recommend that biomedical educators should conduct a review of their teaching materials to ensure that these, including case studies, reflect the diversity and heterogeneity of patient populations.

Although we have taken care to suggest that on one side of the argument, racially nuanced diagnostics could help ethnic minorities, we also acknowledge that, on the other side and as noted above, racial profiling of diagnostic methods that do not critically evaluate the data they are based upon for racist assumptions, or utilizing data from structurally racist healthcare institutions, may perpetuate discriminations that are ingrained and hidden in healthcare infrastructures (Cerdeña, Plaisime, and Tsai 2020).

Decolonizing Reflective Practice

Before systemic changes can occur, educational reflection must first facilitate reflexivity around the concept of "power" in health care, as well as its sources, concentrations, and distributions to prompt political will and collective actions, referred to as *critical consciousness* (Freire 1973; Wong et al. 2021). In the UK, The Academy of Medical Royal Colleges and the Conference of Postgraduate Medical Deans (2018:1) define "reflective practice" as "the process whereby an individual thinks analytically about anything relating to their professional practice, with the intention of gaining insight and using the lessons learned to maintain good practice or make improvements where possible." In addition, we suggest that the overturning of unconscious biases imprinted through the hidden curricula of global health education and training should be facilitated through a deeper process of transformational learning (Lokugamage et al. 2021). This facilitation should involve providing the time and space for learners to comprehend and evaluate their own biases and the structural discriminations within their institutions via the concept of Cultural Safety (see Table 6.1 above).

As Kathryn Curtis and colleagues described in 2012, Cultural Safety shifts the focus from the culture of the patient as "exotic other" to the culture of the clinician or clinical environment against a broader critique of the positioning of healthcare systems, organizations, and providers in interventions to promote healthcare equity (Wong et al. 2021). At an individual level, the process of providing Cultural Safety would essentially entail that a nurse, doctor, or student as part of their reflective practices prior to a patient encounter quickly reflect on their privileged status and any potential power imbalances between themselves and the patient. This quick reflection should provide insight and situational awareness, aspiring to create a fairer clinical encounter (Richardson and Williams 2007). *Structural reflexivity* is an essential aspect of Cultural Safety that could also be incorporated into *human factors training* to improve patient safety. "Human factors training" is defined as: "Enhancing clinical performance through an understanding of the effects of teamwork, tasks, equipment, workspace, culture and organization on human behavior and abilities and application of that knowledge in clinical settings" (Catchpole and McCulloch 2010; Department of Health 2012; Care Quality Commission, Department of Health, Health Education England et al. 2013:40). These types of reflective practices could be developed within biomedical reflective practice syllabi as healthcare human rights checklists, thereby improving professionalism (Lokugamage 2019).

Cultural Safety is key to the decolonial transformations of institutions. A Cultural Safety Tree Model was outlined within the article "Translating Cultural Safety to the UK" by Amali Lokugamage, Elizabeth Rix, Tania Fleming, and colleagues (2021), which incorporates an infographic that could be customized and utilized in other countries. This model has three essential parts:

1. Understanding a patient-centered experience of care, and generating staff self-reflexivity and structural reflectivity in the context of understanding the power imbalances causing privileges and biases.
2. The core values of human rights: the need for institutions to commit to examining and upending structural biases.
3. Supporting pre-existing activities or services in the UK, such as patient-led initiatives to highlight structural blind spots.

An instance of when these have occurred within the existing framework of biomedical curricula is the organization of diversity theme-related reflective practice "Schwartz Rounds" for medical students, first piloted by the University College of London Medical School in 2015 (Wong et al. 2021). These "Schwartz Rounds" were so named because:

> In 1994, a health attorney called Ken Schwartz was diagnosed with terminal lung cancer. During his treatment, he found that what mat-

tered to him most as a patient were the simple acts of kindness from his caregivers, which he said made "the unbearable bearable." Before his death, he left a legacy for the establishment of the Schwartz Center in Boston, to help to foster compassion in healthcare. (See Schwartz 2016; Wong et al. 2021.)

Led by trained facilitators, these Rounds help to facilitate meaningful conversations and reflections in a confidential forum in which students can share their experiences of racism, discrimination, and bias within health care—either of experiencing these themselves, or of perpetrating them on others (Wong et al. 2021). Thus this form of promoting Cultural Safety, among others, could be adapted to tackle microaggressions that reflect, embody, and perpetuate the existing power hierarchies present in today's biomedical education. (See also Chapter 10, this volume, for descriptions of interprofessional education workshops for biomedical and midwifery students in Aotearoa New Zealand.)

Conclusion:
The Importance of Adopting a Decolonizing Attitude

The adoption of a *decolonizing attitude* by healthcare educators, practitioners, and researchers/funders is a deeper way of improving equality, diversity, and inclusion from professional regulatory bodies as well as from legal imperatives. A system of education that encourages biomedical doctors to reflect on the colonial origins of biomedicine, to challenge their own implicit biases, and to cultivate an attitude of open-minded professionalism (see Davis-Floyd's chapter in Volume II of this series: Davis-Floyd 2023 and the Introduction to this present volume, in which Davis-Floyd's chapter is summarized) is vital to addressing the complex power imbalances of the legacies of colonization within health care. Decolonization includes the tolerance of *medical pluralism*. Healthcare workers can learn from *patients as educators* through active listening. We can acknowledge the emerging field of planetary health, which stretches health care beyond the individual, public health, and global health, and which Indigenous peoples have proposed regarding living harmoniously with the planet:

> The decolonizing movement's intent is to re-centre displaced [I]ndigeneity. In doing this, it seeks to elevate the conversation about living in harmony with nature, which also resonates with debate about climate change, as [I]ndigenous people see climate breakdown as a symptom of non-reciprocal and exploitative relationships

with the planet. With the social tide of interest in climate change, understanding its impact on global health is essential. We note that a decolonial dialogue has entered into climate change conversation. For instance, activist Greta Thunberg (Thunberg, Neubauer, and Valenzuela 2019) has insisted, "After all, the climate crisis is not just about the environment. It is a crisis of human rights, of justice, and of political will. Colonial, racist, and patriarchal systems of oppression have created and fuelled it. We need to dismantle them all." (Lokugamage, Ahillan, and Pathberiya 2020a)

Indeed, the role of decolonization within the field of biomedicine will involve implanting Cultural Safety within the soils of different territories and watching and fostering the ways in which it grows under the unique conditions of each area. This is pertinent in light of the growing phenomenon of human migration as a consequence of a number of factors, including economic opportunities, economic crises, conflicts, and man-made disasters stemming from climate change. The importance of humility and reflexivity should not be understated as we negotiate this rapidly evolving field; by subverting dominant paradigms of what constitutes "meaningful knowledge," we come closer to our goal of humanizing biomedicine, thereby achieving a balance between medicalized and physiologic births.

Acknowledgments

This chapter has been revised and updated from its original publication as: Lokugamage A, Ahillan T, Pathberiya SDC. 2020. "Decolonising Ideas of Healing in Medical Education." *Journal of Medical Ethics* 46(4): 265–272. We thank this journal for permission to reprint the parts of the original article that are included herein.

Amali Lokugamage is a consultant obstetrician and gynecologist involved in biomedical education in London, UK. She has more than 30 years of experience in the specialty. Her primary clinical interests lie in medical gynecology and general obstetrics, with expertise in normalizing childbirth. She has published in the fields of human rights in childbirth, healthcare inequalities, and decolonization.

Tharanika Ahillan is a Junior Doctor working in London, UK. Her main clinical interests lie in the fields of infectious diseases and global health, with an interest in medical education. She has authored articles related to honesty in medical education and on a maternity acupuncture service at a London hospital.

S.D.C. Pathberiya is a lawyer who has published on human rights in childbirth and decolonization.

Note

1. This Figure, on which the authors hold the copyright, is derived from Wong, Gishen, and Lokugamage (2021); https://www.scienceopen.com/document/read?vid=4ca9c88e-f28c-4713-8c27-d329d1263742.

References

Ali I, Davis-Floyd R, eds. 2022. *Negotiating the Pandemic: Cultural, National, and Individual Constructions of COVID-19*. Abingdon, Oxon: Routledge.

American Psychiatric Association. 2013. *Diagnostic and Statistical Manual of Mental Disorders (DSM–5)*. Washington, DC: American Psychiatric Association.

Asakura T, Mallee H, Tomokawa S, et al. 2015. "The Ecosystem Approach to Health Is a Promising Strategy in International Development: Lessons from Japan and Laos." *Globalization and Health* 11(1): 3–10.

Baitmangalkar A. 2021. "How We Can Work Together to Avoid Cultural Appropriation in Yoga." *Yoga International*. Retrieved 12 December 2022 from https://yogainternational.com/article/view/how-we-can-work-together-to-avoid-cultural-appropriation-in-yoga.

Bamrah JS, Mehtam R, Everington S, Esmail A. 2021. "Racism and the General Medical Council." *BMJ Blog*, 29 June. Retrieved 12 December 2022 from https://blogs.bmj.com/bmj/2021/06/29/racism-and-the-general-medical-council/.

BBC World Service. 2019. "Indigenous Communities Talk Climate Change. BBC World Service. Retrieved 31 December 2022 from: https://www.bbc.co.uk/programmes/w172wx8tbxr597b.

Beolen C, Heck JE. 1995. *Defining and Measuring the Social Accountability of Medical Schools*. Geneva: World Health Organization.

Brown DL. 2017. "A Surgeon Experimented on Slave Women without Anesthesia: Now His Statues Are Under Attack." *The Washington Post*, 29 August.

Buse C, Oestreicher J, Ellis N, et al. 2018. "Public Health Guide to Field Developments Linking Ecosystems, Environments and Health in the Anthropocene." *Journal of Epidemiology and Community Health* 72(5): 420–425.

Care Quality Commission, Department of Health, Health Education England, The Parliamentary & Health Service Ombudsman for England, NHS Employers, NHS England. 2013. *Human Factors in Healthcare: A Concordat from the National Quality Board*. London: NHS England.

Catchpole K, McCulloch P. 2010. "Human Factors in Critical Care: Towards Standardized Integrated Human-Centred Systems of Work." *Current Opinion in Critical Care* 16(6): 618–622.

Centers for Disease Control and Prevention. 1929-1972. *Tuskegee Syphilis Study*. National Archives at Atlanta National Archives Identifier 281640, Record Group 442.

Centre for Education Studies. 2018. *What Is Decolonising Methodology?* Coventry UK: University of Warwick.

Cerdeña JP, Plaisime MV, Tsai J. 2020. "From Race-Based to Race-Conscious Medicine: How Anti-Racist Uprisings Call Us to Act." *The Lancet* 396(10257): 1125–1128.

Charles C, Gafni A, Freeman E. 2011. "The Evidence-Based Medicine Model of Clinical Practice: Scientific Teaching or Belief-Based Preaching?" *Journal of Evaluation in Clinical Practice* 17(4): 597–605.

Charles E. 2019. "Decolonizing the Curriculum." *Insights* 32(1): 24.

Chavez-Dueñas NY, Adames HY, Perez-Chavez JG, Salas SP. 2019. "Healing Ethno-Racial Trauma in Latinx Immigrant Communities: Cultivating Hope, Resistance, and Action." *American Psychologist* 74(1): 49–62.

Coleman K, Stewart C, Waitzfelder B, et al. 2016. "Racial-Ethnic Differences in Psychiatric Diagnoses and Treatment Across 11 Health Care Systems in the Mental Health Research Network." *Psychiatric Services* 67(7): 749–757.

Columbia Law School. 2017. "Kimberlé Crenshaw on Intersectionality, More than Two Decades Later." *Columbia Law School*, 8 June.

Council of Europe. 1950. *European Convention on Human Rights*. Strasbourg: Council of Europe.

Cross TL, Bazron BJ, Dennis KW, Isaacs MR. 1989. *Towards a Culturally Competent System of Care: A Monograph on Effective Services for Minority Children Who Are Severely Emotionally Disturbed*. Washington DC: National Institute of Mental Health.

Curtis K, Weinrib A, Katz J. 2012. "Systematic Review of Yoga for Pregnant Women: Current Status and Future Directions." *Evidence-Based Complementary and Alternative Medicine: eCAM* 2012: 715942.

Cushman LF, Delva M, Franks CL, et al. 2015. "Cultural Competency Training for Public Health Students: Integrating Self, Social, and Global Awareness into a Master of Public Health Curriculum." *American Journal of Public Health* 105(Suppl 1): S132.

Davis S. 2017. *Being a Queer and/or Trans Person of Colour in the UK: Psychology, Intersectionality, and Subjectivity*. Ph.D. dissertation, Brighton UK: University of Brighton.

Davis-Floyd R. 2018. "The Technocratic, Humanistic, and Holistic Paradigms of Birth and Health Care." In *Ways of Knowing about Birth: Mothers, Midwives, Medicine, and Birth Activism, Davis-Floyd R and Colleagues*, 3–44. Long Grove IL: Waveland Press.

———. 2022. *Birth as an American Rite of Passage*, 3rd edn. Abingdon, Oxon: Routledge.

———. 2023. "Open and Closed Knowledge Systems, the 4 Stages of Cognition, and the Obstetric Management of Birth." In *Cognition, Risk, and Responsibility in Obstetrics: Anthropological Analyses and Critiques of Obstetricians Practices*, eds. Davis-Floyd R, Premkumar A, 14–50. New York: Berghahn Books.

Department of Health. 2012. *Department of Health Human Factors Reference Group Interim Report*. London: Department of Health.

DiAngelo R. 2019. *White Fragility: Why It's So Hard for White People to Talk about Racism*. New York: Penguin Books.

Downes H. 2020. "Honouring the Slaves Experimented on by the 'Father of Gynaecology.'" *The Conversation*, 20 October. Retrieved 12 December 2022 from https://theconversation.com/honouring-the-slaves-experimented-on-by-the-father-of-gynaecology-148273.

ECHR. 2010. *Jehovah's Witnesses of Moscow v. Russia*. (Application no. 302/02) https://hudoc.echr.coe.int/fre#{%22itemid%22:[%22001-99221%22].

Enkin M, Keirse MJNC, Neilson J, Crowther C, Duley L, Hodnett E, Hofmeyr J. 2000. *A Guide to Effective Care in Pregnancy and Childbirth*, 3rd edn. Oxford UK: Oxford University Press.

Equality Challenge Unit. 2013. *Unconscious Bias in Higher Education: Literature Review*. London: Equality Challenge Unit.

European Court of Human Rights (ECHR-CEDH). 2021. *Guide on Article 9—Freedom of Thought, Conscience and Religion*. Strasbourg: Council of Europe.

Fay J. 2018. "Decolonising Mental Health Services One Prejudice at a Time: Psychological, Sociological, Ecological, and Cultural Considerations." *Settler Colonial Studies* 8(1): 47–59.

Foronda C, Baptiste D-L, Reinholdt MM, Ousman K. 2016. "Cultural Humility." *Journal of Transcultural Nursing* 27(3): 210–217.

Foster-Scales A. 2017. *Rebozos in Birth Work*. Meadville PA: Labor Doulas, Northwest PA Doulas.

Freire P. 1973. *Education for Critical Consciousness*. New York: Seabury Press.

Gaines A, Davis-Floyd R. 2003. "Biomedicine." *Encyclopedia of Medical Anthropology*, eds. Ember C, Ember M, 95–108. New York: Kluwer Academic/Plenum Publishers.

Gandhi S, Wolff L. 2017. *Yoga and the Roots of Cultural Appropriation*. Praxis Center, Arcus Center for Social Justice Leadership. Kalamazoo, Michigan: Kalamazoo College.

Ghui R, Bansal JK, McLaughlin C, et al. 2016. "An Evaluation of the *Guidelines of the Society of Obstetricians and Gynaecologists of Canada*." *Journal of Obstetrics and Gynaecology* 36(5): 658–662.

Gishen F, Lokugamage A. 2019. "Diversifying the Medical Curriculum." *British Medical Journal* 364: 1300.

GMC. 2018a. *GMC Publishes Its Strategy on Equality and Fairness*. London: General Medical Council.

———. 2018b. *Outcomes for Graduates 2018*. London: General Medical Council.

Gopal P. 2017. "Yes, We Must Decolonise: Our Teaching Has to Go Beyond Elite White Men." *The Guardian*, 27 October.

Hoffman KM, Trawalter S, Axt JR, Oliver MN. 2016. "Racial Bias in Pain Assessment and Treatment Recommendations, and False Beliefs about Biological Differences between Blacks and Whites." *Proceedings of the National Academy of Sciences of the United States of America* 113(16): 4296–4301.

Horsch A, Stuijfzand S. 2019. "Intergenerational Transfer of Perinatal Trauma-Related Consequences. *Journal of Reproductive Infant Psychology* 37(3):221–223.

Horton R, Lo S. 2015. "Planetary Health: A New Science for Exceptional Action." *Lancet* 386(10007): 1921–1922.

Hu S. 2011. "Skin Cancer in Ethnic Minorities." *Cutaneous Oncology Today*, December:5–8.

Imperial College London. 2021. *Examining Geographic Bias in Our Curricula.* London: Imperial College London.

Jaung R. 2019. "How Decolonising Health Could Save the Planet." *The Spinoff*, 16 April. Retrieved 12 December 2022 from https://thespinoff.co.nz/soci ety/16-04-2019/how-decolonising-health-could-save-the-planet/.

Johnson KC. 1997. "Randomized Controlled Trials as Authoritative Knowledge: Keeping an Ally from Becoming a Threat to North American Midwifery Practice." In *Childbirth and Authoritative Knowledge*, eds. Davis-Floyd R, Sargent C, 350–365. Berkeley: University of California Press.

Jones AW. 2011. "Early Drug Discovery and the Rise of Pharmaceutical Chemistry." *Drug Testing and Analysis* 3(6): 337–44.

Kleinman A. 1987. "Anthropology and Psychiatry: The Role of Culture in Cross-Cultural Research on Illness." *British Journal of Psychiatry: The Journal of Mental Science* 151(2): 747–751.

Knight M, Bunch K, Tuffnell D, et al. MBRRACE-UK. 2018. *Saving Lives, Improving Mothers' Care—Lessons Learned to Inform Maternity Care from the UK and Ireland: Confidential Enquiries into Maternal Deaths and Morbidity 2014–16.* Oxford: Oxford University Press.

Krieger N, Chen JT, Coull BA, et al. 2014. "Jim Crow and Premature Mortality among the US Black and White Population, 1960–2009: An Age-Period-Cohort Analysis." *Epidemiology* 25(4): 494–504.

Lee DH, Vielemeyer O. 2011. "Analysis of Overall Level of Evidence behind Infectious Diseases: Society of America Practice Guidelines." *Archives of Internal Medicine* 171(1): 18–22.

Linklater R. 2014. *Decolonizing Trauma Work: Indigenous Stories and Strategies.* Halifax: Fernwood Publishing.

Lokugamage A, Ahillan T, Pathberiya SDC. 2020a. "Dissipating Historical Medical Inequity through Decolonising Healthcare Education." *Journal of Medical Ethics Blog*, 9 February. Retrieved 12 December 2022 from https://blogs .bmj.com/medical-ethics/2020/02/09/dissipating-historical-medical-inequi ty-through-decolonising-healthcare-education/.

———. 2020b. "Decolonising Ideas of Healing in Medical Education." *Journal of Medical Ethics* 46(4): 265–272.

Lokugamage A. 2019. "Maternal Mortality—Undoing Systemic Biases and Privileges." *BMJ Opinion*. Retrieved 31 December 2022 from https://blogs.bmj.com/bmj/ 2019/04/08/amali-lokugamage-maternal-mortality-undoing-systemic-biases-and-privileges/.

Lokugamage AU, Pathberiya SDC. 2017. "Human Rights in Childbirth, Narratives, and Restorative Justice: A Review." *Reproductive Health* 14(1): 1–8.

Lokugamage AU, Rix E, Fleming T, et al. 2021. "Translating Cultural Safety to the UK." *Journal of Medical Ethics* published online, 19 July.

Lokugamage AU, Wong SHM, Robinson NMA, Pathberiya SDC. 2021. "Transformational Learning to Decolonise Global Health." *The Lancet* 397(10278): 968–969.

Maridass M, De Britto AJ. 2008. "Origins of Plant Derived Medicines." *Ethnobotanical Leaflets* 12: 373–387. https://opensiuc.lib.siu.edu/ebl/vol2008/iss1/44.

Mbaki Y, Todorova E. 2020. *Decolonising and Diversifying the (Medical) Curriculum: Self-Assessment Questions, Examples, and Resources*. Nottingham: University of Nottingham.

McCarthy AM, Yang J, Armstrong K. 2015. "Increasing Disparities in Breast Cancer Mortality from 1979 to 2010 for US Black Women Aged 20 to 49 Years." *American Journal of Public Health* 105 Suppl(S3): S446–448.

Meekosha H. 2011. "Decolonising Disability: Thinking and Acting Globally." *Disability & Society* 26(6): 667–682.

Montgomery v Lanarkshire Health Board. 2015. UKSC 11. Retrieved 12 December 2022 from https://www.supremecourt.uk/cases/docs/uksc-2013-0136-judgment.pdf.

Mukwende M, Tamony P, Turner M. 2019. "Mind the Gap: A Handbook of Clinical Signs in Black and Brown Skin." Retrieved 31 December 2022 from https://www.blackandbrownskin.co.uk/mindthegap.

Muldoon J. 2019. "Academics: It's Time to Get Behind Decolonising the Curriculum." London: *The Guardian*, 20 March.

Nair M, Knight M, Kurinczuk J. 2016. "Risk Factors and Newborn Outcomes Associated with Maternal Deaths in the UK from 2009 to 2013: A National Case-Control Study." *BJOG: An International Journal of Obstetrics & Gynaecology* 123(10): 1654–1662.

Pan RK, Kaski K, Fortunato S. 2012. "World Citation and Collaboration Networks: Uncovering the Role of Geography in Science." *Scientific Reports* 2(1): 1–7.

Pathberiya S. 2016. "Patient Autonomy and Decision Making: Rapid Response to Making Evidence-based Medicine Work for Individual Patients." *British Medical Journal* 353: i2452.

Porter L. 2018. *Decolonising the Hidden Medical Curriculum: Some Historical Perspectives*. London: University College of London.

Prusova K, Churcher L, Tyler A, Lokugamage AU. 2014. "Royal College of Obstetricians and Gynaecologists Guidelines: How Evidence-Based Are They?" *Journal of Obstetrics and Gynaecology* 34(8): 706–711.

Pyānko B, Haynes S. 2019. "A Brazilian Indigenous Leader Shares His Climate Solutions." *Time Magazine*. Retrieved 31 December 2022 from https://time.com/5676877/indigenous-leader-amazonbrazil/.

Quijano A. 2007. "Coloniality and Modernity/Rationality." *Cultural Studies* 21(2–3): 168–178.

Ramsden IM. 2002. *Cultural Safety and Nursing Education in Aotearoa and Te Waipounamu*. Ph.D. dissertation. Wellington NZ: University of Wellington.

Reverby SM. 2001. "Tuskegee: Could It Happen Again?" *Postgraduate Medical Journal* 77(911): 553–554.

Richardson S, Williams T. 2007. "Why Is Cultural Safety Essential in Health Care?" *Medicine and Law* 26(4): 699–707.

Sabaratnam M. 2017. "Decolonising the Curriculum: What's All the Fuss About?" Retrieved 31 December 2022 from https://study.soas.ac.uk/decolonising-curriculum-whats-the-fuss/.

Schwartz K. 2016. "Ken Schwartz's Story." *The Point of Care Foundation*, 5 April. Retrieved 12 December 2022 from https://www.pointofcarefoundation.org.uk/resource/kens-story/.

Skopec M, Fyfe M, Issa H, et al. 2021. "Decolonization in a Higher Education STEMM Institution: Is 'Epistemic Fragility' a Barrier?" *London Review of Education* 19(1): 1–21.

Smith R. 2013. "Moving from Global Heath 3.0 to Global Health 4.0." *Institute of Global Health Innovation, Imperial College London*, 8 October. Retrieved 12 December 2022 from https://blogs.imperial.ac.uk/ighi/2013/10/08/moving-from-global-heath-3-0-to-global-health-4-0/.

SOAS University of London. 2019. "Applying a Decolonial Lens to Research Structures, Norms and Practices in Higher Education Institutions." London UK: School of African and Oriental Studies (SOAS).

State of Hawaii. 2019. "SB No. 899: A Bill for an Act Relating to the Composition of the State Council on Mental Health." The Senate, State of Hawaii, 31st legislature. Retrieved 31 December 2022 from https://www.capitol.hawaii.gov/session2019/bills/ HB292_. Pdf.

Stone SB, Myers SS, Golden CD. 2018. "Cross-Cutting Principles for Planetary Health Education." *Lancet Planetary Health* 2(5): e192–e193.

Stub ST. 2017. "How Babywearing Went Mainstream." *Sapiens*, 3 May. Retrieved 12 December 2022 from https://www.sapiens.org/culture/babywearing-culture-mainstream/.

Surmitis KA, Fox J, Gutierrez D. 2018. "Meditation and Appropriation: Best Practices for Counselors Who Utilize Meditation." *Counseling and Values* 63(1): 4–16.

Tahmasebi H, Trajcevski K, Higgins V, Adeli K. 2018. "Influence of Ethnicity on Population Reference Values for Biochemical Markers." *Critical Reviews in Clinical Laboratory Sciences* 55(5): 359–375.

The Academy of Medical Royal Colleges and the Conference of Postgraduate Medical Deans. 2018. *Academy and COPMeD Reflective Practice Toolkit*. London: The Academy of Medical Royal Colleges.

The Office of Hawaiian Affairs. 2018. *OHA-4: Addressing Native Hawaiian Mental Health Needs Through Culturally Informed Programs and Services*. Honolulu HI: The Office of Hawaiian Affairs. Retrieved 31 December 2022 from https://www.oha.org/wp-content/uploads/OHA-4-Mental-Health-Council-External-White-Paper-Final.pdf.

Thunberg G, Neubauer L, Valenzuela A. 2019. "Why We Strike Again." *Social Europe*, 2 December. Retrieved 1 January 2023 from https://www.socialeurope.eu/why-we-strike-again.

Towle A, Bainbridge L, Godolphin W, et al. 2010. "Active Patient Involvement in the Education of Health Professionals." *Medical Education* 44(1): 64–74.

UCL (University College London). 2015. *Why Is My Curriculum White?—UCL—Dismantling the Master's House*. London: University College London.

UCL. 2018. "Decolonising the Medical Curriculum." London: University College London.

UCL Anthropology Department. 2019. "Flourishing Diversity Series." London: University College London.

UCL Medical School. 2017. "Blog: Liberating the Curriculum at UCL Medical School." Retrieved 1 January 2023 from: UCL Medical School. Liberating the curriculum at UCL medical school. UCL.

Wellcome Collection. 2017. *Ayurvedic Man: Encounters with Indian Medicine, Exhibition at Wellcome Collection.* London: Wellcome Collection.

White N. 2020. "Black Women Were Tortured to Develop Gynaecology Methods: Midwives Want Them Remembered." *Huffington Post UK*, 29 July.

Wong A, Lokugamage A. 2021. "Just Medicine: Universities Need to Engage with the Historical Forces That Have Shaped the Way Medicine Is Taught, Practiced, and Experienced." *ACU Review*, 26 April. Retrieved 12 December 2022 from https://www.acu.ac.uk/the-acu-review/just-medicine/.

Wong SHM, Gishen F, Lokugamage AU. 2021. "Decolonising the Medical Curriculum: Humanising Medicine through Epistemic Pluralism, Cultural Safety, and Critical Consciousness." *London Review of Education* 19(1).

Wright JM. 2007. "Practice Guidelines by Specialist Societies Are Surprisingly Deficient." *International Journal of Clinical Practice* 61(7): 1076–1077.

Young AE, Nadeau D. 2005. "Decolonising the Body: Restoring Sacred Vitality." *Indigenous Women: The State of Our Nations* 29(2): 13–22.

Youssef NA, Lockwood L, Su S, et al. 2018. "The Effects of Trauma, with or without PTSD, on the Transgenerational DNA Methylation Alterations in Human Offsprings." *Brain Sciences* 8(5): 83.

CHAPTER 7

Teaching Humanistic and Holistic Obstetrics

Triumphs and Failures

Beverley Chalmers

Introduction

As a perinatal health psychologist and social scientist, I have been involved in the education of obstetricians and Health Science students for 50 years. I have taught principles of perinatal care to biomedical and allied health science students in undergraduate university programs. I have implemented combined, joint psychology and obstetrics teaching for clinical year medical students. I have developed and implemented evidence-based, psychosocially and culturally respectful perinatal care training programs on behalf of WHO and UNICEF and served as a Master Trainer on these and on the Baby-Friendly Hospital Initiative (BFHI) educational programs for perinatal health care providers throughout the former Soviet Union and the countries of central and eastern Europe and the Central Asian Republics. I was a founding member and later National President of the Association for Childbirth and Parenthood of Southern Africa—a multidisciplinary and multicultural perinatal health promotion group that ran educational conferences and programs for interdisciplinary perinatacare providers to address the clinical, technological, and humanistic needs of women and their families during their transitions to parenthood. I have researched, documented, and lectured to medical and social science students about specific aspects of abusive perinatal practices such as female genital mutilation and Nazi eugenics and euthanasia programs, exposing the importance of biomedical and cultural ethical issues in clinical perinatal care (Chalmers and Omer-Hashi 2003; Chalmers 2015).

While I have at times despaired that I have achieved little after these decades of work in striving toward an integration of humanistic and holistic approaches to care together with technological advancements, I am also reminded of the progress that has been made and the steps that have been, and still need to be, taken to achieve optimal maternity care. This chapter details the triumphs and failures of these varied and often unique approaches to obstetric education.

Medical School Teaching

Education for a multicultural, psychosocial, and evidence-based approach to health care is a prerequisite for achieving it. Traditionally, the teaching of obstetrics, neonatology, nursing, psychology, and related disciplines in biomedical schools has been separated along disciplinary lines (Chalmers 1999; Ratti et al. 2014). Some important components of care are not included at all, particularly those relating to social science issues such as psychology, social work, and childbirth education. More importantly, a concentration on pathology often overshadows the care of the normal birth and of the normal newborn (Chalmers and Levin 2001). Obstetric caregivers are not trained to be sensitive to the emotional, cognitive, or spiritual aspects of perinatal care—or, if they are, the training is insufficient (Chalmers 2011). Little is done to encourage medical students to take courses in medical humanities or in psychosocial-cultural issues. Adrianna Banaszek (2011) reported that only 69 of 133 accredited biomedical schools in the United States required students to take courses in the medical humanities. Few, if any, of the 17 medical schools in Canada require a similar course, although some offer an elective option (Banaszek 2011). Many of these programs, particularly if they are based in psychosocial or Behavioral Science departments or if they are limited to pre-clinical years and focus on theory rather than application, have failed or are likely to fail. They may be perceived by students as programs to be endured, or as classes that are undemanding "bird courses" (because one "flies" right through them) and not central to their abilities as future doctors. They are perceived as more valuable when offered as students face the challenges of caring for people in clinical practice.

Interprofessional, psychosocial, and cultural issues that are involved in clinical practice should be integrated into mainstream biomedical teaching programs. For example, when the clinical management of a fetal death is taught, both the psychological impact on the parents as well as diagnostic and treatment procedures should be considered. In like manner, teaching should be shared by a physician and social scientist concurrently. Joint teaching programs of this nature, when tried, have shown promise of a new and better model for educational success (Chalmers and McIntyre 1993; see also Daellenbach et al., this volume).

Schools of Psychology do not usually provide training for perinatal psychologists, resulting in a dearth of trained professionals able to fill this teaching void. "Perinatal psychologists" are trained in the essentials of clinical perinatal care and in the multitude of psychosocial issues that accompany a family's transition to parenthood (see Chalmers 2017). In my teaching experiences in South Africa from 1971 to 1992, these programs were offered for psychology, biomedicine, physiotherapy, social work, and occupational therapy students at the undergraduate level, and for graduate-level psychology students. In some centers, this role is termed a "Women's Health Psychologist"; these professionals care for women not only during childbearing but also across all health concerns.

Barriers to interprofessional collaboration in perinatal care have been identified and methods of overcoming these have been proposed (Smith et al. 2009; Siassakos et al. 2010; Avery, Montgomery, and Brandl-Salutz 2012; Homer et al. 2012). Interprofessional perinatal education programs are in place at some universities, showing some success, particularly with regard to improving infants' and mothers' mental health outcomes, such as reduced incidences of postpartum depression (Saxell, Harris, and Elarar 2009; Meffe, Moravac, and Espin 2012; Poleshuck and Woods 2014; Department of Ob/Gyn, Columbia University 2019). Fortunately, those involved in education for healthcare providers are increasingly receptive to new interprofessional developments (D'Amour and Oandasan 2004; Oandasan and Reeves 2005; Poleshuck and Woods 2014; University of Toronto 2015; Department of Ob/Gyn, Columbia University 2019). The World Health Organization (WHO) has taken up the challenge of directing attention to interprofessional models of education, practice, and policy across healthcare specializations, and has developed a framework within which to consider local initiatives for greater and more successful interprofessional practices (D'Amour and Oandasan 2004; Oandasan and Reeves 2005; Poleshuck and Woods 2014; University of Toronto 2015; Department of Ob/Gyn, Columbia University 2019). New developments along these lines, with a particular focus on respectful perinatal care, are to be encouraged and welcomed. The WHO/UNICEF training programs in effective perinatal care and breastfeeding promotion are examples of such developments.

As early as the 1970s, the University of the Witwatersrand, Johannesburg, set a model of integrated education, yet medical students generally scorned taking the courses in Human Behavioral Science that were offered as options. Disillusioned with teaching courses for only a handful of students for a number of years, I eventually refused to continue with this approach. I recommended to the Dean of Health Sciences that the medical school allocate this teaching time to courses that faculty obviously valued more highly, such as Anatomy and Physiology, rather than pay lip service to the idea that they were teaching medical students about the social sciences or about humanistic approaches to care. In response, the school decided that students would be required to take, and to pass, the medical school's Human Behavioral Science course that I taught before being allowed to progress to their fourth year of study and the start of their clinical training. This requirement was implemented, to the mortification of a few students who had to repeat a year, and led to full classes and serious students.

Problem-based learning models require that the somewhat artificial distinctions between disciplines be minimized. For example, a more closely integrated teaching model allows for teaching obstetrics together with neonatology; students learn to care for the mother during birth as well as for the baby after delivery. The traditional distinctions between these disciplines in the classroom allowed for the then-customary separation of mother and baby into postpartum wards for mothers (cared for by obstetricians or midwives and obstetric nurses), and nurseries for the babies (cared for by pediatricians, midwives, and pediatric nurses). The need to integrate these disciplines academically made itself clear in the clinical settings in which mothers were separated from their babies after birth. Combined care requires combined teaching models. Changed maternity care services today encourage immediate contact between mother and baby at birth and rooming-in for all mothers and babies—unless the baby is ill and needs to be in a neonatal intensive care unit, where skin-to-skin contact/kangaroo care is increasingly encouraged. To achieve these goals, close cooperation between obstetricians (or other delivery assistants), and pediatricians and neonatologists is required. It seems logical that the teaching of these disciplines should likewise be closely associated, as it is in the model followed by WHO training programs.

As an international health consultant, I have visited hundreds of hospitals around the world, particularly in low-resource countries. In many, the structural layout of delivery rooms includes a separate area to which the baby is removed almost immediately after birth and cared for by a pediatrician, neonatologist, or neonatal nurse rather than an obstetrician, midwife, obstetric nurse, or the mother. Often this is in a separate room adjacent to the birthing room. The separate teaching model followed for obstetric and pediatric education has, in these settings, become architecturalized into the physical layout of the maternity hospital. In Eastern European settings, this structural divide was taken even further: "women's consultations" (women's hospitals) cared for mothers after delivery, whereas infants were cared for in separate buildings (children's polyclinics) by totally different caregivers.

Priorities in Perinatal Care Conferences

The educational developments in South Africa that increasingly incorporated psychosocial issues into clinical obstetric care teaching were mirrored in the national perinatal care conferences that were held annually in the country. From 1982 onward, Professor Alan Rothberg of the Department of Pediatrics at the University of the Witwatersrand organized a remarkable series of annual conferences called "Priorities in Perinatal Care." These well-respected conferences were attended by perinatal researchers primarily employed in State-funded teaching hospitals from across the country, together with invited international guest speakers (two of these were Iain Chalmers and Murray Enkin, founders of the Cochrane Collaboration, which has provided invaluable sources of evidence on maternity care practices for decades). They offered a pioneering framework for multidisciplinary and multicultural exchanges primarily contributed by researchers and clinicians based in academic clinical care settings. In 1992, I reviewed the proceedings of the conferences held between 1985 and 1991 to assess what proportion of the papers presented were focused on psychosocial or educational aspects of obstetrics and pediatrics compared to purely clinical concerns (Chalmers 1992b). In 1985, only 10% of papers considered psychosocial issues; in subsequent years, this proportion increased to between 22% and 30%. At first, these papers were presented primarily by social scientists—myself being one of the first to do so—but as the years went by, the proportion of obstetricians, pediatricians, midwives, and nurses giving psychosocially focused papers far surpassed the number given by social scientists, reflecting the increased awareness by maternity care practitioners of the importance of such issues as teenage or unmarried mothers; contraceptive or sexual behavior; birth procedures such as support for women during labor and birth; stress; infant feeding; postpartum depression; rural care; stillbirth; newborn anomalies; HIV infection; and education of mothers and midwives. Similarly, these papers were initially relegated to the last section of the conference, termed "Obstetric Miscellany." Later this changed to

"General Perinatology," then to "General," and following this, to "Psycho-social Issues." In 1991, this session was awarded the distinguished title of "Psychosocial Aspects of Perinatal Care"—a conceptual growth indeed, reflecting the growing recognition of social and educational sciences by obstetrics and pediatrics. While presentations were offered by multi-cultural faculty and students of perinatal social sciences, these were the minority of delegates (Chalmers 1992b, 2017). The session also moved from being the last session of the three-day conference to a more valued time slot early in the program.

The Association for Childbirth and Parenthood

The development of increasing psychosocial awareness in perinatal care among various professional groups in South Africa led to a need for a professional body that reflected these shared multidisciplinary and multicultural perspectives. In 1984, an "Association for Childbirth and Parenthood" was established by a mixed group of perinatal care pro-fessionals that was initially stimulated by childbirth educators. It grew rapidly to extend to all caregivers across the country who valued shared knowledge, experiences, and practices across obstetrics, pediatrics, mid-wifery, nursing, childbirth education, and perinatal psychology. Unlike most professional bodies established during the Apartheid era, this Asso-ciation was inclusive of anyone of any racial or ethnic background. This was long before the collapse of Apartheid in 1993–94. When applying to affiliate with the International Association of Psychosomatic Obstetrics and Gynaecology, it held—at my instigation as the National President of the Association from 1989 to 1992—a formal vote of all its members to include in its Constitution a clear statement that it did not discriminate against any people on any grounds. The vote was overwhelmingly in favor of amending the Association's Constitution to incorporate this explicit statement of non-discrimination, leading to its affiliation with the Euro-pean-based International Association of Psychosomatic Obstetrics and Gynecology. Given the international ostracism against the Apartheid-based government of South Africa and the resulting sanctions against any international affiliations with South African academic and institu-tions, this approval and recognition were crucial for acceptance into the global perinatal world. This explicitly multicultural association was a forerunner of what was soon to follow in South Africa after the collapse of Apartheid.

The Association for Childbirth and Parenting undertook a variety of educational and clinical practice developments. In addition to monthly presentations given by multidisciplinary members and an annual conference with invited international guest speakers, the association also undertook clinical challenges. One of these was the evident contradiction between what childbirth educators were advocating in their childbirth preparation courses for parents, and what these parents then encountered in the hospital birth setting. In the 1980s, the emphasis in these classes was on a more "natural" approach to birth, inspired by such doyens of childbearing of that time as Ann Oakley, Niles Newton, Frederick Leboyer, Sheila Kitzinger, Michel Odent, and others with similar birth views, with relaxation and breathing techniques being advocated to achieve as non-interventionist a birth as possible. Yet when faced with the clinical birth setting and the increasing drive from practitioners to use such interventions as induction or augmentation of labor, supine positions for delivery, pharmacological pain relief including epidurals, and the resulting "cascade of interventions" that often ended in operative vaginal deliveries (forceps or vacuum extraction) or cesarean births, women emerged from birth feeling disappointed and like "failures" for not having achieved their desired "natural birth." As a result, the Association for Childbirth and Parenting organized full-day meetings at the major maternity hospitals where childbirth educators who served women in the hospitals' neighborhoods shared what they taught prospective mothers with clinical staff of the hospitals. Caregivers, in turn, shared what happened to women giving birth in their hospitals. Areas of differences or conflicts were highlighted, and discussions were entered into on how to reduce these disparities and how best to prepare women for their birth experiences. In particular, we emphasized what clinical care practices could be eliminated or minimized to reach congruence between women's expectations for a "normal or natural" birth and the realities they would face in the hospital. The resulting collaborations between childbirth educators and hospital birth facilities led to greatly reduced tensions between these services, with fewer complaints about contradictions between women's expectations for their birth experiences and their actual experiences. Lines of communication were established so that childbirth educators could call practitioners and talk to them about individual mothers. These outcomes were so good that other hospitals began to ask us to run these kinds of meetings with them as well.

The Association for Childbirth and Parenting became a well-respected professional association continuing to draw membership from across the country and persisting long after I had emigrated to Canada in 1992. Its multidisciplinary nature was exemplified in the fact that the first Chair of the Association was a childbirth educator. I served as its second Chair for some years as a social scientist, and was succeeded as Chair by an obstetrician. There are few national professional associations serving perinatal care needs that are as grounded in a multidisciplinary approach with its implications for research, teaching, and clinical practice. Most national associations perpetuate a "silo effect"— specific groups serving the specific needs of obstetricians, pediatricians, midwives, and nurses independent of each other: a recipe for conflict.

The Canada-WHO-St. Petersburg Maternal and Child Health Program

In 1996, after immigrating to Canada, I initiated and ran a series of ten week-long training programs in St. Petersburg, Russian Federation, in partnership with the WHO's Regional Office for Europe and the Health Department of St. Petersburg, funded by the Canadian International Development Agency. These trainings were directed toward strengthening prenatal, labor, and birth care and the training of childbirth educators in all the hospitals in the city. A unique feature of these courses was the adoption of a unitary approach to maternity and newborn care, regardless of the professional background of the caregiver. My teaching team consisted of an obstetrician, a pediatrician who was also an epidemiologist, a midwife, and a nurse, as well as myself as a social scientist and breastfeeding consultant. Following an interprofessional teaching model, we structured course participants to be multi-professional, with obstetricians, pediatricians, midwives, and nurses all attending the same courses. This model proved so successful that I extended it into the WHO's Regional Office for Europe training programs that followed from 1998 onward.

One of the challenges facing us at the start of the St. Petersburg program was the lack of evidence-based knowledge in the former Soviet countries. *A Guide to Effective Care in Pregnancy and Childbirth* had been published (Enkin, Keirse, and [Iain] Chalmers 1989). By the early to mid-1990s, that extremely useful book had not yet been translated into Russian (or any other Eastern European language), and there was no local knowledge of this new, revolutionary approach to assessing the value of interventions through scientific evidence. Instead, tradition, custom, experience, and the writings of a few Russian professors served as the guiding principles for practice. As the former Soviet counties had been almost totally isolated from the Western world, there was little or no access to developments in Western scientific knowledge available to local caregivers or educators. In fact, one of the additional developments that became necessary during the Canada-WHO-St. Petersburg Maternal and Child Health Program was the offering of special sub-courses in evidence-based knowledge and practice for senior academic staff of perinatal care faculty at universities to expose them to the ideas underlying evidence-based care. Just as these concepts had been shocking in the West when first brought to attention—along with their support for a demedicalized, less interventionist approach to maternity care—so too were these ideas almost heretical in the face of traditional, highly medicalized and rigid approaches to care that characterized many aspects of Soviet obstetrics (Chalmers 1997, 2005). Ragner Tunell, a Swedish neonatologist, and I received funding to translate the first edition of the *Guide to Effective Care in Pregnancy and Childbirth* into Russian, and we were able to distribute this translated version widely.

Dissemination of educational materials in Russian was another major component of the Canada-WHO-St. Petersburg Maternal and Child Health Program. I had learned that, due to the scarcity of Western biomedical knowledge in the Soviet Union, the occasional rare copies of articles published in English might find their way to the offices of the Chief of Obstetrics or Pediatrics, but usually never went beyond their doors. Nor did they widely share this new information; at that time, English was not commonly understood or spoken in the Russian Federation, making dissemination of English language information problematic. We therefore arranged for the translation into Russian of hundreds of recent journal articles on perinatal care, and provided course participants with copies of each one. We believed that putting the knowledge into the hands of all caregivers was essential if new concepts and practices were to be considered in maternity care settings.

The outcomes of our program were proof of the success of our approach to teaching obstetricians and their perinatal colleagues about alternate, evidence-based, psychosocially sensitive, respectful, and less interventionist ways to provide care. Clinical outcomes showed marked changes over the five years of our program. There was an overall decline in maternal mortality in St. Petersburg from 61.8/100,000 live births in 1994 to 34.4 in 1996, and in perinatal mortality from 16/1,000 live births in 1994 to 12.7 in 1996 (Stephenson et al. 1997). The number of preterm births remained reasonably low (7.1% and 7.4% in the two time periods), as did the number of low-birthweight babies (6.7% and 6.4%, respectively). These improvements in maternity care were not achieved with the increased use of technology; cesarean birth rates remained low (11.9% to 12.8%), and operative vaginal delivery was rare. In addition, a more humanistic approach to care was introduced. In particular, changes regarding family-centered care services were becoming widely accepted, including hospital visiting by family members, increased breastfeeding, more favorable attitudes toward an increasing role for fathers in labor and delivery, and a decrease in some of the more "unacceptable" obstetric interventions, as described below.

Nevertheless, some routine interventions, frowned upon in the West, persisted, such as pubic and perineal shaving and enemas, contrary to evidence. These interventions were also contrary to the wishes of most women, based on surveys of women undertaken as part of the Canada-WHO-St. Petersburg program, despite obstetricians' beliefs that mothers desired them. The fact that *any* deviation from rigidly enforced procedures occurred over such a short period of time indicated a growing awareness of the numerous additional factors that needed to be considered in implementing effective care in pregnancy and childbirth. Of significance was that maternity care practices were changing and moving toward a decreased use of technology without any locally feared, negative consequences for mothers and babies materializing.

Teaching with WHO in the European Region

Concern over the excessive use of technology in perinatal care led WHO to undertake a survey of birth practices in the European region. In 1985, WHO published the book *Having a Baby in Europe* (WHO 1985b) as well as an article in *The Lancet* entitled "Appropriate Technology for Birth" (WHO 1985a). These publications were controversial, as they challenged the existing emphasis on the technological management of birth. They aroused debate throughout the European region and stimulated 43 birth conferences in 23 member states of the region, as well as in Canada, the United States, Australia, and China. Three interregional conferences (European and American) covering appropriate technology for perinatal care were also held. Despite the extensive underlying research, debate and discussion, readers in technologically sophisticated countries such as the United States, the UK, the European nations, and others remained skeptical about the WHO recommendations for reduced interventions in childbirth. Questions were raised regarding their scientific basis, implying that these were simply the conclusions of left-wing, radical, or extremist "natural birth" advocates.

With the publication of *Effective Care in Pregnancy and Childbirth* in 1989, it soon became possible to address the question of whether the WHO recommendations that emerged from discussion and debate at consensus conferences were supported by "evidence-based" research. In reality, almost identical recommendations for reductions in the use of many traditional interventions in pregnancy and childbirth emerged in both the WHO recommendations for birth and the outcomes of randomized controlled trials, leading me to conclude at that time, when comparing the two documents, that "The WHO recommendations for appropriate technology for birth, as developed through survey research, discussion and debate, are strongly endorsed by the findings of carefully controlled, and critically evaluated, randomized controlled trials" (Chalmers 1992a:709). More than 30 years later, most countries and, indeed, many individual obstetricians and perinatal caregivers could still benefit from an examination of their perinatal services in light of evidence-based knowledge and the WHO recommendations for perinatal care. In 1998, this process of reassessment commenced in Europe with a Perinatal Care Workshop that I assisted the WHO Regional Office for Europe to implement, which led to the development of principles that should underlie perinatal care in the future (WHO 1998a, 1998b). At that time, 10 Principles of Perinatal Care were listed by WHO (Chalmers and Mangiaterra 2001). These were:

1. Care for normal pregnancy and birth should be de-medicalized, meaning that essential care should be provided with the minimal interventions necessary and that less rather than more technology should be applied whenever possible.
2. Care should be based on the use of appropriate technology, which is defined as a complex of actions that includes methods, procedures, techniques, equipment, and other tools, all applied to solve a specific problem (WHO 1998b). This point is directed toward reducing the overuse of technology or the application of sophisticated or complex technology when simpler procedures may suffice or indeed be superior.
3. Care should be evidence-based, meaning supported by the best available research, and by randomized controlled trials where possible and appropriate.
4. Care should be regionalized and based on an efficient system of referral from primary care centers to tertiary levels of care.
5. Care should be multidisciplinary, involving contributions from such professionals as midwives, obstetricians, neonatologists, nurses, childbirth and parenthood educators, and social scientists.
6. Care should be holistic and should be concerned with the intellectual, emotional, social and cultural needs of women, their babies and families, and not only with their biological care.
7. Care should be family centered and should be directed toward meeting the needs of not only the woman and her newborn but also of her partner and significant family or friends.

8. Care should be culturally appropriate and should consider and allow for cultural variations in meeting these expectations.
9. Care should involve women in decision-making.
10. Care should respect the privacy, dignity, and confidentiality of women.

These principles strongly endorsed protection, promotion, and support for effective family-centered perinatal care, which I later incorporated into the technical materials as well as into the monitoring and evaluation tools of the WHO's European regional office. The WHO developments reflected a growing acknowledgement of the need for an evidence-based, family-centered approach incorporating psychosocial and culturally sensitive perinatal care. Principles 5 through 10 clearly emphasize these aspects of pregnancy and birthing care, while evidence-based care remains the cornerstone of all.

Implementing the WHO Principles of Perinatal Care

I was integrally involved in the development of the WHO's 10 Principles of Perinatal Care, and was asked to assist with the planning and implementing of two Perinatal Care Workshops. At the first Perinatal Task Force workshop, it was proposed that a training program be developed by the WHO Regional Office for Europe in collaboration with UNICEF to implement their Principles of Perinatal Care into practices across the European region. To disseminate their ideas, two Perinatal Care courses were developed by the Child Health and Development Unit of the WHO European office. One course was devoted to obstetric care (Chalmers, Mangiaterra, and Porter 2001; WHO 2002) and the second course to neonatal care and breastfeeding (WHO 1997). In addition, the Baby-Friendly Hospital Initiative, for which I served as a Master Trainer, was launched in St. Petersburg in 1992 by WHO and UNICEF, and multiple courses on this Initiative were offered throughout the former Soviet Union in the following decade.

I was asked by the WHO Regional Office for Europe to develop the obstetric course and to integrate into it my approach to evidence-based obstetrics combined with psychosocially sensitive care. I did so, and this course was then offered from 1998 onward throughout the European region. I remained a course trainer or team leader on this program for many years and in many countries, while also contributing to the neonatal care program.

Like the Canada-WHO-St. Petersburg Maternal and Child Health Program that I had previously developed, a distinctive feature of the WHO courses was the adoption of a unitary approach to maternity and newborn care, regardless of the professional background of the caregiver. These courses were not designed specifically for midwives, or for obstetricians, or for family practitioners, but for all caregivers involved in the care of women during pregnancy and birth. For this reason, these courses were taught to mixed professional groups. Both the WHO and the St. Petersburg programs were based on the philosophy that care should be rooted in the principles of evidence-based practice, together with a family-centered and respectful approach, regardless of who the caregiver is. This approach balances not only good practice but also good care.

The training programs for the WHO/UNICEF courses were, similarly to my previous program offered in St. Petersburg, run by three trainers: an obstetrician, a midwife, and a perinatal psychologist. For example, when demonstrating alternative positions for women to adopt in birth, we would customarily role-play a birth situation, with the obstetrician playing the father and supporting the mother by sitting behind her and holding her in his arms while she "gave birth" in an upright, seated position, with her open legs bent and resting on the bed. The midwife in the team was always responsible for attending the "birth." The image thereby created served to reinforce the importance of midwifery care, the value of an upright birth position without the use of stirrups, and the value of companionship in labor—all evidence-based, psychosocially sensitive practices.

The WHO/UNICEF obstetric, neonatal, and breastfeeding promotion courses were offered across the countries of the former Soviet/European region. I served, primarily as a team leader, for courses offered in the Russian Federation, Hungary, Poland, Georgia, Armenia, Belarus, Moldova, Lithuania, Latvia, Estonia, Kazakhstan, Tajikistan, Uzbekistan, Kyrgyzstan, and Azerbaijan. In addition, I was also asked to prepare and offer courses on psychosocial issues in pregnancy, birth, and postpartum, which, in Moldova, led to the decision to appoint perinatal psychologists in every maternity hospital in the country. When offering these courses, as well as those provided by the Canada-WHO-St. Petersburg Maternal and Child Health Program, participants initially divided themselves up by profession: obstetricians and neonatologists sat together on one side of the room and midwives and nurses on the other. By the final day of these five-day programs, participants mingled easily, with barriers to communication being shed through recognition of a shared approach to caregiving that was not congruent with their hitherto rigidly held, silo-based hierarchy, which had placed physicians at the apex and nurses at the base, with mothers' or families' perceptions hardly being considered at all.

To What Extent Did Our Programs Succeed?

I conducted surveys of women's experiences of their perinatal care in a number of cities and countries in the former Soviet Union where the WHO/UNICEF programs were introduced, including St. Petersburg, Azerbaijan, Moldova, and Lithuania (Chalmers 2012). In St. Petersburg, I was able to examine perinatal practices at both the early stages of our programs (1995) and two years later (1997). While cesarean rates increased slightly over this period, from 10.2% to 12.2%, most other rates of interventions decreased, such as inductions (from 39.2% to 30.4%); shaving (from 84.0% to 62.2%); artificial rupture of membranes (from 52.6% to 33.6%); and episiotomies (from 49.1% to 46.2%). Rooming-in of mothers and babies increased from 67% of mother-baby pairs to 80.2%; more mothers were discharged (after seven days) still breastfeeding (increasing from 87.5% to 89.5%), and fewer babies were given fluids other than breastmilk during their hospital stays (from 41.5% to 28.1%). At that time, no epidurals were offered in the city for either vaginal or cesarean births, and electronic fetal monitoring (EFM) was just being introduced to replace the (optimal) handheld fetal stethoscope that was the standard of Russian fetal monitoring practice. EFM use rates increased over the study period from 18.8% to 32.2%, indicating how vulnerable these knowledge-hungry professionals remained for novel interventionist approaches. The longer-term effects of my work are described in *Pregnancy and Birth in Russia: The Struggle for Good Care* by Russian authors Anna Temkina, Anastasia Novkunskaya, and Daria Litvina (2022; See also the following chapter by Anna Ozhiganova and Anna Temkina, this volume.).

Midwives and Obstetricians

There have long been conflicts between midwives and obstetricians regarding their value or place in maternity care, with family doctors providing an intermediate role offering some elements of both professions (Chalmers and Levin 2001). In some parts of the world, such as Aotearoa New Zealand, the Netherlands, the Scandinavian countries, and other parts of Europe, the midwife's role is well-recognized, and midwives are responsible, as WHO advocates, for the care of normal birth. Obstetricians in this context provide specialized care for complications—an entirely appropriate use of resources. Yet in other parts of the world, particularly in North America, battles have long raged over the place of professional midwifery in perinatal care (see, e.g., Cheyney, Burcher, and Vedam 2014). Midwives have been excluded and sometimes persecuted for their humanistic and holistic approaches to care, and many obstetricians perceive them as insufficiently trained and too prone to making mistakes or missing important diagnoses. In turn, many midwives—especially those who attend home births—perceive obstetricians as too prone to intervene and as insufficiently trained in normal, physiologic birth (see, for examples, Cheyney 2011; the chapters in Volumes I and II of this series [Davis-Floyd and Premkumar 2023a, 2023b]; and other chapters in this present volume). Yet midwives are welcomed by most mothers who use them, as they generally provide continuity of caregiver and humanistic, supportive care. In Canada, for example, almost three-quarters of women cared for by midwives rated their overall pregnancy and birth experience as "very positive," compared to a little over half cared for by obstetricians, family doctors, or nurses (Public Health Agency of Canada 2009).

Although many hospital-based midwives practice in highly technocratic ways, ideally, midwives offer a personal and holistic approach to perinatal care. They regard themselves as responsible for preparing the woman and her family, both emotionally and intellectually, for all aspects of birth and parenting, in addition to providing clinical care, whereas physicians do so to a much lesser extent. Family doctors provide continuity of caregiver, particularly if they offer care at birth and after birth as well as during pregnancy, but usually take a less holistic, albeit humanistic, approach to care than midwives. (See the Introduction to this volume, and Davis-Floyd 2018, 2022, for descriptions of the technocratic, humanistic, and holistic paradigms of birth). Obstetricians (57%) and family doctors (36%) are most likely to regard birth as dangerous; few midwives agree (4%) (Ratti et al. 2014). Randomized trials have clearly shown that intervention rates for similar kinds of mothers, and levels of risks and complications, are far higher among physicians than among their midwifery colleagues. Not surprisingly, outcomes of midwife-managed births tend to be better than outcomes for physicians (Hueston and Rudy 1993; Harvey et al. 1996; Cheyney et al. 2014). Despite this, in some countries, including Canada and the United States, only around 10% of women are able to access professional midwifery care—whether community- or hospital-based—though that percentage varies widely by region (Canadian Association of Midwives 2015; Davis-Floyd 2018b, 2022).

The conclusion to be reached is not necessarily that midwives should care for all normal births, but that *the quality of care that is needed by women is the same, no matter who the caregiver is* (Chalmers and Levin 2001; Chalmers 2017). Humanistic, sensitive, caring support, together with respectful treatment that is considerate of the biological, emotional, and intellectual needs of childbearers and their family members should be offered by all caregivers to all pregnant and birthing women, regardless of the degree of normality of their birth experiences or the degree of complications they develop. There is no theoretical or practical justification for condoning differences in this regard. And it is crucial that all caregivers be competent and highly skilled, and thus able to avoid disasters.

The Written Teaching Model

Another approach to educating obstetricians and other perinatal caregivers is the written word. This may take the form of journal publications, books, training programs, national guidelines, or global principles of perinatal care. I have tried them all and remain concerned that these formats depend not only on the ability or willingness of practitioners to read them but also on peer pressure, long-held practice conventions, the legal consequences of their actions (or inactions) to implement current knowledge, or the lack of any follow-up assessment of their applications in practice. When, for example, perinatal guidelines are promoted in a country, or principles of perinatal care are published for global consumption, who monitors which caregivers are introducing changes in their practices as a result? Or what consequences follow for caregivers who do not change their practices when this is advised? Very few, if any.

In Canada, I co-chaired a national Maternity Experiences Survey on behalf of the Public Health Agency of Canada (Chalmers et al. 2008). We interviewed more than 6,000 women—a randomly selected sample drawn from a national census survey—about their recent pregnancy, birth, and postpartum experiences. This remarkable survey resulted in more than 40 academic journal articles being published utilizing data collected in this publicly available dataset. The findings also contributed substantially to the revision of Canada's national perinatal care guidelines, called "Family-Centred Maternity and Newborn Care." I served as a member of the Steering Committee for this revision and was responsible for writing (together with a supportive team) the "Principles of Perinatal Care" that form the overall perspective on perinatal care to be followed in Canada and that are outlined in Chapter I of this document (Chalmers, Aziz, et al. 2017). These principles are outlined more fully in my book *Family-Centred Perinatal Care: Improving Pregnancy, Birth and Postpartum Care* (Chalmers 2017). In addition, I have over 300 publications in journals or books that address perinatal care issues in differing social, cultural, economic, and political contexts, and have given more than 460 presentations on these subjects globally. There is no way to assess the actual impacts of these activities on perinatal practices, although the more than 15,000 citations that these have received, as listed by Google Scholar, suggest that some have at least read them, if not applied their findings. At the very least, they provide some evidence to substantiate my perinatal care advocacy for humanizing childbirth.

As I noted near the beginning of this chapter, I have recently looked back at my past 50 years of teaching obstetricians with feelings of despair, thinking that I had achieved little despite—to my mind—my heroic efforts, as many of the problems I have sought to solve remain ever-present. But then my always-supportive husband reminded me of how far we had come since I embarked on this Sisyphean task. When I gave birth to my first baby in 1977, I had to obtain written permission from the matron of the South African maternity hospital where she was born for my husband to accompany me during the birth. This "privilege" was only granted to a few; it was granted to me because I was a doctoral researcher in this maternity hospital at the time, and my husband also has a graduate degree. He was, therefore, thought to be responsible enough not to arrive in the delivery room intoxicated or to faint at the sight of birth. Rooming-in was also a privilege granted to only a few, and although breastfeeding was encouraged, there were no breastfeeding counselors to support it. Episiotomies and perineal shaving were routine, as were pharmacological pain management, supine delivery, induction of labor, visual inspection of the cervix after delivery (routine examination of the mother's cervix after birth by the insertion of a speculum, together with the grasping and visualization of the cervix with forceps to check for tears or bleeding) and a myriad of other fairly standard and (today regarded as) unnecessary interventions, making birth a long-lasting nightmare.

In contrast, around 45 years later, at least in higher-income countries, companionship during labor and birth is regarded as essential (except, horrifically, in the era of COVID, during which, for many months, childbearers were not allowed labor companions [see Davis-Floyd, Gutschow, and Schwartz 2020]); many practitioners understand the benefits of laboring and birthing in upright positions; episiotomies, enemas, and pubic shaving are no longer routinely performed; the cervix is not routinely visualized after birth; and we know more about how to support, promote, and protect breastfeeding. Sadly, far too many inductions and augmentations of labor, continuous electronic fetal monitoring, and cesareans are still performed, and attempts are made to encourage child-bearers to have epidurals. Nevertheless, we can celebrate the many humanistic inroads that have been made into technocratic approaches to birth (see Davis-Floyd 2022), although there is still much to be done.

What Succeeds and What Fails in Teaching Obstetricians?

In retrospect, there are a number of factors that appear to have contributed to whether my/our teaching approaches have been successful or less so. These include:

- *A Teachable Moment:* Whether any educational approach will have a positive impact will depend on whether the knowledge to be gained is what students often refer to as "being relevant." For example, healthcare students, and particularly medical students, become far more interested in the human side of care when they see patients in their clinical years, compared to when such courses as "Human Behavioral Science" are offered in their pre-clinical years. Similarly, in the former Soviet countries, courses on breastfeeding promotion were welcomed after the collapse of the Soviet Union because women were struggling to breastfeed successfully due to inappropriate clinical practices, and caregivers had no idea how to support and facilitate this optimal, invaluable method of newborn feeding. Courses for obstetricians and pediatricians were also welcomed, as it was realized that WHO and UNICEF had much to offer them in comparison to their limited exposure to new knowledge during the Soviet years.
- *Combined Clinical, Technological, and Humanistic Care:* Information is far more readily accepted when a combined approach incorporating evidence-based knowledge, psychosocially sensitive care, and appropriate use of technology is advocated. This approach has proven to be the most logical and acceptable manner in which to teach or to learn about perinatal care, and formed the basis of the activities of the Association for Childbirth and Parenthood, as well as the foundation upon which the educational courses that I developed during my decades of work with WHO and UNICEF were based.
- *Multidisciplinary Teaching and Participation:* Involving obstetricians, pediatricians, midwives, and nurses in both the teaching team and

as course participants provides an opportunity for caregivers from diverse professional backgrounds to find common ground and to develop collaborative approaches for the care of women and their families. This principle held true when undergraduate medical students were offered combined psychosocial and obstetric training during their obstetric rotations, or when offering courses in the Canada-WHO-St. Petersburg Maternal Child Health Program, the WHO/UNICEF Effective Care in Pregnancy, Birth and Postpartum courses, the Psychosocial Issues in Perinatal Care courses, or the BFHI programs.

- *A Respectful Approach:* Throughout all my years of teaching, research, and health promotion, I have always maintained a respectful approach to working with obstetricians, pediatricians, midwives, nurses, and childbirth educators, acknowledging the remarkable knowledge, skills, and abilities that each profession has to offer. Perhaps because of my non-biomedical professional status, I was able to suggest change without threatening their own professional territories. The temptation to criticize caregivers in the former Soviet Union was always present among those consultants who undertook the challenges of offering global teaching programs under extremely difficult—and occasionally dangerous—settings and conditions. I was careful to remind my teams that the caregivers we met in clinical settings as course participants, or as hosts in the multiple hospitals we visited—no matter how outdated their obstetric or perinatal care practices—were offering the best care they knew how to give. None were intentionally harming women or their babies, even if their actions resulted in care that we would today regard as disrespectful, harsh, uncaring, cruel, or even as violence against women. Yet this was not their intention: the kinds of care they gave were based on their education; the ideologies instilled in them by their teachers; a lack of access to alternate knowledge; and by the biomedical customs and traditions prevalent at the time. Their care was not deliberately harmful, even if it did result in adverse clinical or psychological outcomes. It was our role as consultants to understand their own situations and to provide optimal and respectful knowledge for them in the same ways in which we were advocating that they provide optimal and respectful care to their patients. This principle applies in the technologically sophisticated world just as much as it did in the former Soviet Union countries.

- *What's Best for Mothers, Babies, and Families:* Underlying all the above is a genuine intention to do what is best for mothers and babies and to strengthen caregivers' abilities to provide optimal care. In what was a truly holistic approach, I always advocated for providing the most optimal clinical, psychological, social, and spiritual care for women and families, regardless of the practitioners' professional backgrounds.

Change comes slowly. It takes time, respect, support, repetition, patience, and determination. It requires a multidisciplinary, multimodal, and multifaceted approach. The development of evidence-based care and its evolution into the Cochrane Collaboration Database resulted in a seismic revolution in the assessment of the appropriateness of obstetric care. Concurrently, the availability of online information has resulted in increased knowledge regarding medical care being moved into the hands (and minds) of clients. While the impacts of this change have been slower to see than those experienced after the publication of *Effective Care in Pregnancy and Childbirth*, the result has been an increasing need for caregivers to listen to, understand, respect, and consider the perspectives of their now more knowledgeable clients. The outcome of this revolution in the sources of authoritative knowledge regarding perinatal care is, and will continue to be, a welcome, more humanistic approach to caring for women, their babies, and their families in their transition to parenthood. Education for obstetricians and other perinatal caregivers will need to reflect and enact this new worldview, which, over time, will become widely shared, simply because it is better for mothers, babies, and families.

Beverley Chalmers (Canada) has two doctoral degrees: a PhD in Psychology and a DSc (Med) in Multicultural Childbirth. Her research examines the birth experiences of women in difficult religious, social, political, and economic situations. She has over 300 publications, including 57 book chapters and 11 books. She has given over 460 conference presentations globally and has undertaken 141 international health promotion activities in 26 countries. Her book *Family-Centred Perinatal Care: Improving Pregnancy, Birth and Postpartum Care* (Cambridge: Cambridge University Press, 2017) integrates her decades of work in perinatal care. Her books *Birth, Sex and Abuse: Women's Voices under Nazi Rule* (2015) and *Betrayed: Child Sex Abuse in the Holocaust* (2020) have together won 14 book awards. They expose neglected and often taboo topics in Holocaust studies. Other publications include *African Birth: Childbirth in Cultural Transition* (1990); *Female Genital Mutilation and Obstetric Care* (2003); *Humane Perinatal Care* (2001) and *Child*

Sex Abuse: Power, Profit, Perversion (2022). Her book *Obstetric Abuse* is forthcoming in 2023.

References

Avery MD, Montgomery O, Brandl-Salutz E. 2012. "Essential Components of Successful Collaborative Maternity Care Models: The ACOG-ACNM Project." *Obstetrics & Gynecology Clinics of North America* 39(3): 423–434.

Banaszek A. 2011. "Medical Humanities Becoming Prerequisites in Many Medical Schools." *Canadian Medical Association Journal* 183(8): c441–c442.

Canadian Association of Midwives. 2015. "Midwifery in Canada Is Growing." *The Pinard: Newsletter of the Canadian Association of Midwives* 5(1): 5–6.

Chalmers B. 1990. *African Birth: Childbirth in Cultural Transition.* Sandton: Berev Publications.

———. 1992a. "WHO Appropriate Technology for Birth Revisited." *British Journal of Obstetrics and Gynaecology* 99: 709–710.

———. 1992b. "Psychosocial Components of Priorities in Perinatal Care Conferences." *South African Medical Journal* 82: 77–78.

———. 1997. "Childbirth in Eastern Europe." *Midwifery* 13: 2–8.

———. 1999. "Multicultural, Multidisciplinary, Psychosocial Obstetric Care." *Journal of Obstetrics and Gynaecology of Canada* 21: 975–979.

———. 2005. "Maternity Care in the Former Soviet Union." *British Journal of Obstetrics and Gynaecology* 112: 495–499.

———. 2011. "Shame on Us!" *Birth* 38(4): 279–281.

———. 2012. "Childbirth across Cultures: Research and Practice." *Birth* 39(4): 276–280.

———. 2015. *Birth, Sex and Abuse: Women's Voices Under Nazi Rule.* London: Grosvenor House Publishers.

———. 2017. *Family-Centred Perinatal Care: Improving Pregnancy, Birth and Postpartum Care.* Cambridge: Cambridge University Press.

———. 2020. *Betrayed: Child Sex Abuse in the Holocaust.* London: Grosvenor House Publishers.

———. 2022. *Child Sex Abuse: Power, Profit, Perversion.* London: Grosvenor House Publishers.

———. 2023. *Obstetric Abuse.* London: Grosvenor House Publishers. (Forthcoming)

Chalmers B, Aziz K, Ciofoni L, LeDrew M, Menard L, Miller K, Nemrava J. 2017. "Philosophy and Principles of Care." In *Canadian National Guidelines for Family-Centred Maternal and Neonatal Care,* Chapter 1. Ottawa, ON: Public Health Agency of Canada.

Chalmers B, Dzakpasu S, Heaman M, Kaczorowski J, for the Maternity Experiences Study Group. 2008. "The Maternity Experiences Survey: An Overview of Findings." *Journal of Obstetrics and Gynaecology of Canada* 30: 217–228.

Chalmers B, Levin A. 2001. *Humane Perinatal Care.* Tallinn, Estonia: TEA Publishers.

Chalmers B, Mangiatterra V. 2001. "Appropriate Perinatal Technology: A WHO Perspective." *Journal of the Society of Obstetricians and Gynaecologists of Canada* 23: 574–575.

Chalmers B, Mangiaterra V, Porter R. 2001. "WHO Principles of Perinatal Care: The Essential Antenatal, Perinatal and Postpartum Care Course." *Birth* 28: 202–207.

Chalmers B, McIntyre J. 1993. "Integrating Psychology and Obstetrics for Medical Students: Shared Labour Ward Teaching." *Medical Teacher* 15(1): 35–40.

Chalmers B, Omer-Hashi K. 2003. *Female Genital Mutilation and Obstetric Care*. Vancouver, BC, Canada: Trafford Publishers.

Cheyney M. 2011. "Homebirth as Ritual Performance." *Medical Anthropology Quarterly* 25(4): 519–542.

Cheyney M, Burcher P, Vedam S. 2014. "A Crusade against Home Birth." *Birth* 41(1): 1–4.

D'Amour D, Oandasan I. 2004. "Interprofessional Education for Patient-Centred Practice." In *Education for Collaborative, Patient-Centred Practice: Research & Findings Report*, eds. Oandasan I, D'Amour D, Zwarenstein M et al. Ottawa, ON: Health Canada.

Davis-Floyd R. 2018a. "The Technocratic, Humanistic, and Holistic Paradigms of Birth and Health Care." In *Ways of Knowing about Birth: Mothers, Midwives, Medicine, and Birth Activism*, Davis-Floyd R and Colleagues, 3–44. Long Grove IL: Waveland Press.

Davis-Floyd R. 2018b. "American Midwifery: A Brief Anthropological Overview." In *Ways of Knowing about Birth: Mothers, Midwives, Medicine, and Birth Activism*, Davis-Floyd R and Colleagues, 165–188. Long Grove IL: Waveland Press.

Davis-Floyd R. 2022. *Birth as an American Rite of Passage*, 3rd ed. Abingdon, Oxon: Routledge.

Davis-Floyd R, Gutschow K, Schwartz DA. 2020. "Pregnancy, Birth, and the COVID-19 Pandemic in the United States." *Medical Anthropology* 39(5): 413–427.

Davis-Floyd R, Premkumar A, eds. 2023a. *Obstetricians Speak: On Training, Practice, Fear, and Transformation*. New York: Berghahn Books.

———. 2023b. *Cognition, Risk, and Responsibility in Obstetrics: Anthropological Analyses and Critiques of Obstetricians' Practices*. New York: Berghahn Books.

Department of Ob/Gyn, Columbia University. 2019. "Columbia Ob/Gyn Launches New Integrated Clinical Care Program, Centered on Mental Health. New York." *Columbia University Irving Medical Center*, 12 July. Retrieved 12 December 2022 from https://www.columbiaobgyn.org/news/columbia-ob-gyn-launches-new-integrated-clinical-care-program-centered-mental-health.

Enkin M, Keirse M, Chalmers I. 1989. *A Guide to Effective Care in Pregnancy and Childbirth*. Oxford: Oxford University Press.

Harvey S, Jarell J, Brant R, Stainton C, Rach D. 1996. "A Randomized Control Trial of Nurse-Midwifery Care." *Birth* 23: 128–135.

Homer CS, Griffiths M, Brodie PM, et al. 2012. "Developing a Core Competency Model and Educational Framework for Primary Maternity Services: A National Consensus Approach." *Women & Birth: Journal of the Australian College of Midwives* 25(3): 122–127.

Hueston W, Rudy M. 1993. "A Comparison of Labour and Delivery Management between Nurse-Midwives and Family Physicians." *Journal of Family Practice* 37: 449–454.

Meffe F, Claire Moravac C, Espin S. 2012. "An Interprofessional Education Pilot Program in Maternity Care: Findings from an Exploratory Case Study of Undergraduate Students." *Journal of Interprofessional Care* 26(3): 183–188.

Midwives Alliance North America. 2015. "What Is a Midwife?" Retrieved 12 December 2022 from http://mana.org/about-midwives/what-is-a-midwife.

Oandasan I, Reeves S. 2005. "Key Eelements of Interprofessional Education. Part 2: Factors, Processes and Outcomes." *Journal of Interprofessional Care* Supplement 1: 39–48.

Poleshuck E, Woods J. 2014. "Psychologists Partnering with Obstetricians and Gynecologists." *American Psychologist* 69(4): 344–354.

Public Health Agency of Canada (PHAC). 2009. *What Women Say: The Maternity Experiences Survey*. Ottawa, ON: Public Health Agency of Canada.

Ratti J, Ross S, Stephanson K, Williamson T. 2014. "Playing Nice: Improving the Professional Climate between Physicians and Midwives in the Calgary Area." *Journal of Obstetrics & Gynaecology Canada* 36(7): 590–597.

Saxell L, Harris S, Elarar L. 2009. "The Collaboration for Maternal and Newborn Health: Interprofessional Maternity Care Education for Medical, Midwifery, and Nursing Students." *Journal of Midwifery and Women's Health* 54(4): 314–320.

Siassakos D, Draycott TJ, Crofts JF, et al. 2010. "More to Teamwork than Knowledge, Skill and Attitude." EBM Reviews—Cochrane Central Register of Controlled Trials. *British Journal of Obstetrics and Gynecology* 117(10): 1262–1269.

Smith C, Brown JB, Stewart M, et al. 2009. "Ontario Care Providers' Considerations Regarding Models of Maternity Care." *Journal of Obstetrics & Gynaecology Canada* 31(5): 401–408.

Stephenson P, Chalmers B, Kirichenko V, et al. 1997. "Reducing Maternal Mortality in St Petersburg." *World Health Forum* 18: 189–193.

Temkina A, Novkunskaya A, Litvina D. 2022. *Pregnancy and Birth in Russia: The Struggle for "Good Care."* Abingdon, Oxon: Routledge.

University of Toronto. 2015. "U of T IPE Curriculum." Retrieved 12 December 2022 from https://ipe.utoronto.ca/u-t-ipe-curriculum.

WHO. 1985a. "Appropriate Technology for Birth." *Lancet* 8452: 436–437.

———. 1985b. *Having a Baby in Europe*. Copenhagen: World Health Organization.

———. 1997. *Essential Newborn Care and Breastfeeding*. Copenhagen: WHO Regional Office for Europe.

———. 1998a. "Second Meeting of Focal Points of Reproductive Health/Health of Women and Children in the European Region." Copenhagen: World Health Organization.

———. 1998b. "Workshop on Perinatal Care Proceedings: Venice." Copenhagen: World Health Organization.

———. 2002. *Essential Antenatal, Perinatal and Postpartum Care Course*. Copenhagen: WHO Regional Office for Europe.

CHAPTER 8

The Inconsistent Path of Russian Obstetricians to the Humanization of Childbirth in Post-Soviet Maternity Care

Anna Ozhiganova and Anna Temkina

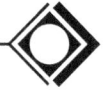

Introduction: The Post-Soviet Bureaucratic Legacy and the Commercialization of Maternity Care

In this chapter, we consider the professional strategies of Russian obstetricians leading to the *partial humanization* of post-Soviet maternity care. By "humanization," we mean the process of progressive changes aimed at relieving maternity care from *obstetric aggression* or "obstetric iatrogenesis" along the UHDVA spectrum first delineated by Kylea Liese and colleagues (2021); this spectrum ranges from unintentional harm (UH) to overt disrespect, violence, and abuse (DVA) as described in the Introduction to this volume. Three paradigms of obstetric practice delineated by Robbie Davis-Floyd (2001, 2018a, 2018b, 2022)—the technocratic, humanistic, and holistic models (also described in the Introduction to this volume) are applicable to Russian conditions, except that instead of the technocratic and holistic approaches, the concepts of "medicalized" and "natural" childbirth are used, and the State bureaucracy has an especially strong influence. The humanistic approach has been widely used by Russian perinatal specialists in recent years, and to them it means a model of care focused on the needs of women and newborns and on shared decision-making between maternity care providers and childbearers. It is important to note that in Russian obstetric care, a specific model of medicalization was formed in which the routine stimulation of labor with artificial oxytocin and the use of dangerous obstetric manipulations—in particular, "squeezing out" the child through heavy fundal pressure (the Kristeller maneuver)—was widespread, while the rate of cesarean births (CBs) remained relatively low for many years (around 8%), only reaching around 30% in 2018 (Federal State Statistics Service 2019.).

We conceptualize the post-Soviet system of maternity care as a *hybrid* of the legacy of Soviet bureaucratic paternalism and neoliberalism in contemporary reformations. By "paternalism," we mean a system positing that those in authority "know best" (from top State bodies to physicians in hospitals) and act in condescending or controlling ways; this leads to an asymmetrical balance of power and to expectations that physicians will obey controlling institutions, and that childbearers will obey physicians (Temkina, Novkunskaya, and Litvina, 2022). Soviet health care was characterized by socialized and centralized medicine; monopolized direct control of the Soviet State; limited resources; powerless patients with equal access to care but with a lack of proper care and a lack of trust in their caregivers; and poorly paid, politically inert State-employed physicians with a lack of autonomy and also with a lack of independent professional status. Russian maternity care was (and still is to some extent) highly biomedicalized, with many interventions yet few resources. In Soviet times, it was also characterized by a rude and authoritarian emotional style called *khamstvo* (Field 1967, 1988; Rivkin-Fish 2005a; Saks 2015; Temkina 2019; Temkina and Rivkin-Fish 2020). In her ethnographic research in St. Petersburg maternity hospitals from 1990 to the early 2000s, Michele Rivkin-Fish showed that Soviet health-care providers were responsible for fulfilling the interests of the State, not those of the individual patient. Providers often felt helpless in the rigid State paternalistic hierarchies; since they lacked decision-making autonomy, they re-established their power in interactions with patients using crude and cruel techniques of domination—*khamstvo*. Patients remained docile, as obstetricians threatened any women whom they perceived as challenging their authority. This situation called for changes in obstetricians' positioning (Rivkin-Fish 2005a, 2005b).

Beverley Chalmers, who—as she describes in the preceding chapter in this volume—worked in the 1990s as a consultant for WHO/UNICEF on maternal and child health in Russia and other countries of Eastern Europe, noted that "Russian medical workers recognize that change is important and long overdue, and they are ready for a 'transition of authoritative knowledge'" (Chalmers 1997:275). She pointed to the factors that can trigger the process of transforming the authoritative knowledge (Jordan 1997) of obstetricians (and their positions) in the former Soviet countries where, unlike in the United States and Western

Europe, the women's movement is weak and unable to promote women's struggles for the rights to choose how, where, and with whom to give birth. Chalmers saw factors that could lead to changes: the spread of evidence-based medicine; exposing the inadequacies and even harms of routine procedures that previously had been considered to be useful for women and newborns (see Liese et al. 2021 and the Introduction to this volume, in which that article is described); and the influence of midwives, who represent alternative authoritative knowledges yet are also capable of compromising with the biomedical approach.

From the early 1990s, attempts to reform and improve health and maternity care were carried out through decentralization and marketization (Novkunskaya 2019). Official payments in private, marketized hospitals and departments became legitimate in the 1990s, private care and commercial services in public hospitals developed, and affluent women could officially pay in cash. Previously, such payments had been unofficial "gifts" (Temkina 2019; Temkina and Rivkin-Fish 2020). However, in general, providers continued to be inattentive to women' needs in conveyor-like services and overburdened wards.

In 2006, the National Project for Health led to significant changes in health care, and especially in maternity care, which was announced as a State priority related to the State's desire for population growth. Reforms were aimed at improving the quality of care, the provision of more biomedical obstetric facilities, and raising the salaries of maternity care providers (Sheiman and Shishkin 2010). Pregnant women, who had previously had no choice in where they gave birth, became free to choose whichever publicly funded maternity hospital they wished, but not their obstetrician or midwife. The promotion of patient choice in both State and commercial services opened more possibilities for women in maternity care, involving a mix of State (public) and private institutions (Saks 2015). The paid services offer patients improved conditions (e.g., a remodeled room) and the possibility to choose an obstetrician and a midwife; thus new opportunities were opened for the humanization of care. Marketization and the possibility of choice led to several significant shifts in the organization of maternity care: from a centralized system partly compensated by informal welfare payments to a less rigid market-driven system; from authoritarian state employees to market-driven providers; and from powerless obedient women to empowered consumers-clients. The State, however, has not left the stage, continuing direct regulation of maternity care. Bureaucratic paternalist and commercial principles in this new hybrid system coexist, often contradict each other, and lead to inconsistency in care, even where it has become more humanized.

This hybrid system entails requiring obstetricians to fulfill top-down rules and orders, to obtain and report "proper" statistical indicators of their clinical practices, and to expect childbearing women to follow their instructions. New challenges appeared as consumer-oriented clients who expected to get what they wanted entered the scene, necessitating special efforts from obstetricians to cope with both State top-down rules and control and the growth of women's demands. According to the Investigative Committee of the Russian Federation, obstetrics traditionally leads in the number of patient complaints (Petrova 2017), and according to forensic experts, this profession ranks first in the number of established errors in biomedical care provision (Loban et al. 2015). Obstetricians and their associations generally have no significant influence on changes in post-Soviet maternity care. While liberalization and commercialization open new possibilities for client-oriented and more women-friendly humanistic care, providers, most especially obstetricians (obs) find themselves between "a rock and a hard place"—a situation of pressure both from the State and from the market of consumer-oriented women. Obs are limited in their autonomy and agency, and often express their feelings of vulnerability (Litvina, Novkunskaya, and Temkina 2020). Many providers are not satisfied with their positions and have become very critical of the overall maternity care situation. Victor Radzinsky, Doctor of Medical Sciences and Corresponding Member of the Russian Academy of Sciences, is well known for his strong critiques of current birth practices and his call for reform of the obstetric care system. He considers practices such as unnecessary cesarean births, labor inductions, and more to be "obstetric aggressions," as these practices not only have no evidence base, but also directly contradict medical research data, including those set out in obstetric practice standards (Radzinsky and Kostin 2007; Radzinsky 2011).

Our questions here are: What have obstetricians done and what can they do to provide more humanistic maternity care almost 20 years since researchers first noticed a tendency to shift from a Soviet paternalistic approach to more progressive and humane practices? What roles could obstetricians play in coping with new obstetric institutional conditions or in challenging them?

Methods and Materials

The data on which this chapter is based include Anna Temkina's 19 interviews with maternity care practitioners (2018) and 35 childbearing women (2015–16), and her two years of ethnographic fieldwork

(2018–19) in a high-tech maternity hospital in a large Russian city (see Temkina 2019); she calls this hospital simply "the Hospital." Temkina carried out this work together with social scientists Daria Litvina and Anastasia Novkunskaya (see Temkina, Litvina, and Novkunskaya 2021; Temkina, Novkunskaya, and Litvina 2022). Such tertiary care hospitals, which have emerged in most large cities according to the National Project (2006), provide specialized biomedical treatments for high-risk pregnancies and births, low-weight newborns, assisted reproductive technologies, and gynecological treatments and surgeries. Women who are routed to the Hospital usually have complicated pregnancies and do not expect a natural birth. Treatment is free of charge, but there are also commercial wards and paid services. Additionally, interviews conducted with women who paid for maternity services in the 2010s in different hospitals are used.

The other dataset on which this chapter is based derives from Anna Ozhiganova's empirical materials on the reforming of an ordinary public maternity hospital in Moscow, which she calls "the Center." These include in-depth interviews with the Chief obstetrician and Chief midwife, eight interviews with individual midwives and doulas who attended births in this hospital, and four interviews with homebirth midwives who had informal relationships with the Chief obstetrician (2018–2021). Some public speeches by the Chief obstetrician of this hospital (2018–20) are also included in Ozhiganova's empirical materials.

Humanization by Default: Obstetricians Adapting to New Conditions in Maternity Hospitals

Obstetricians' Strategies

In looking at different cases, we are interested in what strategies are employed by obstetricians to improve and to humanize maternity care, and how obstetricians maneuver between State and market (consumer) demands. We ask, how do obs interact with childbearers and accept—or don't accept—their agency, needs, and knowledge, and what are the result of obs' strategies in relation to the humanization of maternity care?

Taking requests for changes toward humanization into account, we now delve further to analyze two types of obstetricians' strategies: (1) *Coping strategies* in maternity hospitals connected to commercialization, emotional labor, and hands-on "manual management" in the Hospital— that is, personal, informal efforts to make conditions in maternity care workable and to offer more woman-centered care; (2) The strategy of *reforming the system* at the Hospital and in the Center: reorganization of all departments—prenatal, maternity, and postnatal; cooperation with individual midwives who have practiced as homebirth midwives; births with partner and doula support; rejection of routine medicalization; and a benevolent emotional style in opposition to the Soviet-style *khamstvo* (again, a highly authoritarian style that involves extreme rudeness).

The Commercialization of Maternity Care: Humanization Due to Clients' Demands

As Anna Temkina has shown in previous research (Temkina 2019; Temkina and Rivkin-Fish 2020), the commercialization that has been sweeping throughout the country has generally changed clients' demands and maternity care standards, and overall, care has become more humanized. As previously mentioned, the commercialization of childbirth provides women who can afford them with many options: a woman in paid care can choose specific attendants—an obstetrician and a midwife—who will provide her with individual personalized care during labor, birth, and the postpartum period; an individual delivery room and guaranteed partner participation (a separate suite is necessary for this, and none of this is guaranteed in free-of-charge public wards). Pregnant women who choose paid maternity care make an agreement with their chosen doctor and midwife in advance by signing an official contract guaranteeing that they will pay for these services, and that such services will be provided to them. Women expect the chosen obstetrician to provide high-quality maternity care and emotional support; they also expect attention to their needs and relevant comprehensive information and explanations during labor. In general, such women expect an approach that is much more humanistic than the Soviet-style authoritarian *khamstvo* approach, which lingers on in the attitudes of some obstetricians toward the women they attend.

In paid care, conditions have also changed for providers. Not only have obs' salaries significantly increased, but they have also gained more autonomy and individual responsibility in their decisions and cooperations with the chosen midwife. This new situation is opposed to the Soviet-style collective-oriented work in "conveyor-belt" childbirth, and to the post-Soviet organizational context of a regular department with its "anonymous" crowds of participants. In paid services, obstetricians know women in advance; they take into account their individuality and needs, as well as clinical indicators, thereby gaining the opportunity to plan the labor and manage the process of delivery from beginning to end. This continuity of care contrasts with the rigidly organized 24-hour shifts in free public hospitals, where one team may leave the delivery room and another team will appear to replace them with new tactics, or the original team may try to artificially augment labor in order to complete the births they are attending before their shifts end. Many obs appreciate the more personal approach and continuity of care that can take place in paid commercial wards, along with more flexible times and techniques.

Communication with women and communicative skills during labor and birth have by now become important for obs and other care providers. Many obs are no longer conceptualizing the care receivers as objects, but as individual human beings requiring respect (at least ideally) and emotional care. Previously, obstetricians did not think reflexively about their communications with childbearers, but saw themselves purely as medical experts with authoritarian knowledge (Rivkin-Fish 2005a). Reflexivity has now begun to soften paternalism and helps obstetricians to humanize childbirth.

Today's Russian obs recognize that they are located within market competition, and that their income depends on their reputations, created by internet reviews and word of mouth. These conditions are radically changed in comparison to those that characterized birth and maternity care during Soviet times, when obs were never held to account by their patients who, knowing that they had no other choice, passively submitted to obs' orders and procedures. Today, obstetricians—even those who work in public hospitals—have to be more attentive to client needs; however, they still insist on foregrounding their expertise and practicing paternalistically. Obstetricians accuse women of being too demanding and service-oriented when their behavior becomes aggressively consumeristic; one ob interlocutor complained, "Some patients treat [us] as their personal servants." Obs try to explain to women that this is not a "shopping" for maternity care, and that they provide a professional expertise, not a service. But generally, in commercial departments under market pressure, providers accept clients' requests/demands, and their approaches to childbirth have generally become more humanistic and women-centered.

Emotional Labor: Ambivalent Humanization

As we found in both of our research sites, providers—most especially obstetricians—have to perform a great deal of *emotional labor*—the process of managing feelings and their expressions connected to work duties (Hochschild 1983) to meet the demands of consumer-oriented women who expect polite service with a *smile*—which was almost never given during the Soviet *khamstvo*-style era. Our ob interlocutors told us that this style had first changed in commercial departments, but because often the same providers work in both private paid and public free services, this style slowly changed everywhere. Emotional labor and attentive care are requested not only by consumer-oriented clients, but also by those women who have complications, feel themselves miserable, and/or are unsatisfied with hospital care and file complaints. Obstetricians have told us that it is very important to communicate with women, explain their health conditions to them, and try to calm them down by listening to them and addressing their issues: "They [some women] are very unhappy. They often cry, just cry, here . . . Yes, we ourselves have already become psychotherapists."

Obstetricians, though with ambivalent attitudes, have gradually accepted that they should "sell" their expertise and manage not only the emotions of the women they attend, but also their own emotions. They have slightly changed their paternalistic, authoritarian positionings, as the new conditions are conducive to the new emotional "smiling" style (Temkina et al. 2021, 2022). As one ob interlocutor put it, "No matter how regrettable it may sound, in order to sell yourself, you need to do something for this, and somehow slightly change your view of things. You need to learn, and you need to somehow control yourself, learn to smile, learn to address patients [kindly]."

Though obstetricians have become more reflexive due to the emotional demands of service users, we also observed a great many episodes in which the rude style of *khamstvo* was still in use, especially when obstetricians are forced by their hospitals—or choose on their own—to subordinate childbearers to rigid rules and instructions, without desire or possibility to take their needs and desires into account. Providers maneuver between different emotional styles—*khamstvo* and smiling—to meet patients' demands and desires but also to make patients conform to institutional conditions.

Obs understand that unsatisfied women's complaints can lead to problems, including follow-up investigations by members of State regulatory bodies. Thus they realize that they have to be emotionally sensitive during their patient interactions. This newfound sensitivity makes conditions for women more humane in comparison to the rude and authoritarian Soviet style. Emotional labor has become part and parcel of obstetric professionalism. But, as Anna Temkina showed in her previous research, obstetricians do not become much more egalitarian with the development of consumer culture and the smiling emotional style; they still remain authoritarian figures in childbirth (Temkina 2019; Temkina and Rivkin-Fish 2020; Temkina et al. 2022). Maternity hospitals remain highly biomedicalized, and women can only accept this high level of medicalization, even in the commercial departments with better conditions and more attention from personnel. These conditions lead to the "obstetric paradox": intervene in birth to keep it safe, thereby causing harm (Cheyney and Davis-Floyd 2019:8). In Russia, obstetricians interfere in the normal physiologic process of birth according to top-down instructions supposedly designed to keep women and newborns safe; they make women obey these norms, still often in rude ways, thereby causing discontent and suffering.

Yet interestingly, many pregnant women feel that they have taken control of their births and exercised their agency by choosing their obs and their midwives; after that, they tend to *choose* to give over control of their birthing bodies to those practitioners, still believing, in this highly paternalistic society and its maternity care system, that "the doctor knows best." Said one such childbearing interlocutor, "You choose your practitioners, and then you do what they tell you. You have to just trust that they know best."

"Manual Management": Humanization by Default

In this section, I (Anna Temkina) refer to the ethnographic research my colleagues, Anastasia Novlunskaya and Daria Litvina, and I carried out in the Hospital (Temkina, Novlunskaya, and Litvina 2022). We found that to cope with new demands, obstetricians and other physicians in the Hospital have to do some special work that has unintended influences on childbirth care. We named this work "manual management" (*ruchnoe upravlenie*) as an analogy to "manual control"—a term used in political science to describe the manual interference of the Russian State top bodies into both routine and urgent problems all around the country on the operational level (Monaghan 2012). The lack of autonomy of local actors causes problems to be solved not by them according to legal procedures, but by systematic "manual management" from the top. Similarly, in a large and complex high-tech hospital, many special "manual" (individual, hands-on) efforts must be made to meet the demands of the State and of newly consumeristic women under contradictory rules. Such work has to be done in every maternity hospital in Russia, but here I focus on a particular institution, the Hospital, in which, due to the complexities of this very large institution, systematic personalized regulation and coordination are needed.

Discontinuity in maternity care, rigid State and institutional control, and consumer needs provoke numerous challenges for obstetricians. As clients, childbearing or ill women, or women with sick children, expect more care; should they become dissatisfied with their care, they report their dissatisfaction to various official bodies, which then carry out inspections, and negative sanctions follow. Such punitive actions are what every hospital wants to prevent. Working under rigid formal hierarchical rules and controls, maternity care providers—most especially obs—have to negotiate informally and to hybridize their daily work when clinical necessity does not fit into official rules, or rules do not exist, or they are outdated and unhelpful, or contradict each other; needed resources are lacking; or the trajectory of a patient is unclear; or inspection is expected, and so forth. This non-clinical manual labor through systematic personal informal regulation and coordination in-between formal regulative rules is aimed at navigating women through organizational inconsistencies and making conditions suitable for all participants. Providers must maintain the institutional order of the Hospital, meet women's expectations, and prevent their discontents, thereby preventing the dreaded government body inspections and the negative sanctions that may ensue.

In the Hospital, practitioners must be personally involved in the coordination of different care providers and receivers, specialists, departments, equipment, and resources. For personalized coordination in the Hospital (as well as in other hospitals), both vertical and horizontal connections are needed to maintain formal rules on the operational level. Obstetricians and other physicians, especially Chiefs of different wards, coordinate their decisions personally with each other. Providers should not violate laws and rules, as institutional control over these is total and rigid, and so providers, including obs, look for solutions in the "grey" zone of personal communications with colleagues, Chiefs, and subordinates.

My colleagues and I (Temkina, Novkunskaya and Litvina 2022) often observed situations in which something was going awry. For example, one woman came to the Hospital without appropriate papers; she had come from another city, and her providers there were not familiar with these requirements (the regulations are very complicated). She waited for hours in the emergency room while the Chief obstetrician tried to solve the problem by negotiating with those involved, both from the Hospital and from outside facilities. Finally, at the end of the shift, we saw that the problem had been solved—the woman had received the necessary permission, which had taken the Chief several hours to obtain.

As my colleagues and I observed entire working shifts in different wards, we saw how much coordination work had to be done by the Chiefs of departments, their teams, and other providers. One particular obstetrician solves numerous problems during regular patient care or in the regulation of clinicians, and, in her words, systematically constructs logistical "chains" of different actors to achieve goals, as I described in a fieldnote:

> Working the shift with the Chief. "Manual management." [During the day I observe how the] "Chain" combines different practitioners—that is, permanent coordination of different cases, between physicians, and obstetricians and patients—the construction of "chains." This work has little to do with formalized rules . . . I ask whether everything is coordinated like this? Yes—she is smiling—this are real "chains." Women, obstetricians, nurses come to her to clarify personally, call personally, ask personally. She has about 40–50 incoming and outgoing calls per working day, mostly about coordination. (Fieldnote, 6 February 2019)

My colleagues and I observed various problematic situations in which manual management was required, such as when providers had to find places for women in the overcrowded maternity wards, or make personal efforts to find urgent medications, or to personally coordinate consultations for patients with complications. They activated their personal connections each time a woman did not want to follow their instructions, or had special demands, or intended to complain, or wanted to leave the hospital against medical advice. They asked colleagues for help; they called other doctors and hospitals to find solutions. This sort of "manual management" is part and parcel of coordination within inflexible healthcare systems regulated by contradictory rules and having to cope with multifaceted demands.

In such high-ranking and technologically advanced hospitals in Russia, there are many non-standard situations, as the most complicated cases from across the country are routed there. Providers have to use all their resources and connections to help women, but at the same time must do their best not to be sanctioned by the multiple controlling institutional and State bodies when there is a mismatch between their actions and "the rules," and for this they have to implement a great deal of ad hoc coordination work—manual management.

In non-standard situations, providers are often not supplied with sufficient resources and relevant information (protocols or scripts). For example, a Chief doesn't know what to do in a critical situation, such as a demand for early discharge from the Hospital (before the whole treatment is provided) or a demand from a woman intent on changing her ob. In trying to find a solution, the Chief consults with the hospital lawyer, to no avail. Then, in these and similar cases, she will negotiate (manually manage) with a Director of the Hospital, with patients, their relatives, social services, Chiefs, and physicians in different wards to find an individual solution to this individual problem. But when the final, individualized, decision has low formal legitimacy, the decision-maker faces the risk of punishment for not following the standard protocols or the woman for whom she is doing all this might anyway formally complain to different state bodies, including the President's office, if she is unsatisfied with the ultimate solution.

The working lives of obstetricians in the Hospital consist of dozens of details that demand their personal involvement in coordination, which, again, is manual management. We observed informal exchanges of equipment and drugs between wards (when they agreed with each other), with practitioners running from one ward to another or through negotiations with Chiefs. In all such cases, providers had to initiate negotiations with colleagues and patients, and their success often depended on personal skills, personal relationships, and networking.

The obstetricians and midwives we observed managed problems manually, often to navigate a woman through the complicated organizational system of the Hospital, and to help her to receive all the services that she needed. This is a hidden layer of the work it takes to humanize care. For such humanization, obs must do a great deal of extra-clinical work. Their manual managements humanize and personalize maternity care, making it more acceptable to women—despite the fact that often, the main intention of the providers is not to humanize care, but rather to maneuver between different rules and demands. So, the care provided in some cases continues to be technocratic, but, in this hybridized system, becomes more humanistic in others.

Humanization as a Project: Obstetricians Are Personally Reforming Maternity Hospitals

Guidelines for Restructuring: Privacy, Connection, and Attentive Care

In this section, I (Anna Ozhiganova) consider the case of a Moscow maternity hospital that I call "the Center," which for almost four years (2014–2018) served as an exemplar of the humanistic approach to maternity care. This humanization became possible due to the efforts of a new Chief of the Center, Dr. Olga Vladimirovna (her real name), who managed to carry out a comprehensive reorganization and to assemble a team of like-minded specialists.

Vladimirovna's professional path as an enthusiastic promoter of the humanistic approach was not easy. She faced obstetric aggression when giving birth to her first child in the mid-1990s while still a medical student. The birth "by agreement with a good doctor" was induced by the infusion of artificial oxytocin, which was common practice at the time, and became traumatic for her newborn. Later, in clinical residency, Olga learned that induced or "programmed" labor was to be considered as "prophylaxis" for all kinds of complications: "The professor told us: 'It's not the birthing process that should guide you, but you should guide the birth.'" Although she wrote her PhD dissertation on the theme "Programmed Childbirth in Post-Term Pregnancy," she noticed that this approach did not give good results. However, she did not see a solution, since she observed only highly medicalized births in her training and practice, and it seemed to her that women no longer could give birth naturally.

However, Olga had other teachers and sources of information. She visited the Netherlands and studied the experiences of Dutch homebirth midwives. She was very impressed by the ideas of the renowned French obstetrician and natural childbirth enthusiast Michel Odent. In 2014, she took part in his "Author's Workshop," which was organized especially for Russian obstetricians, midwives, and doulas. She asked Odent a question: "How could you conduct natural childbirth if we needed prophylaxis for overmaturity and weak labor?" and received the answer: "You just have to wait, monitoring the condition of child," and then he added: "You make so many people unhappy simply for prevention reasons." As Olga often repeats in her public speeches, these words became a turning point in her career. Taking the position of the Chief of the Center in 2014, she began to implement the basic principles of the humanistic approach: a non-intervention strategy and favorable conditions for women and newborns.

This Center was located in an older building of the 1960s with an outdated layout—large prenatal and delivery rooms for several women at once, separation of newborns, and so on—and considerable disrepute. Olga said, "Everybody knew that this was a bad place, where it is better not to come." With the support of Chief Midwife Elena Petrovna (also her real name), Olga started with the restructuring of the interior space: they made individual delivery rooms and postnatal rooms where mothers stayed with their newborns. While such transformations have been a common trend in obstetric care innovations under the National Project of 2006, there have also been many initiatives from below to humanize care. The homelike birthing suites were arranged in accordance with the principles of natural birthing as outlined by Michel Odent: darkness, silence, and warmth. Noisy consultations were transformed; ob/gyns and midwives learned to speak in whispers. It was twilight, thanks to blackout curtains and night lamps. Women were allowed to bring bedding from home, clothes, candles, and aromatic oils, and even to listen to music.

These conditions were created for all women free of charge, and the Center received a large flow of women in labor arriving by ambulance. In total, about 5,500 births took place there per year; according to my interlocutors, there were shifts with 40 births per day. There was also an opportunity to pay a contract for a more comfortable suite, some of which had bathtubs, and water birth was acceptable. However, Olga wanted these opportunities to be available to everyone. My interlocutors recalled the cases when women came by ambulance without a contract and got a comfortable room with a bathtub: "Just imagine, she was transferred to a room with a bathtub, the light was turned off. The midwife of the brigade on duty came in, quietly sat down, and began to softly murmur the text from the hypno practice: 'Things are good . . . You have very good contractions . . . You give birth very well . . .'"

All my interlocutors noted that the emotional style in the Center was very "pleasant and inspiring—everyone greeted each other and smiled." Olga organized a kitchen where doulas, midwives, and even dads could have tea and rest. She also fought the ingrained rudeness (*khamstvo*) of medical personnel: "For a long time, we still had nurses who would say something rude or unpleasant to women. But now everyone has really become friendly and smiling." A humanistic model of women-centered care was in fact fully implemented in this maternity hospital, although the Chief Midwife thinks they weren't doing anything special: "We just want to make a maternity home where women are not afraid to come. We just want to turn to people, see and listen to what they want, and do as they want. It is not difficult at all, I can tell you honestly."

Changes in Obstetric Practice: "Break Away from the Outdated Approach"

The changes initiated by the new Chief, Olga Vladimirovna, were not only improvements in the conditions and the emotional style of the hospital. Obstetric practice also radically changed: Olga implemented "wait and see" tactics, freedom of behavior during labor, vertical births, births in water or on a special birthing chair. She has always explained in her public statements that all these innovations had a rational basis confirmed by medical research: "If a woman chooses a position for herself in childbirth, as it is convenient for her, she thus protects the baby, since the blood flow in this case does not decrease so much during each contraction. This is a natural defense mechanism." From these positions, she opposed the use of epidural anesthesia ("blood flow decreases, a child receives less oxygen"), as well as routine amniotomy (breaking the amniotic sac), and talked about the cases of the births of babies "in a shirt" (in the amniotic sac), which basically does not occur in contemporary Russian clinical practice but began to happen in this hospital.

Olga abandoned the practice of planned cesarean operations and supported women with babies in the breech position, women with twins, as well as women with one or even two cesarean scars to give birth naturally. With this approach, the rate of cesarean births (CBs) was only 18%, which was one of the lowest rates in the country; 50% of women with babies in the breech position and 40% with prior cesareans gave birth physiologically. Even more optimistic were the data when the births took place with individual midwives (under a contract): here the total rate of CBs was only 12%, and of the women having vaginal births after cesarean (VBACs), 52% gave birth physiologically. As Olga explained in in a public lecture at the Moscow Childbirth Preparation Center in 2017, these data demonstrate that "women can give birth naturally, if only they are not disturbed and do not come up with imaginary indications for a cesarean. When they give birth quietly, in a friendly atmosphere, with the midwives they trust, the results are very good." Olga also believes that surgical interventions when they are really needed should be humane. She introduced the practice of what is called in Russia a "soft" cesarean, which enables a woman to go through labor and even push the baby out through a small incision in the uterus after the ob elevates the fetal head (see also the chapter by Irene Maffi, Caroline Chautems, and Alexandre Farin in Volume II of this series on "The Introduction of the 'Gentle Cesarean' in Swiss Hospitals: A Conversation with One of Its Pioneers" [2023]).

The practice of the "golden hour," when a newborn spends the first hour after birth on the mother's breast, has recently been widely implemented in Russian maternity hospitals and is usually done formally: obstetricians and pediatricians first conduct routine examinations, measurement and weighing, and only then the newborn, already in diapers and tightly wrapped, is handed over to the mother. In contrast to this standardized practice, Olga implemented the rule that a newborn spends two hours after birth on the mother's chest, and a pediatrician conducts a full examination only after that.

Olga also extended the principles of the humanistic model to the cases of perinatal loss. The situations when a non-viable child is expected or a fetus dies in utero are often treated very harshly in Russian hospitals, with multiple violations of human and patient rights. Women who experience such losses are not given the opportunity to say a final farewell to their baby and are subjected to humiliation and insults (see a 2017 documentary novel by Anna Starobinets called *Look at Him*; also see Temkina, Novkunsakya, and Litvina [2022]). In addition, hospitals usually try not to admit such women, since they worsen their perinatal statistics. According to my interlocutors, women in such cases often decide on home birth regardless of all kinds of medical and legal risks. Thus, it took courage for Olga and her staff to open their hospital doors to such "quiet births," as they became called at Olga's suggestion. Women with perinatal losses were provided with an individual postpartum room, and even with an individual midwife, free of charge. One of these individual midwives said that Olga personally asked her to attend bereavement births: "All at the hospital understood that it was not worth interfering, that it was necessary to give parents time to say goodbye to their baby, and that there was no need to put him in a yellow bag [a medical waste disposal bag] in front of his parents."

All these innovations were made possible by the support of the maternity care providers who shared the principles of the humanistic approach. The Chief Midwife, Elena Petrovna, was responsible for monitoring compliance with medical protocols, sanitary and epidemiological requirements, and other prescriptions. Surprisingly, unlike many maternity care providers, she spoke positively about the official recommendations:

> We have very good protocols [methodical recommendations of the Ministry of Health]. Everyone always says: "What bad protocols!" and prevent a midwife from doing what is written in them. The protocols recommend free behavior in labor, they say that the most unfavorable is the position on the back, that breastfeeding is a priority. The protocols say that it is recommended to attach the baby to the breast immediately after the operation if there was cesarean. And much more. It's just that no one reads them.

Thus, Elena Petrovna is in solidarity with Victor Radzinsky (2011), who noted that the main obstacle to the humanization of birth is that many ob/gyns do not understand the physiology of childbirth well and act in the ways they were taught, not relying on evidence-based medicine (see also Davis-Floyd 2022, other chapters in this present volume, and the chapters in Volumes I and II of this three-volume book series (Davis-Floyd and Premkumar 2023a, 2023b). Overall, the changes in obstetric practice were aimed at abandoning obstetric iatrogenesis and implementing the principle of RARTRW care (the right amount at the right time in the right way) (Cheyney and Davis-Floyd 2020).

Formalized and Informal Interactions
with Doulas and Homebirth Midwives

The Center was also one of the first maternity hospitals in Moscow (and in Russia) where doulas could provide support to women in labor by official agreement with the Association of Professional Doulas (APD). APD is the first and the largest professional association of Russian-speaking doulas, created in 2008 via alliances with international doula associations (Ozhiganova 2021b). Doulas provided free-of-charge support to their clients as part of a volunteer project: one or two doulas came every day and offered their help to laboring women.

Another humanizing practice has become the integration of homebirth midwives with formal medical education into hospital work. Although home birth is illegal in Russia, some homebirth midwives are quite successful at integrating into obstetric care, thanks to various, semi-formalized practices (Ozhiganova 2019). Twenty of these midwives worked officially at a quarter of the working rate and had the status of "individual" midwives, which means that they did not work on shift, but only with their individual clients, by contract. This model is not something new; since the middle of the first decade of the 21st century, it has been proven to be successful and has by now been implemented in many maternity hospitals, not only in Moscow, but also in other cities in Russia.

However, the level of interaction between individual midwives and the Center staff was unique. Typically, midwives who do not work in the healthcare system experience great difficulties in hospitals: they don't know exactly where the instruments are located; they are not familiar with the specific type of CTG/EFM (cardiotocography/electronic fetal monitoring) apparatus used; they don't know how to fill out papers correctly, and so on. My interlocutors explained that this often gave rise to conflicts, which were avoided in the Center only thanks to the efforts of the Chief, Olga: "She explained to the doctors that these specialists need help, that there is nothing wrong with showing how the necessary device works or placing a catheter in a vein. But they [the midwives] will do a lot of work on their own."

Individual midwives were in demand in the Center because they were able to attend vaginal births in challenging situations—with VBACs, twins, and breech presentations—without resorting to biomedical manipulations or cesareans. These midwives could also offer non-pharmaceutical methods of pain relief, knew how a woman's posture affects the progress of childbirth, and so supported laboring and birthing in upright positions. Unlike the midwives of the maternity hospital, these individual midwives are accustomed to acting independently, providing the woman and the newborn with comprehensive care, including emotional support.

At the same time, Olga has a negative attitude toward home birth, which she called "Russian roulette." She is convinced that if all the necessary conditions are created in hospitals, women will not be afraid to come there, and the number of home births will decrease. Nevertheless, both Olga and Chief Midwife Elena Petrovna considered it their duty to help women when a home birth went awry. They did not intimidate the transferring midwife, and would even allow her to accompany the woman in childbirth at the Center, "in order to help us and be a participant in all further actions."

Interactions with doulas and homebirth midwives were facilitated by the fact that Olga was well acquainted with many of them through Michel Odent's seminars and other events for natural childbirth enthusiasts. All of them recall this period of fruitful teamwork with great gratitude: "Those were the golden times, because on the basis of a public hospital with public funding, you could see a great example of progressive obstetrics."

Under Olga's leadership, the Center achieved good medical results and commercial efficiency: health indicators improved, the number of complaints decreased, and women came to that hospital not only from Moscow but also from other cities. But, in 2018, Olga was dismissed for a formal reason related to the reorganizations in the Center; this reason was a personal conflict with the Chief Physician, who did not support Olga's changes, and the Center as a whole (not counting its maternity ward, of which I have been speaking here) was far from a patient-oriented approach. (In the Russian hierarchical hospital structure, the Chief of the maternity unit is subordinate to the Chief Physician of the hospital). With Olga's dismissal (and the departure of the Chief Midwife who left with her), the Center's maternity ward lost its attractiveness, the flow of patients dropped sharply, and soon it was closed "for repairs." Together with a midwife, Olga went to work at another public hospital, which immediately became a center of attraction for women seeking natural childbirth. However, the progressive practices that were available to *everyone* in the Center have now become possible only on a paid contract basis.

Olga continues to participate in the reforming of Russian obstetrics "from the inside," by sharing her experiences of maternity hospital reorganization and its reconciling with current sanitary and epidemiological regulations. She also participates in the activities of a newly created (in 2019) professional non-profit association, Midwifery Union. This organization brings together not only midwives, but also various perinatal specialists—ob/gyns, doulas, childbirth educators and others—who are interested in promoting the (humanistic and holistic—see the Introduction to this volume) midwifery model of care. Its creation demonstrates a noticeable shift from a binary model of competing forms of authoritative knowledge (Jordan 1997) to a new synthesis of different (biomedical and alternative) approaches and more effective, safe, and humane maternity care (Ozhiganova 2020).

This case of the comprehensive reorganization of the Center's maternity ward and obstetric practices was unique in Russia. The fact that the Chief, Olga, was the initiator and leader of this radical reform reveals how dissatisfied some ob/gyns are with the current state of affairs in Russian maternity care. This case also illustrates the reasons that contribute to the fact that obs *can* revise generally accepted practices and become supporters of the humanistic approach; these reasons are, first, personal experience of motherhood and a resultant disillusionment with obstetric practice; and second, gaining familiarity with the humanistic approach/midwifery model in foreign clinics and during internships and seminars, as Olga had done.

Conclusion: Inconsistent Humanization in Post-Soviet Russian Maternity Care

The cases presented in this chapter show that many obstetricians are dissatisfied with the current situation in Russian maternity care as they face bureaucratic control and market demands. But they also understand the complexity of the "obstetric paradox": intervene in birth to keep it safe, thereby causing harm (Cheyney and Davis-Floyd 2019), which, as many obs have come to realize, they (often unwittingly) implement in their practices. For some years now, such obs have been and are striving to make Russian maternity care more humanized.

Maternity care providers can choose among varying strategies to humanize obstetric practices: some of them try to cope with new demands by default, meaning that they have to respond to women's consumer demands, even if the bureaucratic conditions of the hospital are far from favorable for such responses; others seek to elaborate special innovative projects as Olga did. In this chapter, we have demonstrated the great differences between the strategies of a tertiary-level high-tech hospital (the Hospital) aimed at providing care in complex medical cases, and those of a smaller maternity hospital unit (the Center) focused on facilitating normal, physiologic birth. As we have previously noted, high-tech systems guided by the authoritative knowledge of ob/gyns are usually less likely to accept childbearing women's agency, whereas low-tech systems more often value the experience-based knowledge of midwives and the bodily experiences of women (Sargent and Bascope 1997:202; Cheyney 2011; Davis-Floyd et al. 2021; Davis-Floyd 2022). Our data confirm that this pattern is also found in Russian realities. The highly humanistic model that Olga and her colleagues implemented in the Center demonstrates how hierarchical structures can give way to horizontal forms of knowledge distribution as a result of the "mutual accommodation" (Jordan 1997:73) of the different approaches presented by ob/gyns, independent midwives, and doulas.

However, in both cases—*copying* and *reforming* strategies—we could see positive results; these included declines in or rejections of obstetric aggression and inappropriate biomedicalization, the implementation of a friendlier emotional style in obs' communications with women, and significant improvements in conditions—in particular, a respect for privacy. Intentionally and unintentionally, these obstetricians' strategies have led to positive changes in childbirth practices in general. This trend has already been reflected in existing biomedical protocols, which demonstrate a commitment to evidence-based medicine and humanistic approaches voiced by such influential actors as WHO (2018).

We have shown that reforms and the commercialization of maternity care have led to ambiguous and ambivalent results. On the one hand, these contribute to increasing inequality in access to medical care, as optimal humanistic care must often be paid for. On the other hand, commercialization opens opportunities for humanization: progressive innovations tend to spread from paid departments to free public facilities as women and healthcare providers begin to embrace newer, more humanistic practices. However, such changes place obstetricians in the difficult situations of having to maneuver among bureaucratic oversight, the requirements of commercial efficiency, and the growing demands of women for humanistic care. As a result, obstetricians face multiple institutional tensions and must compensate for these tensions with numerous personal efforts—manual managements—and additional work.

Progressive achievements very often turn out to be local, unstable, and unsustainable, since they always arise and develop within rigid systems, despite their pressures and thanks to the efforts and enthusiasm of individual actors in such rigid situations. As our data show, during the COVID-19 pandemic, the situation in Russian maternity hospitals became much worse. As State control increased, obstetricians became discontented, and mostly assumed that they could do nothing to create change, given the pandemic-induced restrictions on women's rights and the pre-existing excessive biomedicalization of birth (Ozhiganova 2021a).

The path to humanizing changes in Russian maternity care is very complicated, full of twists and turns, as the horizontal distribution of knowledge and the development of egalitarian relationships have been inconsistent, while the State still promotes its interests and imposes its vertical rules. The reforming and humanizing projects are also inconsistent, and authoritarian biomedical knowledge is challenged only by some actors and in some situations. Barriers to humanization and changes in the distribution of knowledge include not only the lingering Soviet industrial conveyor-belt approach, but also include the Soviet legacy of bureaucratic-paternalistic medicalized health care and the contradictory consequences of market and Statist post-Soviet reforms. It remains to be seen whether the localized humanistic changes that we have described in this chapter will eventually develop into overall system reform.

Anna Ozhiganova is a medical anthropologist and Senior Researcher at the Institute of Ethnology and Anthropology, Russian Academy of Sciences, Center of Medical Anthropology. Her research interests include the intersections of religion, health, reproduction, and alternative social movements. She is currently studying the late- and post-Soviet Russian homebirth movement and changing maternity care in Russia. Anna is the author of *New Religiosity in Modern Russia: Teachings, Forms and Practices* (2006) and of more than 50 articles and book chapters on the Russian New Age and homebirth movements, water birth, midwifery, and obstetrics.

Anna Temkina is Professor and Chair in Health and Gender Studies, European University at St. Petersburg, Department of Sociology, and co-director of the Gender Studies Program. She is the author of books in Russian on *Russia in Transition; Women' Sexuality: Between Subordination and Freedom*; co-author of *Gender Sociology: 12 Lectures*; and lead author of *Pregnancy and Birth in Russia: The Struggle for "Good Care"* (2022), co-authored by Anastasia Novkunskaya and Daria Litvina. Temkina has also authored or co-authored hundreds of publications on gender studies and feminist research, the sociology of health, and qualitative methods of sociological research. Her most recently published articles address the consumerization of maternity care, changes in the organization and management of childbirth, and the sensitivities of healthcare professionals.

References

Chalmers B. 1997. "Changing Childbirth in Eastern Europe: Which Systems of Authoritative Knowledge Should Prevail?" In *Childbirth and Authoritative Knowledge: Cross-Cultural Perspectives*, eds. Davis-Floyd R, Sargent C, 263–286. Berkeley: University of California Press.

Cheyney M. 2011. "Homebirth as Ritual Performance." *Medical Anthropology Quarterly* 25(4): 519–542.

Cheyney M, Davis-Floyd R. 2020. "Birth and the Big Bad Wolf: A Biocultural, Co-Evolutionary Perspective, Part 2." *International Journal of Childbirth* 10(2): 66–78.

Davis-Floyd R. 2001. "The Technocratic, Humanistic, and Holistic Paradigms of Childbirth." *International Journal of Gynecology & Obstetrics* 75: S5–S23.

———. 2018a. "The Technocratic, Humanistic, and Holistic Paradigms of Birth and Health Care." In *Ways of Knowing about Birth: Mothers, Midwives, Medicine, and Birth Activism*, Davis-Floyd R and Colleagues, 3–44. Long Grove IL: Waveland Press.

———. 2018b. "The Rituals of Hospital Birth: Enacting and Transmitting the Technocratic Model." In *Ways of Knowing about Birth: Mothers, Midwives, Medicine, and Birth Activism*, Davis-Floyd R and Colleagues, 45–70. Long Grove, IL: Waveland Press.

———. 2022. *Birth as an American Rite of Passage*, 3rd ed. Abingdon, Oxon: Routledge.

Davis-Floyd R, Lim R, Penwell V, Ivry T. 2021. "Sustainable Birth Care in Disaster Zones: Low-Tech, Skilled Touch." In *Sustainable Birth in Disruptive Times*, eds. Gutschow K, Davis-Floyd R, Daviss BA, 261–276. New York: Springer.

Davis-Floyd R, Premkumar A, eds. 2023a. *Obstetricians Speak: On Training, Practice, Fear, and Transformation*. New York: Berghahn Books.

———. 2023b. *Cognition, Risk, and Responsibility in Obstetrics: Anthropological Analyses and Critiques of Obstetricians' Practices*. New York: Berghahn Books.

Federal State Statistics Service. 2019. "Health Care in Russia", *Statistical Digest*. Moscow: ROSSTAT. https://resursor.ru/statisticheskij-sbornik-zdravooxranenie-v-rossii-2019-polnaya-versiya/zdorovye-naseleniya-vzroslye/#15856873648 17-72d37041-725d.

Field M. 1967. *Soviet Socialized Medicine: An Introduction*. New York: The Free Press.

———. 1988. "The Position of the Soviet Physician: The Bureaucratic Professional." *The Milbank Quarterly* 66: 182–201.

Hochschild AR. 1983. *The Managed Heart: Commercialization of Human Feeling*. Berkeley CA: University of California Press.

Jordan B. 1997. "Authoritative Knowledge and Its Construction." In *Childbirth and Authoritative Knowledge: Cross-Cultural Perspectives*, eds. Davis-Floyd R, Sargent C, 55–79. Berkeley: University of California Press.

Liese KL, Davis-Floyd R, Stewart K, Cheyney M. 2021. "Obstetric Iatrogenesis in the United States: The Spectrum of Unintentional Harm, Disrespect, Violence, and Abuse." *Anthropology & Medicine* 28(2): 188–204.

Litvina D, Novkunskaya A, Temkina A. 2020. "Multiple Vulnerabilities in Medical Settings: Invisible Suffering of Doctors." *Societies* 10(1): 5.

Loban IE, Isakov VD, Lavrentyuk GP, et al. 2015. "Statistical Characteristics of Examinations in Cases of Professional Offences and Crimes of Medical Workers (On Materials of St. Petersburg Bureau of Forensic Medicine, 2009–2014)" [in Russian]. *Medical Law: Theory and Practice* 1(1): 264–274.

Maffi I, Chautems C, Farin A. 2023. "The Introduction of the 'Gentle Cesarean'" in Swiss Hospitals: A Conversation with One of Its Pioneers." In *Cognition, Risk, and Responsibility in Obstetrics: Anthropological Analyses and Critiques of Obstetricians' Practices*, eds. Davis-Floyd R, Premkuar A, Chapter 5. New York: Berghahn Books.

Monaghan A. 2012. "The Vertical: Power and Authority in Russia." *International Affairs* 88(1): 1–16.

Novkunskaya A. 2019. "Institutionalized Fragmentation of Care in Russian Maternity Care" [in Russian]. In *Social Care: Professions and Institutions*, eds. Borozdina E, Zdravomyslova E, Temkina A, 58–87. St. Petersburg: European University Press.

Ozhiganova AA. 2019. "Official (Biomedical) and Alternative (Home) Obstetrics: Formalized and Informal Interactions" [in Russian]. *Journal of Economic Sociology* 20(5): 28–52.

———. 2020. "Authoritative Knowledge of Childbirth and Obstetrics: Analysis of Discursive Practices of Russian Perinatal Specialists." *Population and Economics* 4(4): 74–83.

———. 2021a. "'Soldiers of the System': Maternity Care in Russia Between Bureaucratic Instructions and the Epidemiological Risks of COVID-19." *Frontiers in Sociology* 6: 611374.

———. 2021b. "Doula's Work, Public and Intimate: Professional Care, Self-Organization and Activism" [in Russian]. *Monitoring of Public Opinion: Economic and Social Changes* 3: 200–225.

Petrova TN. 2017. "Features of Investigation of Crimes Related to Poor Quality Medical Care in Childbirth" [in Russian]. *Consilium Medicum* 19(6): 9–31.

Radzinsky VE. 2011. *Obstetric Aggression* [in Russian]. Moscow: Status Praesens.

Radzinsky VE, Kostin IN. 2007. "Safe Obstetrics" [in Russian]. *Obstetrics and Gynecology* 5: 12–16.

Rivkin-Fish M. 2005a. *Women's Health in Post-Soviet Russia: The Politics of Intervention*. Bloomington: Indiana University Press.

———. 2005b. "Gifts, Bribes, and Unofficial Payments: Towards an Anthropology of Corruption in Russia." In *Corruption: Anthropological Perspectives*, eds. Haller D., Shore C, 47–64. London: Pluto Press.

Saks M. 2015. *Professions, State, and the Market: Medicine in Britain, the United States and Russia*. Abingdon, Oxon: Routledge.

Sargent CF, Bascope G. 1997. "Ways of Knowing about Birth in Three Cultures." In *Childbirth and Authoritative Knowledge: Cross-Cultural Perspectives*, eds. Davis-Floyd R., Sargent C, 183–208. Berkeley: University of California Press.

Sheiman I, Shishkin S. 2010. "Russian Health Care." *Problems of Economic Transition* 52(12): 4–49.

Starobinets A. 2017. *Look at Him* [in Russian]. Moscow: Corpus.

Temkina A. 2019. "'Childbirth Is Not a Car Rental': Mothers and Obstetricians Negotiating Consumer Service in Russian Commercial Maternity Care." *Critical Public Health* 30(5): 521–532.

Temkina A, Rivkin-Fish M. 2020. "Creating Health Care Consumers: The Negotiation of Un/Official Payments, Power and Trust in Russian Maternity Care." *Social Theory & Health* 18: 340–357.

Temkina A, Litvina D, Novkunskaya A. 2021. "Emotional Styles in Russian Maternity Hospitals: Juggling between *Khamstvo* and Smiling." *Emotions and Society* 3(1):1–19.

Temkina A, Novkunskaya A, Litvina D. 2022. *Pregnancy and Birth in Russia: The Struggle for "Good Care."* Abingdon, Oxon, UK: Routledge.

WHO. 2018. "WHO Recommendations: Intrapartum Care for a Positive Childbirth Experience." WHO, 7 February. Retrieved 12 December 2022 from https://www.who.int/publications/i/item/9789241550215.

CHAPTER 9

The Paradigm Shifts of Humanistic and Holistic Obstetricians
The "Good Guys and Girls" of Brazil

Robbie Davis-Floyd and Eugenia Georges

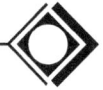

Introduction: The Movement to Humanize Birth in Brazil

> Question: *Where does your passion come from?*
> João Batista: *From my heart. I believe in justice and rights, and women in Brazil have neither, and their rights are most violated during childbirth . . . I want every ob professor to teach this to his residents: "The woman is the center of care!"*

Throughout Latin America, "humanization" is the unifying concept around which social movements to demedicalize and transform childbirth have coalesced. Although a diverse project, humanization at its core is grounded in the principle that safe, respectful, and supportive maternity care free of unnecessary medical interventions, is a *childbearer's human right*. To ensure that such unnecessary interventions are eliminated, the humanization movement also insists that the care of mother and infant should consist exclusively of "best practices" that are supported by up-to-date, evidence-based medicine (see Irvine 2022). Thus, the objectives of humanization are simultaneously ethical (promoting the view of childbearers as persons with the right to respect and autonomy and of doctors as committed to protecting those rights) and instrumental (improving the quality of care), and thereby improving both physical and psychological outcomes for mothers and babies.

Brazilian birth activists, including a significant number of obstetricians, have long been in the forefront of attempts to humanize birth practices. In 1993, ReHuNa (*Rede pela Humanização do Parto e Nacimento*; the Network for the Humanization of Childbirth) was officially formed as an NGO to advocate for women's rights to humane and respectful childbirth experiences grounded in scientifically sound practices. ReHuNa is composed predominantly of obstetrician/gynecologists, public health doctors, nurses, professional midwives, and other highly educated professionals. In this chapter, we focus on Brazilian humanistic and holistic obstetricians, almost all of whom are members—and some, founders—of ReHuNa, describing their motivations to humanize their practices and their processes of transformation. In order to understand what their "paradigm shifts" were from and to, see Davis-Floyd (2018a, 2022) and the Introduction to this volume for descriptions of the "the technocratic, humanistic, and holistic paradigms of birth and health care."

How This Research Project Was Born: The I International Congress on the Humanization of Childbirth

Robbie's idea for this research project began in November of 2000 when she delivered a keynote speech on those three paradigms at ReHuNa's I International Congress on the Humanization of Childbirth, held in Fortaleza, Ceará, Brazil. The conference was predominantly funded by the Japan International Cooperation Agency (JICA), which has close ties to many projects in Brazil, and was co-sponsored by many other agencies and local and national ministries. Around 600 attendees were initially expected, but as Day 1 of the Congress progressed, the auditorium kept filling up until there was standing room only—in the end, more than 1,800 attendees from multiple Latin American countries had registered, and everyone there realized that they were witnessing the full-fledged emergence of a national and international social movement for the humanization of birth. And indeed, following this Fortaleza conference, most other countries in Latin America held their own conferences on birth humanization, some of which continue at regular intervals.

As Robbie turned to step down from the podium after her talk, she found a group of good-looking young men waiting for her, all enthusiastically holding copies of her books for her to sign. "Who are you?" she asked. "We are the good guys!" was their response. "The bad guys are the ones who do the routine cesareans. We are humanistic and holistic obs who work hard to put the woman first! We have read all your books, and we try to put your ideas into practice. We call ourselves 'the Floydettes,' and we compete with each other to see who can quote you the most!" Beyond delighted, Robbie happily signed the books, but had no time in the moment to find out who these obs were—what their names were, where they lived, how they practiced, and most of all, why had they chosen to practice humanistically and holistically in a country with one of the highest cesarean rates in the world? At subsequent ReHuNa conferences, Robbie found opportunities to meet these "good guys and girls" and to get to know many of them. Eventually, Robbie, joined by Eugenia (Nia) Georges, undertook a research project to answer the questions above; in 2012, we interviewed (in English) 32 of these "good guys and girls" (as they happily continue to call themselves) at great length, in the cities in which they lived and practiced. For the purposes of this chapter, in January 2022, Robbie collected updated information from 10 of the original interlocutors, almost all of whom are still in practice.

Tracing Transformative Trajectories

Herein, we trace the transformative trajectories of these 32 interlocutors, who have been pioneers in radically reshaping how women are cared for during childbirth. We explore how and why these obstetricians, trained and credentialed in high-status and authoritative modes of knowledge and practice, undertook the decision to reject their deeply embodied technocratic orientations and to retrain/re-embody themselves in less-prestigious, professionally stigmatized—and even sometimes legally persecuted humanistic and holistic approaches. One of them, Ricardo Jones (2023) tells his own story of transformation and resultant persecutions in Chapter 7 of Volume I of this three-volume series (Davis-Floyd and Premkumar 2023). We examine the processes by which the obs we interviewed managed to re-socialize and recraft themselves into different sorts of humanized practitioners. What narratives, discourses, norms, and techniques did they deploy to guide their transformations and stay the course in the face of the criticism and opprobrium of their colleagues?

About the Interlocutors

The 32 obstetricians we interviewed, whom we call by their real names at their requests, are a cosmopolitan and diverse group of people with varying hues of skin. Half are women and half are men. For some, the preponderance and clarity of the scientific evidence in favor of supporting normal physiologic birth was most important in their decision to transform their practices; for others, it was allegiance to humanistic values rooted in their intersecting affiliations with feminism, left-wing politics, liberation theology, environmentalism, and midwifery, as well as a variety of New Age or older spiritual beliefs. Despite their differences, they typically shared an ethos that blended, or at least honored, all these dimensions to varying degrees. Some of these interlocutors had private practices that catered to a select group of highly motivated middle- and upper-class women—those who, in the words of one "good guy," were "100% to 10,000% committed to normal birth." This group of interlocutors attended home births almost exclusively and had cesarean rates of 7–10%. Others had cesarean rates of 14–30% because they chose to care for all who came to them, believing that every woman has the right to a humanized birth, whether that is a natural birth at home or in hospital, or a scheduled cesarean birth (CB). Others worked in the public health system, providing care primarily for women in conditions of precarity. Some interlocutors occupied influential positions in the national or regional Ministries of Health. Others held faculty positions at some of Brazil's most prestigious universities, and some were hospital directors. For example, two interlocutors, Dr. Ivo Lopez de Oliveira and Dr. João Batista (whom we quote at the beginning of this chapter), work as Clinical Directors of Hospital Sofia Feldman in the city of Belo Horizonte, state of Minas Gerais, which is the subject of our next section.

Hospital Sofia Feldman: An Exemplar of Humanistic Practice

According to Clinical Director João Batista, during the mid-1980s, he and some fellow medical students:

> were looking for some real experience outside medical school. And we realized that here at this hospital, something was beginning, because the people of the community were building the hospital with their own resources [and its focus would be maternity care] . . . So, I decided to be an ob, and when I graduated, I did my residency at the Federal University Hospital, a very conservative ob/gyn department . . . But we had some ideas about natural birth because we studied here at Sofia Feldman separately from the school. We gathered medical students and nurses and had discussions about birth. [Roberto] Caldeyro-Barcia made a presentation in Japan in 1979 about the humanization of birth, and it was published here in an ob journal . . . in 1981 or 1982. We read it and began to discuss that we have to implant this here, to start here with *these* ideas, not what they are teaching us in medical school and residency.

Sofia Feldman is a high-risk public hospital providing tertiary-level care that is available to all childbearers in the state. At the time of our visit in 2012, more than 50 nurse-midwives practiced there, along with 20 obs and 14 doulas, who are provided by the hospital for those women who bring no companion. They have long had very low rates of forceps, vacuum extraction, and episiotomy (around 8% for each); electronic fetal monitoring is used only intermittently; and delayed cord-clamping and vertical births are the norms. Sofia Feldman is widely regarded as an exemplar of sustainable humanistic practice in the international childbirth movement. In December 2012, Clinical Director João Batista stated:

> Our cesarean rate is 24%, the lowest rate in Minas Gerais and one of the lowest in Brazil—but last year it was only 20%—it went up 4% in one year! That year there was a huge increase in high-risk women sent to us from all over the state, including malformations, et cetera. They are from other cities or towns in the state of Minas Gerais who were transferred to Hospital Sofia Feldman weeks before birth and can stay for a week or two afterward in shared rooms with their babies always present. Mothers and babies are *never* separated in this hospital unless the baby is truly ill and needs NICU care. And even in our NICU, mothers and their babies are together as much as possible and we focus on kangaroo care.
>
> We are a high-risk hospital with a 42-bed NICU—the biggest one in the state, so our PNMR [perinatal mortality rate] is 14.4/1000; 10% of our babies are preterm. More than 50% of the women who give birth here are from other cities. Maybe we are doing the best we can. Hypertension, preterm labor, premature rupture of membranes are the most common—hypertension is the really big one, a lot of preeclampsia. If they come to us early, we can stop it, but most are sent late.

In 2012, said João, "we had 20.8% of women with high-risk conditions." By early 2022, that percentage had risen to over 35%, due to another increased influx of high-risk pregnant women from around the state. Thus Sofia Feldman's 2021 cesarean rate rose to 28%—still one of the lowest in Brazil—and their PNMR rate rose to around 18/1000—the same as for the state as a whole. In 2012, the practitioners of Sofia Feldman attended 9,909 births. In 2021, they attended 11,200 births, and their NICU now has 55 beds. Being financially stable, they have been able to hire more practitioners, some of whom they have had to re-socialize into their humanistic model of care—another reason for the higher CB rate.

When we asked João, "Are you afraid of birth?" he responded, "No. I am afraid of not doing all I can for women!"[1]

Now we turn to an examination of the tools and resources that the "good guy and girl" interlocutors found helpful in their processes of self-transformation. These include guidance from books and films, from midwives and doulas, and from social movements and their networks.

Tools and Resources for Self-Transformation 1: Guidance from Books and Films

Working in relative isolation because they did not know of each other at the time, they began their new trajectories (mostly during the late 1980s and the 1990s) and feeling "alone and lonely," these humanistic—and often holistic—obs nevertheless undertook a process of self-education to effect their personal and professional transformations. In almost all instances, this process was profoundly influenced and guided by a common corpus of resources that served as guides. Particularly influential were books written by international advocates of childbirth reform. Among the authors they most frequently cited were the French doctors and reformers Frederick Leboyer and Michel Odent (whom Jones [2009:277] described as "open[ing] new doors of perception for me about the miracle of birth"); the Uruguayan obstetrician and former President of FIGO (the French acronym for the International Federation of Gynecology and Obstetrics) Roberto Caldeyro-Barcia; British authors and activists Sheila Kitzinger and Janet Balaskas; and the US writers Marsden Wagner, Penny Simkin, Marshall Klaus, Ina May Gaskin, Henci Goer, Elizabeth Davis, and Robbie Davis-Floyd. "Good girl" Melania Amorim explained:

> I started my Masters of Science Program [in 1993]. And I was introduced to evidence-based medicine. I also had to read philosophy of science and I was introduced to Thomas Kuhn and research on scientific revolutions. And I began to think, "Oh! It can be different!" And I started to read about the [standard obstetric] procedures . . . and I could realize that they were not necessary! That there was *no evidence* to support my practices. But I couldn't realize, why, with so much evidence against these procedures, they always have been performed by other obstetricians . . . And so finally I encountered Robbie's book *Birth as an American Rite of Passage*, and I could understand what evidence-based medicine didn't explain—why these procedures have been maintained for decades with no scientific evidence—because they are *rituals* that reflect deep cultural values.

And that's why her book changed my life. Because before I had books, I was changing my practice, but I didn't understand *why* all the others continued to maintain the old procedures.

Almost all of these interlocutors said that Robbie's first book, *Birth as an American Rite of Passage* ([1992] 2003) had taught them that they needed to change, and *From Doctor to Healer: The Transformative Journey* (Davis-Floyd and St. John 1998) had shown them how. [*Author's note:* It is a distinct thrill for an anthropologist to find her work useful to and applied by practitioners!]

The critiques of conventional childbirth that the interlocutors pored over and took to heart have deep domestic roots as well. Moysés Paciornik's book *Aprenda a Nascer com os Índios: Parto de Cócoras* (*Learn to Give Birth like the Indians: Squatting Birth*) and classic film *Birth in the Squatting Position*,[2] released in 1979, have had significant impacts on birth activists, not only in Brazil, but internationally as well. (For example, Robbie, who lives in the US state of Texas, vividly remembers the sense of enlightenment she experienced upon first seeing that film sometime in the 1980s—an experience she shared with multiple other birth scholars and activists across the country.) Paciornik also designed his own birthing chairs to provide the benefits of the squatting position (*parto salvagem*; savage birth) that he used in his private hospital in Curitiba and sold to other obstetricians and hospitals throughout Brazil (for the equivalent of around 200 USD). These birth chairs (which can be laid flat at the childbearer's request) have a bar for holding onto while squatting, and an indentation underneath the birthing woman on which a hot water bottle, covered with a sterile towel, can be placed so that the newborn can "float" there until the mother reaches down, in her own time, to tentatively explore and then pick up her baby. The practitioner needs only to receive the baby and to gently lower the newborn onto the towel.

Hugo Sabatino, a Professor of Obstetrics at UNICAMP, was also one of the early pioneers whose teachings and writings on squatting birth were highly influential in stimulating the movement for humanized birth. And the early work during the 1970s and 1980s of Dr. José Galba de Araújo in the state of Ceará in humanizing hospital birth and providing effective and culturally appropriate support to the rural traditional midwives in his catchment area was so influential that today, ReHuNa gives an annual award in his name to the hospital that has made the greatest strides toward humanization in that year. (Unsurprisingly, Hospital Sofia Feldman was the first winner.)

Not only did the texts and individuals we mention above serve as exemplars, but also some of their international authors, such as Michel Odent, Marsden Wagner (now deceased), Robbie Davis-Floyd, and Ina May Gaskin, themselves developed close ties to the humanization movement, visiting Brazil on numerous occasions, offering workshops, attending conferences, and delivering keynote speeches.

Tools and Resources for Self-Transformation 2: Guidance from Midwives

Another source of guidance in reshaping the interlocutors' views toward childbirth was the recuperation/revaluation of midwives. By 1970, schools that had trained direct-entry professional midwives, called *obstetrizes*, had been shut down and were replaced by nurse-midwifery programs. Yet nurse-midwives (*enfermeiras obstetras*[3]) have made few inroads into Brazilian birthing culture to date; according to Daphne Rattner (personal communication, September 2021)—a physician and epidemiologist who formerly worked in the national Ministry of Health and is now a Professor at the University of Brasilia—nurse-midwives (as of 2021) attend only 10% of Brazilian births—up slightly from 8% in 2017—some of which take place at home or in freestanding birth centers. Meanwhile, the *obstetriz* has been reinvented in a direct-entry (non-nursing) midwifery program at the University of São Paulo, which was founded in 2005 by one of the few remaining original *obstetrizes*, Dulce Gualda, and by 2020 had graduated approximately 500 *obstetrizes*, about half of whom have entered obstetric practices around the country or attend births at home or in birth centers—some of which are in hospitals and some are freestanding. Others wait to begin practicing until they have completed academic studies in related fields or for various other reasons (Ana Cristina Duarte, *obstetriz*, personal communication, November 8, 2021).

All the interlocutors believe that, ideally, professional midwives should be the primary birth attendants in Brazil—indeed, in every country—because, again ideally, midwives are or should be the experts in normal physiologic birth. When there are professional midwives in their cities, the "good guys and girls" are generally happy to work with them as a team, support them however they can, and back them up when needed. They often wistfully lament the small number of Brazilian nurse-midwives (in 2021, according to Rattner, there were only 6,008 *enfermeiras obstetras* practicing in Brazil) and the even smaller number (again, around 500) of *obstetrizes*. (In dramatic contrast, Daphne found that there were precisely 35,587 obstetrician/gynecologists practicing in Brazil in 2021.) All interlocutors wish that there were many thousands of professional midwives in their country attending the vast majority of births, and many actively work to create new midwifery programs within universities, to support and expand the existing ones, and to develop birth centers in which the "midwifery model of care" can be actively implemented. In the meantime, they try themselves to practice the midwifery model (which is based on keeping the woman at the center and on understanding and facilitating normal physiologic birth with a minimum of interventions; see Davis-Floyd 2018b for a full description). For example, Carla Polido noted:

> After concluding my Master's degree, I began to teach at the new medical school. I found out about humanization—it hit me like a bomb—I couldn't think of anything else! This friend of mine was the first step—she was an obstetric nurse and now she is a nurse-midwife. [She taught me about normal birth and now] I attend home births with her.

Those who do have professional midwives in their communities not only support those midwives, but also receive support and encouragement from them, and from doulas as well—in fact, given their general ostracism by their technocratic colleagues, these obs generally receive their *primary* emotional and psychological support from their local midwives, doulas, and birth activists. Some call themselves "midwife-obstetricians," yet Carla Polido noted, "I would like to say I'm a midwife, but I can't say that because I have this little monster in my head saying, 'Oh shouldn't I do an episiotomy?' I'm an obstetrician, I'm a teacher."

Yet until more contemporary times (and today in some rural areas, most especially the Amazon region), Indigenous midwives still attended childbirths. Some of the older obs we interviewed acknowledged the midwives who had assisted their mothers in childbirth and expressed respect and appreciation for their skills, as did others who were raised in rural areas and had witnessed the midwife-assisted home births of relatives. Two interlocutors, Claudio Paciornik (son of Moysés) and Bernadette Boussada, had in fact learned directly from Indigenous or traditional midwives. Claudio and his father spent years observing the birth practices of the Kaigang and Guarani tribes on tribal reserves in Ibirama and Xanxare in South Brazil during the 1970s, applying what they learned to their own practices, and making the previously mentioned film *Birth in the Squatting Position*.

Learning from Midwives: Bernadette Boussada

Bernadette first met traditional midwives when she was assigned after residency to a hospital in the remote city of Coração de Jesus in Minas Gerais for one year (1997–98). She was the only ob in the only maternity hospital there. There were two *parteiras tradicionais* (traditional midwives) working in that hospital as auxiliary nurses; they became both her assistants and her guides. She told us that the two most important things these midwives taught her were: (1) respect for the woman; and (2) respect for the physiology of birth. She watched them treating women with kindness, attending labors without interfering, and encouraging movement, upright positions, squatting, no episiotomy, and so forth. She slowly started to practice more and more like they did. The first intervention she gave up was the Kristeller maneuver (forceful pushing on the abdomen), then forced pushing (yelling at the woman to "push, PUSH!"), then episiotomy, "then all the rest of it all at once!" When we asked Bernadette if she was afraid of birth, she exclaimed, "Yes, I am afraid of birth. But I am a woman of courage!"

After leaving Coração de Jesus, in 2001 Bernadette opened a private practice in the city of São Sebastião in the state of São Paulo, and also worked shifts in the public hospital there. In her hospital practice, Bernadette kept all the women she was responsible for—often five at a time—in one room, where she attended them during labor and received their babies. She stayed until they all had given birth and did not allow any other practitioners in the room to preserve the holistic integrity of the space—what Ricardo Jones (2009) calls the *psychosphere* of birth. Bernadette told us that her patients posted their positive birth experiences widely on Facebook, making the other nine obs in that hospital angry because their own patients started demanding from them the kind of humanistic treatment that Bernadette provided. Her personal CB rate was 10%, while that of her hospital was over 70%. The other nine obs there thought she was "crazy" and talked about her behind her back, but were nice to her and respected her. They were aware that her perinatal mortality rate was much, much lower than theirs. In her 12 years there, she had two perinatal deaths—one from "fetal suffering" and the other from a congenital malformation. They had many more. In 2008, Bernadette started searching around on the internet, found ReHuNa, joined it, and started going to their conferences. She was "absolutely delighted" to finally be part of a group; she said, "I had felt so alone for so long!"

In late 2012, feeling a need for change, Bernadette returned to Rio de Janeiro, her hometown where she had done all her professional training. She wrote in an email to Robbie (November 12, 2021):

I returned to my job at the Federal University, a teaching hospital, where I have the opportunity to train new obstetricians, residents, and undergraduate students. I was very well received back by my colleagues. With love and determination, I have been showing that doing obstetrics with respect and science is possible.

In 2018, my daughter Giovanna entered obstetric residency; today she is a humanistic reference in obstetrics here in Rio and in Brazil. (My other daughter, Giulianna, is a doula trainer.) We've been a team that practices quality obstetrics. When I returned to Rio, the maternity ward we work in now was called "the Temple of Cesarean Sections," with a cesarean rate close to 100%. Today it can be called "the Temple of Childbirth!" We have managed to cut the cesarean rate to 50% and are working on lowering it more. I increasingly understand that obstetric care must be individualized, and I continue to respect the individuality of each family and their choices, always based on scientific evidence.

Tools and Resources for Self-Transformation 3: The Importance of Doulas

Doulas have long existed in Brazil, and the doula movement there continues to grow. Perhaps the very first Brazilian doula is Maria de Lourdes da Silva Teixeira, affectionately known as Fadynha (Little Fairy). She has practiced for around 40 years and is still in practice at the time of writing (March 2023), supporting hundreds of women during labor and birth and working as a doula trainer. Fadynha is also one of the founders of the humanization movement in Brazil and an active member of ReHuNa; she has organized many conferences herself and has spoken at many others.

The doula movement in Brazil was given a large boost in January of 2003 when Debra Pascali-Bonaro, a renowned doula and doula trainer from New Jersey, was brought to Brazil by humanistic ob Maria Helena da Silva Bastos. (Robbie had connected them, suggesting to Maria Helena that she bring Debra to develop doula programs for Brazil.) Interlocutor Marcos Diaz helped to start the first doula program at the Municipal Secretariat of Rio de Janeiro at the Leila Diniz Hospital, a large public maternity hospital attending 300–400 births per month. Until 1998, this was the only public hospital in Rio that allowed a laboring woman to bring a labor support companion. For the program, Fadynha and Maria Helena recruited volunteers from community centers to be trained as doulas, naming their program *Amigas na Luz* (Friends in Light—because the Portuguese way to say "give birth" is *dar à luz*—

to give to light). Resistant at first, the obs and nurses at that hospital quickly warmed to the doulas as they proved their abilities to soothe and support birthing mothers, and women increasingly began to ask for these hospital-provided doulas at their births.

As we previously noted, most of the humanistic and holistic interlocutors are the only such obs in their cities. Many told us that they could not practice as holistically as they do without the doulas who are there for that one-on-one continuous support long proven to be extremely beneficial (see, e.g., Kennell et al. 1991; Klaus, Kennell, and Klaus 1993; Scott, Klaus, and Klaus 1999; Scott, Berkowitz and Klaus 1999; and Hodnett et al. 2003).

Ricardo Jones, Cristina Guimares, and the Mystery of Page 128

Far away in the south of Brazil, in the city of Porto Alegre in the state of Rio Grande do Sul, obstetrician Ricardo Jones had already made his paradigm shift and was working hard to keep reducing his intervention rates, as he found, over and over, that *the less he intervened, the better were his outcomes*. But despite his efforts, he could not get his cesarean rate below 25%. His goal was the 10–15% rate long recommended by WHO. Frustrated and unsure as to why he seemed unable to lower that rate (in a city with a CB rate of 75%), one day while attending a course on homeopathy in Buenos Aires, he entered a bookstore and discovered a tattered copy of the famous *Birth Reborn* (1994) by world-renowned holistic obstetrician Michel Odent. The full-page picture on page 128 captivated Ric's attention: it showed a midwife at Pithiviers—the hospital in France where Odent first began attending water births—in a full-bodied embrace with a naked laboring woman. "Well," thought Ric, "if that's what it takes to get my cesarean rate down, I'm never going to succeed—I'm a Brazilian male, and if I tried to do that, my client's husband would kill me!"

Some weeks later, a woman named Cristina Guimares (her real name) came to Ric to ask him to attend her natural childbirth in the hospital, which he did. Two weeks after the birth, she came back to his office for a postnatal exam and announced, "You need me and I need you, and we are going to work together!" "Oh?" said Ric. "And what is it that you do?" "I'm a doula," she replied; Ric's answer, of course (this was many years ago), was "What's a doula?" As soon as Cristina explained the doula's role in birth, Ric immediately saw that here was the answer to what he had been thinking of as "the mystery of page 128." He felt that, as a man, he could not embrace a naked woman who was not his wife, but Cristina as a doula could do precisely that, and much more.

As Ric describes in his chapter "Teamwork" (Jones 2009), he and Cristina began to work together almost immediately. Ric's wife Zeza began to go with them, at first out of curiosity, and soon became "hooked on birth" herself. Already a trained pediatric nurse, it took her only one year to complete a nurse-midwifery program, and so the three became a team—the obstetrician, the midwife, and the doula. This teamwork model they created together carried on for 34 years, until Ricardo unjustly lost his medical license in 2016, as he poignantly describes in his chapter (Jones 2023) in Volume I of this three-volume book series (Davis-Floyd and Premkumar 2023a, 2023b, 2023c). After Cristina married and moved away, he and Zeza trained other doulas. Part of the doula's job was to arrive at the home of the laboring couple shortly after labor began. If it was a planned home birth, the doula called the midwife and doctor to tell them when they should come. If a transport and a cesarean birth were required, Ric performed the CB, providing complete continuity of care. If a planned hospital birth, the doula provided support in the family's home during early labor, and then accompanied the couple to the hospital, where they were met by Ric and Zeza and cared for by the team. To preserve the integrity of the "psychosphere" of birth, like Bernadette, they did not allow any other hospital practitioners into the birthing room (except for the pediatrician, who was required by law to come in soon after the baby was born). By the time Ric lost his license due to persecution by the obstetric establishment in his city (see Jones 2023), more than half of their births were home births, and their cesarean rate had long stood at 16.5%.

Ric believes that midwives and doulas should be the primary attendants at birth; he only used to go to home births to provide legal protection for the team. There he mostly confined his role to taking photos, and afterward created a beautiful slide show of the labor and birth, set to the music of the couple's favorite song, as a special gift. The day after the birth, the team would go to the couple's home to give them the DVD, and they all would watch the slide show together.

Tools and Resources for Self-Transformation 4: Social Movements and Networks

In addition to books, midwives, and doulas, the interlocutors credited ReHuNa (which, again, some of them were instrumental in founding) and other activist networks as critical sources of knowledge, support, and guidance. Many of them met each other for the first time at ReHuNa conferences (which started in 2000 and have continued every five years since—except for the year 2020 due to COVID-19), and, like Bernadette, were beyond delighted to discover that they were part of a community of like-minded alternative practitioners previously unknown to them. Today, Brazil's "good guy and girl" obs keep in regular touch via Facebook and other social media, where they engage in vigorous dialogues and debates over such issues as whether it is wise and safe to assist a woman with two or more previous cesareans to give birth vaginally, how best to turn a breech baby, and what constitutes optimal nutrition during labor, among many other issues. "Good girl" Melania Amorim described her discovery of the Internet chat group *Parto Nosso* (Our Birth) as "magic . . . It was a revolution in our lives because you could find persons whose thoughts were similar to ours. We were not 'crazy.' We were accepted, we were stimulated." When they experience ostracism or outright persecution from their technocratic colleagues (often called *cesaristas* for their routine use of cesareans, as opposed to *vaginalistas*—another term by which these good guy and girl interlocutors identify themselves), they turn not only to midwives and doulas, but also to these activist networks for both advice and support.

The Process of Transformation

Pivot Points

Ricardo Jones: The Epiphany
One bright day in the first year of Dr. Ricardo Jones's obstetric residency (1986), a nurse came bounding into the residents' lounge where he was hanging out with his colleagues, saying directly to him, "Please doctor, come quickly—there is a woman who has just come in from the street with no prior prenatal care, and she is having her baby in the emergency room!" Realizing that he was the senior resident in the room, Ric rushed downstairs to the ER. Pushing the door open, he was shocked to see the delivery table empty, and turned angrily toward the nurse, thinking she was playing a trick on him. "No, doctor," said the nurse, "please push the door further!" And there, Ric was "horrified" to see a "peasant woman" squatting on the floor in the corner of the room. He yelled at her to stand up immediately and get onto the table, but, as he told us years later, "She was in another world, and she simply looked right through me, as if I were made of glass." Lifting her skirt, Ric saw the baby's head crowning. No time even to put on gloves, so he knelt and caught the slippery body with his bare hands, handing the baby off to the nurse as quickly as pos-

sible with a shudder of disgust—he had never before touched a newborn without wearing gloves. Then he scolded the woman, who continued to "look right through me," for making such a bloody mess on the floor as the placenta emerged. The baby was whisked off to the NICU because "it" was considered "contaminated," while the mother, who finally did climb onto the table, was rolled away to a postpartum recovery ward.

All day Ric felt bothered by that birth but couldn't pinpoint why, until later in the afternoon the nurse exclaimed to him, "Doctor, what a good thing you were there! Only think what might have happened had you not been there!" And suddenly it hit him "with the force of a strong blow" that if he had not been there, that mother would in fact have had a perfect birth. She would have caught her own baby; she had not needed him for anything—indeed, everything he had done was to spoil, not enhance, her birth experience. And with that realization began his long journey from technocratic to holistic practice, which he has described in Portuguese in his books *Memórias do Homem de Vidro* (*Memories of a Man made of Glass*) (Jones 2010) and *Entre as Orelhas: Historias do Parto* (*Between the Ears: Birth Stories*) (Jones 2012), and in English in his chapter "Teamwork: An Obstetrician, a Midwife, and a Doula in Brazil" (Jones 2009) in *Birth Models That Work* (Davis-Floyd et al. 2009).

Roxana Knobel: The Evidence

During her residency, Roxana Knobel, an obstetrician from Florianopolis, state of Santa Catarina, read a study about the iatrogenic effects of episiotomies to enlarge the perineum during birth; she found the evidence so compelling that she immediately stopped performing them. And just as immediately, her colleagues and superiors began to chastise her for that. This chastisement for stopping what she now understood to be a completely unnecessary procedure in the vast majority of cases made her suspicious of everything else she was being taught, so she began to read more studies, until she finally understood the detriments she was causing to the normal physiologic process of birth with all those interventions—in what Melissa Cheyney and Robbie Davis-Floyd (2019:8) call the "obstetric paradox": intervene to keep birth safe, thereby causing harm. Once Roxana entered private practice, she completed her paradigm shift. Since 2007, she has been teaching obstetrics at the Universidad Federal, focusing on women-centered care. In 2017, she left private practice and now works shifts in the public Hospital Universitário da Universidade Federal de Santa Catarina (see below), where she provides deeply humanistic care to those most in need of it. (See the Introduction to this volume for an explanation of the differences between "superficial" and "deep" humanism in birth.)

Paulo Batistuta: The First Vertical Birth

Paulo Batistuta's turning point came when he accepted a scholarship to study normal birth in Sweden. Having performed over 1,000 cesareans by then, he realized that he knew little about normal birth and decided to take this opportunity to learn. In Sweden, he watched midwives attend normal births, but never did so himself. Upon his return to his city of Vitória, he was approached by a French woman who informed him in no uncertain terms that she wanted "a vertical birth." Feeling empowered by his experiences in Sweden, he agreed, and was a bit shocked during labor to find himself on the floor underneath the laboring woman, who was standing, attempting at her request to ascertain her cervical dilation. But he was unable to interpret what his fingers were feeling, as he had never before performed a vaginal exam "from below." So, not wanting to appear incompetent, he just took a guess and said "4 centimeters." His experience shows us how deeply embodied biomedical knowledge becomes (see Smith-Oka and Marshalla 2023); his fingers, used to assessing cervical dilation "from above," simply did not know what they were feeling in that unfamiliar position. The birth turned out beautifully, and he was "hooked," quickly becoming an expert on normal birth and empowering some of his patients to birth on their own. Nevertheless, his CB rate was 40% "because I have a very busy hospital practice, the cesarean rate in my hospital is 75%, and I can only provide that kind of holistic care to the few women who truly want it." Paulo made a gorgeous and sensual video of couples giving untrammeled birth in his hospital called *Sagrado* (*Sacred*) subtitled in English, Spanish, and French.[4]

In an email to Robbie on January 4, 2022, Paulo wrote that he still attends births, and currently works at the Federal University of Espírito Santo:

> where we teach medical students and ob/gyn residents our humanistic practice. These practices are now routine at the University Hospital: freedom to choose a companion and positions during childbirth; episiotomy as an exception; a policy for reducing c-sections; and a multidisciplinary team, among others. In addition, currently more than 30 obstetricians are dedicated to humanized childbirth in the city of Vitória where I live. Several private and public hospitals now honor humanizing practices in childbirth care. I believe they are echoes of the work I carried out two decades ago, step-by-step.

"Step-by-Step" along the Transformation Spectrum

As we came to understand during our interview process, even for inter-locutors like Ric, Roxana, and Paulo, whose narratives of transformation highlight a pivot point—an "aha! moment" in which their perspectives abruptly shifted—changing their day-to-day practices was in almost all cases a slow and painful process that required the conscious choice to dissociate themselves from their habitual forms of thinking and acting. Changing deeply embodied knowledge and habits typically occurred "step-by-step" (Paulo Batistuta) and could take years to complete. As Ric eloquently put it, "between rationality and fear, there was a considerable space still to cross" (Jones 2009:292).

For many, the episiotomy was one of the hardest routine procedures to give up. Carla Polido noted:

> [As a student at UNICAMP], I saw squatting births with Dr. Hugo [Sabatino] but it didn't influence me—the other professors said he was a lunatic, "That's for savages!" At the time, I also thought that those women were too demanding. Today I *want* women to have demands, but at the time, I was Dr. House—I was The Boss. We didn't value the woman—we thought that *we* were the stars of the show, not her. From there was a whole process, one birth after an-other. The toughest thing for me to stop doing was the episiotomy. I had this fear of the perineum blowing up!

Carla also said that the first thing she started to change was the epidural:

> I didn't want to attend women under drugs anymore because the ba-bies didn't cry, their muscle tones were bad, they were floppy. Then induction, and the due date—"Oh it is magic, 40!" No, we can wait to 42 weeks. The ultrasound for estimating baby's weight—that's a big fat lie that we tell women—"Oh, your baby's too big to come vagi-nally." The vaginal exam, sweeping the membranes—that was terri-ble. I did that on a woman once without telling her, and she was very angry at me, and I thought, "Why did I do that?" So I looked in my books and I didn't find anything that justified this kind of maneuver. So I did that because I was *taught* to do that—and it was very discom-forting for the woman. Then position—I demanded that the hospital buy a birthing stool because I wouldn't attend the birth on the gy-necological table anymore—300 *reais* [52.00 USD] was all it cost.

The step-by-step nature of this transformative process was further elaborated by Marilena Pereira. Even once convinced that a procedure was unnecessary, finally relinquishing it was sometimes still a struggle, as Marilena described:

> I filled in at the last moment for a colleague to do a home birth, but I arrived late, just as the woman was giving birth . . . I didn't do anything; she was doing it all. I had the intuition to shut my mouth, not to tell her what to do. That's when the light went on for me, when I understood what was happening. [Yet] many times, I still couldn't believe it would be ok not to cut. When the birth would start, I'd say to myself, "It's going to tear, it's going to tear," and I would cut. Sometimes I would succeed in not cutting, but I was afraid—really afraid—so many times I would cut. [It took me] the next two years to give up doing episiotomies.

Yet give them up she did, soon discovering, as the other interlocutors did, that upright positions were much more likely to prevent vaginal tears. Attending women who are upright—sitting on a birthing chair or ball, squatting, standing, and including down on hands and knees[5]—of course requires the ob to be below her, perhaps sitting on a low stool or kneeling in front of the laboring woman—or, if she is on all fours, sitting, squatting, or kneeling at her "butt." This sort of status reversal was a challenge for some, while others took to it easily. Quick to go was the routine use of Pitocin to speed labor; hard to learn was the patience it takes to attend births without artificially rushing the process. Interlocutor Helio Bergo noted:

> When I started with squatting birth, with the woman in a vertical position, I saw that there was no need anymore for forceps and other aggressive and invasive methods. Because this is natural! . . . Little by little I was learning to watch the rhythms, and this is what enchanted me. Do not intervene. [Just] watch. I would just be there, observing and learning. I learned in this way from attending home births. To respect the rhythm was the hardest thing to learn. And it's what brought me the most benefits. When I learned how to do that, things became easy. But it was hard to let go, to respect the rhythm, to not intervene. Because there are moments when, without any doubt, it is necessary to intervene. To know, to decide which moment it is, without intervening prematurely, is difficult.

During residency, Carla Daher found herself shocked and horrified that thirsty laboring women were not allowed to drink, even though they were working so hard and sweating. She began to offer them water (and later food) during labor and to encourage them to move around and walk. Carla said, "I learned that the essence of a healthy labor is movement, not being imprisoned in a supine position." Like Helio, she learned from a sympathetic colleague "to be patient, to just watch women work, to be nice." She gave up manual extraction of the placenta (still a common practice in Brazil for vaginal births) because she saw it as "unnecessary and cruel." As a result, her ob Chief called her practice "messy," and so made sure that she was the only resident in her cohort who was not hired by the hospital from which she graduated. She happily went into private practice.

For these interlocutors, giving up routine interventions meant placing great emphasis on treating their patients as individuals, which in turn entailed getting to know them as such. Banished were the five-minute standard question and answer sessions, which they replaced with prenatal visits lasting an hour or more, with childbirth education classes they often taught themselves, and with discussion sessions in which their patients could come together in groups and ask all the questions they wished (see Rising and Jolivet 2009). Those in private practice made conscious decisions to limit the number of patients they accepted to be able to provide the high-quality humanistic care they now offered. They found themselves happy to accept lower salaries, and often ostracism from their technocratic colleagues, as small prices to pay for the much greater levels of satisfaction they experienced via providing that high-quality care.

On the spectrum technocratic—humanistic—holistic, which Robbie (Davis-Floyd 2022) has redefined as "technocratic—superficially humanistic—deeply humanistic—holistic" (see also the Introduction to this volume), all interlocutors placed themselves very much on the deeply humanistic side (centering the woman, and facilitating what Robbie calls the *deep physiology* of birth) merging into holism (perceiving the body as energy and birth as a spiritual process) (see Davis-Floyd 2018a, 2022, and this volume's Introduction). Some vacillated between the terms; for example, João Batista explained:

> I don't consider myself a holistic ob, but Andrea [one of the Sofia Feldman midwives] is. She is holistic—she believes in energy, in everything that's supernatural. Sometimes I believe, sometimes I don't—I'm in the middle. She is a spiritualist. I don't consider myself one—but my wife says I am. Sometimes I'm technocratic because I need to be. Most of the time I'm a humanist, sometimes I'm holistic too.

Characteristics of Holistic Obstetricians

As we poured over our interview transcripts, we became able to pin-point certain characteristics of the ob interlocutors who practiced in fully holistic ways. (Many of these also apply to the humanistic obs we interviewed.) These characteristics include:

- Trust in women and birth.
- Respect for women and love of the birth process.
- Passion.
- A spiritual orientation.
- Recognition of birth as a spiritual process, of the body as an energy field, and of their responsibility to keep the psychosphere of birth clear and clean.
- Sensitivity to women's desires and choices and a desire to fulfill them.
- Critical thinking.
- Thinking before acting.
- A science and research orientation: many interlocutors conducted research and wrote scientific articles and books.
- An emphasis on educating women about perinatal issues through classes—weekly, bi-weekly, or monthly.
- Supporting the normal physiology of birth by encouraging lots of movement, eating, and drinking at will during labor, any and all birth positions, and water labor and birth if possible.
- Willingness to wait until 42 weeks of gestation, and sometimes longer.
- Deep appreciation for midwives and doulas.
- Spending lots of time with laboring women.
- Longer prenatal consults—60 minutes or more.
- In their private practices, taking only 4–10 clients per month to conserve their energy to do the best they can for each mother and family.
- Working shifts in public hospitals when possible to provide more women with access to their care. (For example, Bernadette Bous-sada attended around 17 births per month because she worked shifts in a public hospital.)
- Receiving support from midwives and doulas to help them deal with the persecutions that many of them experienced.
- Happiness and fulfillment in their practices.
- Acceptance of making less money than their technocratic peers in return for that happiness and fulfillment.

- Political involvement and participation in the social movement for the humanization of birth because of their desire to make birth better not just for their own patients, but for all birthing people.

The Loss of Obstetrician-Attended Home Births in Brazil: The CREMERJ Regulations

Although their numbers are still small—though they are growing—the obs we describe in this chapter and their like-minded colleagues have managed to provide options for humanistic maternity care in nearly every major city in Brazil. Sadly, most of them are no longer able to offer the homebirth option, due to highly restrictive regulations from CREMERJ (the Medical Board of the State of Rio de Janeiro). Ricardo Jones (personal communication 2016) has translated and summarized these regulations for us as follows:

- Article 1. The participation of doctors in the so-called domiciliary actions related to birth and perinatal assistance is forbidden.
- Article 2. Doctors are forbidden from providing supervision to other professionals attending home births.
- Article 3. An exception can be made in the case of an obstetric emergency/urgency, but notification to the Medical Board of Rio de Janeiro (CREMERJ) is compulsory.
- Article 4. When obstetricians working on shift in the hospital assist in births transported to hospitals from homes or birth centers, they must report that assistance to CREMERJ.
- Article 5. Non-compliance with these resolutions is considered an ethical infraction and can result in disciplinary action.

These regulations were generated by CREMERJ in 2014, in part because of a film that gave huge impetus to the movement for the humanization of birth, O *Renacimento do Parto* (*The Rebirth of Birth*, or *Birth Reborn*).[6] This film was shown in movie theaters all over the country for five months, was watched by more than 30,000 people, and helped to generate large marches in 30 Brazilian cities (and one in Italy) supporting the humanization of birth. These CREMERJ regulations were part of a strong obstetric establishment backlash against that film and against the humanization movement. Strictly speaking, these regulations are not legally binding, but have been influential enough to make most obstetricians afraid of attending home births. So as of 2014, almost all home births in Brazil are attended by midwives—either nurse-midwives (*enfermeiras obstetras*) or direct-entry (non-nurse) midwives (*obstetrizes*). As we mentioned above, collectively these professional midwives attend around 10% of births nationwide, mostly in hospitals, but sometimes in homes and birth centers. The "good guy and girl" obs back these midwives up when possible, and a very few of these obs still do attend home births. They have also succeeded in creating several institutionalized humanistic practices in Brazil, such as Hospital Sofia Feldman, the Federal University of Espírito Santo in Vitória where Paulo Batistuta works, the Hospital Universitário da Universidade Federal de Santa Catarina (see below), and others.

The Obstetrician as the "Hero of the Hospital"

For humanistic ob Marcos Leite, his "pivot point" had come when his young son got robbed for the fifth time while walking home from school, and he realized that, to provide a safer life for his children, he had to get out of Rio de Janeiro, where he had been enjoying a highly lucrative practice attending the births of movie stars and other extremely wealthy women. So he and his family moved to the more laid-back and much safer small city of Florianopolis in the state of Santa Catarina. There, accepting a far lower salary than he had enjoyed in Rio, he joined the maternity care practice at the Hospital Universitário da Universidade Federal de Santa Catarina. Having read many books and articles on the benefits of humanistic care by then, but unable to figure out how to change his practice while in Rio, he took this move as that opportunity and convinced some of his new colleagues to make a paradigm shift to humanistic practice. Their first step was to send some of the labor and delivery nurses to a nurse-midwifery training program. Once they returned one year later, Marcos and some of his colleagues turned the care of normal pregnancies and births over to the nurse-midwives, reserving themselves for the higher-risk cases. Thus Marcos's cesarean rate, for as long as he practiced at that hospital, was 75%. How, you might ask, could a humanistic ob like Marcos have a CB rate that high? And the answer, of course, is that all of the women he attended were referred to him by the midwives, so he dealt only with true pathologies that the midwives could not handle. And he was very proud that nevertheless 25% of the births he attended were vaginal—he didn't just take "the easy way out" by performing cesareans on all his patients. Marcos said, "I think the obstetrician should be the hero of the hospital, swooping in to save the day when truly needed, while all the rest of the births should be attended by midwives who practice the midwifery model of care." Marcos is now in private practice in Florianopolis with his obstetrician son

Pablo. The two of them see all clients, so that if one leaves—for example to attend a conference or to take a vacation—the other can attend and the care can be continuous.

As "good guy" Carlos Miner noted about the hospital where Marcos had worked, and where Roxana Knobel now practices:

> Some of our residents are from Santa Catarina, and there I think they are . . . more advanced . . . Last night I was on duty . . . with some residents who were my students two or three years ago, and they accepted everything—they were practicing like me—and so I think there is going to be a change.

And indeed, although Brazil's national CB rate stubbornly remains at 56% (Rudley, Leal, and Rego 2020), many members of the up-and-coming generation of obs have joined ReHuNa and are doing their best to practice humanistically. According to the two younger obs whom we interviewed fresh out of residency, they don't bother to read any of the books that were so important to the now-older generation of good guys and girls; rather, they get all their information from the members of the ReHuNa listserv and via Facebook communication. For example, one of them, Braulio Zorzella, told us that during many of the births he attended, if he had a question about how to proceed, he simply used his iPad to get on Facebook, and always received immediate answers from more experienced humanistic obs.

The "Good Guys" on the "Bad Guys"

According to Braulio Zorzella, Bernadette Boussada, and others of the good guys and girls, in Braulio's words:

> There are two groups of techno-obs. Those in the first, smaller one truly believe that cesareans are best—their wives all have cesareans and they *cannot* change. Those in the second, larger group know that vaginal birth is better [and their wives have vaginal births] but do cesareans anyway because they can't be bothered—they are unethical and immoral, but *could* change—they would do vaginal births if they were paid more for them.

And according to Bernadette, "They are very materialistic—they like to acquire things, more and more things—houses, boats, cars, clothes, trips. They are always looking for something and they never find it."

In Conclusion: The Humanization of Birth

To synthesize the concept of humanization as applied to childbirth, Ric (Jones 2012:223) noted that "humanized birth" is characterized by:

1. The protagonism it gives to women, without which we would be merely further entrenching the dependence of women on men imposed over millennia by patriarchy.
2. An integrative and interdisciplinary view of birth focused on a deep understanding of the characteristics of the biological process and its emotional, social, cultural, and spiritual aspects, which must all be equally valued and attended to.
3. A visceral connection with evidence-based medicine, making clear that the humanization of childbirth movement works under the aegis of reason.

Ric said that his objective in creating the above synthesis was to offer a simple vision of the movement's proposals. "More than general indignation at the excess of intervention," he said, "we needed a very clear idea of what we wanted for birth."

Acknowledgments

This chapter has been significantly revised and updated from its original appearance by the same title in *Ways of Knowing about Birth: Mothers, Midwives, Medicine, and Birth Activism* by Robbie Davis-Floyd and Colleagues, 141–164 (Long Grove IL: Waveland Press, 2018). We sincerely thank Tom Curtin of Waveland Press for granting permission to reprint large portions of the original chapter herein.

Robbie Davis-Floyd, Adjunct Professor, Department of Anthropology, Rice University, Houston, Fellow of the Society for Applied Anthropology, and Senior Advisor to the Council on Anthropology and Reproduction, is a cultural/medical/reproductive anthropologist interested in transformational models of maternity care. She is also a Board member of the International MotherBaby Childbirth Organization (IMBCO), in which capacity she helped to wordsmith the *International Childbirth Initiative: 12 Steps to Safe and Respectful MotherBaby-Family Maternity Care* (www.ICIchildbirth.org). The ICI has been translated into more than 30 languages and has been implemented in birth facilities, small and large, around the world, showing that transformative change is indeed possible. Hospital Sofia Feldman, described in this chapter, is an ICI implementation site. Researchers are needed to study the processes and effects of ICI implementation in multiple sites around the world; if you are interested, please contact Robbie at davis-floyd@outlook.com.

Eugenia Georges is a Professor in the Department of Anthropology at Rice University. She has conducted research on the implications of transnational migration for gender and class hierarchies in the Dominican Republic and on the political mobilization of Dominican immigrants in New York City. Her research in Greece examines the medicalization of reproduction, with a focus on the historical processes through which pregnancy and Greek obstetric practice have been shaped in interaction with a range of reproductive technologies. She is the author of multiple articles and book chapters and of *The Making of a Transnational Community: Migration, Development and Cultural Change in the Dominican Republic* (1992), and *Bodies of Knowledge: The Medicalization of Reproduction in Greece* (2008).

Notes

1. Over the years, the practitioners at Hospital Sofia Feldman have faced multiple challenges from their Regional Medical Council (which is like a state Medical Board in the United States) whose members do not approve of their humanistic model of care. These challenges have included a recent set of "ethical trials" at the Minas Gerais State Medical Regional Council against three of its doctors—Dr. Ivo, Dr. Batista, and Dr. Lucas—for allowing the hospital nurse-midwives to perform ultrasounds. As a result of these trials, disciplinary actions were issued against these three obstetricians. The penalty to Dr. Ivo was to have his medical license revoked, and to Dr. Batista and Dr. Lucas, a public reprimand. They have appealed to the Federal Council and are waiting for the results.

2. This historic film—one of the first to be made on normal births—shows a series of births in the squatting position taking place in the clinic originally built and run by Brazilian obstetric pioneer Moysés Paciornik and now operated by his son Claudio Paciornik. All you see of the obstetrician, Moysés, is his hand receiving a baby and lowering it down to the soft pad underneath, and at one point you see him turning sideways and crying at the beauty of birth. Available in English. Varik K. 2013. "Birth in Squatting Position." *Youtube*, uploaded 26 February. Retrieved 12 December 2022 from https://www.youtube.com/watch?v=aAF5n3GBkPA.

3. The term *enfermeira obstetra* translates literally as "obstetric nurse," so there is some confusion over whether or not it should be translated as "nurse-midwife." *Enfermeiras obstetras* follow much the same educational pathway as US nurse-midwives, but they do not have "midwife" in their titles and don't have edu-

cation in "midwifery" per se but rather in nursing and obstetric nursing. They differ from general nurses in that they have higher level of training; after obtaining their BA in Nursing (which takes 4–5 years), they undergo 1–2 years of specialized training in obstetric nursing. Most of them practice in hospitals under the supervision of obstetricians; some attend home births or work in birth centers—in-hospital or freestanding. According to midwife Paloma Terra, who has practiced both in Brazil (alegally) and in the US as a CPM (certified professional midwife):

> *Enfemeiras obstetras* can do vaginal exams, electronic fetal monitoring, medication monitoring under doctors' orders, catch babies, suture, etc.—everything obstetrics related (except for performing cesareans, vacuum extractions, and forceps). So basically, most *enfermeiras obstetras* in Brazil can and do act the same way as US nurse-midwives [although sometimes they function simply as obstetric nurses].

Thus, for the purposes of this chapter, we translate *enfermeira obstetra* as "nurse-midwife." We also note that the actual translation of "midwife" in Brazilian Portuguese is *parteira*, but professional midwives—*enfermeiras obstetras* and *obstetrizes*—are not called *parteiras* because that term is associated with traditional or Indigenous midwives, who still practice mostly in rural regions of the Northeast and the Brazilian Amazon and are culturally regarded in wider Brazilian society as illiterate and premodern vestiges of the past. Yet in Brazil, Paloma practiced as a *parteira prática*, which is an occupation recognized by the Brazilian Code of Occupations and therefore not illegal. *Parteiras* in general are not illegal in Brazil, but they do not have a legal professional practice framework as do *enfermeiras obstetricas* and *obstetrizes*, whose practice is restricted in private hospitals due to insurance concerns, yet in public hospitals, there are guidelines and protocols that allow nurse-midwives and *obstetrizes* to attend labors and births from beginning to end. Many of the *obstetrizes* with whom we spoke wished to reclaim the word *parteira* by calling themselves *parteiras profesonais*, as Mexican professional midwives, who call themselves *parteras professionales* (see Davis-Floyd 2001) have done, but were outvoted on that issue.

4. The film *Sagrado* (*Sacred*) can be ordered directly from Paulo Batistuta at WhatsApp +55 27 99981 7040 or by E-mail: paulobatistuta@terra.com.br.

5. This all-fours position, known as the "Gaskin Maneuver," opens the pelvis to its maximum outlet (see Bruner et al. 1998; Kovavisarach 2011), and thus is ideal for shoulder dystocias and breech deliveries. World-renowned holistic midwife Ina May Gaskin learned this position from traditional midwives in Guatemala, who themselves learned it from watching laboring women instinctively get on their hands and knees to give birth. Wanting this maneuver to carry the name of a midwife, and not knowing the names of the traditional midwives who taught it to her during a group conversation, she chose to name it after herself.

6. This film, O *Renacimento do Parto* (*The Rebirth of Birth*, or *Birth Reborn*) was produced by Érica de Paula and Eduardo Chauvet in 2013. Robbie is one of the "talking heads" in this film, as are Michel Odent, Ricardo Jones and others of our "good guys and girls" interlocutors. Chauvet E, dir. 2013. O *Renacimento do Parto* [*The Rebirth of Birth*, or *Birth Reborn*] Brasília: Chauvet Filmes. It is available on Netflix at https://www.netflix.com/il-en/title/80995575).

References

Bruner JP, Drummond SB, Meenan AL, Gaskin IM. 1998. "All-Fours Maneuver for Reducing Shoulder Dystocia during Labor." *Journal of Reproductive Medicine* 43(5): 439–443.

Cheyney M, Davis-Floyd R. 2019. "Birth as Culturally Marked and Shaped." In *Birth in Eight Cultures*, eds. Davis-Floyd R, Cheyney M, 1–16. Long Grove IL: Waveland Press.

Davis-Floyd R. 2001. "*La Partera Profesional*: Articulating Identity and Cultural Space for a New Kind of Midwife in Mexico." *Medical Anthropology* 20(2–3): 185–243.

———. (1992) 2003. *Birth as an American Rite of Passage*, 2nd ed. Berkeley: University of California Press.

———. 2018a. "The Technocratic, Humanistic, and Holistic Paradigms of Birth and Health Care." In *Ways of Knowing about Birth: Mothers, Midwives, Medicine, and Birth Activism*, Davis-Floyd R and Colleagues, 3–44. Long Grove IL: Waveland Press.

———. 2018b. "The Midwifery Model of Care: Anthropological Perspectives." In *Ways of Knowing about Birth: Mothers, Midwives, Medicine, and Birth Activism*, Davis-Floyd R and Colleagues. Long Grove IL: Waveland Press, 323–338.

———. 2022. *Birth as an American Rite of Passage*, 3rd ed. Abingdon, Oxon: Routledge.

Davis-Floyd R, Barclay L, Daviss BA, Tritten J. 2009. *Birth Models That Work*. Berkeley: University of California Press.

Davis-Floyd R, Premkumar A, eds. 2023a. *Obstetricians Speak: On Training, Practice, Fear, and Transformation*. New York: Berghahn Books.

———. 2023b. *Cognition, Risk, and Responsibility in Obstetrics: Anthropological Analyses and Critiques of Obstetricians' Practices*. New York: Berghahn Books.

———. 2023c. *Obstetric Violence and Systemic Disparities: Can Obstetrics Be Humanized and Decolonized?* New York: Berghahn Books.

Davis-Floyd R, St John G. 1998. *From Doctor to Healer: The Transformative Journey*. New Brunswick NJ: Rutgers University Press.

Hodnett ED, Gates S, Hofmeyr GJ, Sakala C. 2003. "Continuous Support for Women during Childbirth" (Cochrane Review). *The Cochrane Library* 3(3): CD003766.

Irvine LC. 2022. "Selling Beautiful Births: The Use of Evidence by Brazil's Humanised Birth Movement." In *Anthropologies of Global and Maternal Reproductive Health: From Policy Spaces to Sites of Practice*, eds. Wallace LJ, MacDonald MM, Storeng KT, 199–220. Switzerland: Springer Nature.

Jones R. 2009. "Teamwork: An Obstetrician, a Midwife, and a Doula in Brazil." In *Birth Models That Work*, eds. Davis-Floyd R, Barclay L, Daviss BA, Tritten J, 271–304. Berkeley: University of California Press.

———. 2010. *Memórias do Homem de Vidro* [*Memories of a Man Made of Glass*]. Porto Alegre, Brazil: Editora Ideias a Granel.

———. 2012. *Entre as Orelhas—Histórias de Parto* [*Between the Ears: Birth Stories*]. Porto Alegre, Brazil: Editora Ideias a Granel.

———. 2023. "The Bullying and Persecution of a Humanistic/Holistic Obstetrician in Brazil: The Benefits and Costs of My Paradigm Shift." In *Obstetricians Speak:*

On Training, Practice, Fear, and Transformation, eds. Davis-Floyd R, Premkumar A. Chapter 7. New York: Berghahn Books.

Kennell J, Klaus M, McGrath S, et al. 1991. "Continuous Emotional Support during Labor in a US Hospital: A Randomized Controlled Trial." *Journal of the American Medical Association* 265: 2197–2201.

Klaus MH, Kennell J, Klaus P. 1993. *Mothering the Mother: How a Doula Can Help You Have a Shorter, Easier, and Healthier Birth.* Boston: Addison Wesley.

Kovavisarach E. 2011. "Gaskin Maneuver 'All Fours' for Coping with the Obstetric Nightmare 'Shoulder Dystocia.'" *Thai Journal of Obstetrics and Gynaecology* 35–36.

Odent M. 1994. *Birth Reborn.* London: Souvenir Press.

Paciornik M. 1979. *Aprenda a Nascer com os Índios: Parto de Cócoras* [Learn to give birth like the Indians: Squatting birth]. Brasília, Brazil: Editora Brasiliense.

Rising SS, Jolivet R. 2009. "Circles of Community: The Centering Pregnancy Group Prenatal Care Model." In *Birth Models That Work*, eds. Davis-Floyd R, Barclay L, Daviss BA, Tritten J, 365–384. Berkeley: University of California Press.

Rudey EL, Leal MDC, Rego G. 2020. "Cesarean Section Rates in Brazil: Trend Analysis Using the Robson Classification System." *Medicine* (Baltimore) 99(17): e19880.

Scott KD, Berkowitz G, Klaus M. 1999. "A Comparison of Intermittent and Continuous Support during Labor: A Meta-Analysis." *American Journal of Obstetrics and Gynecology* 180(5): 1054–1059.

Scott KD, Klaus PH, Klaus M. 1999. "The Obstetrical and Postpartum Benefits of Continuous Support during Childbirth." *Journal of Women's Health and Gender Based Medicine* 8(10): 1257–1264.

Smith-Oka V, Marshalla MK. 2023. "Crossing Bodily, Social, and Intimate Boundaries: How Class, Ethnic, and Gender Differences Are Reproduced in Medical Training in Mexico." In *Cognition, Risk, and Responsibility in Obstetrics: Anthropological Analyses and Critiques of Obstetricians' Practices*, eds. Davis-Floyd R, Premkumar A. Chapter 8. New York: Berghahn Books.

CHAPTER 10

Interprofessional Education for Medical and Midwifery Students in Aotearoa New Zealand

Rea Daellenbach, Lorna Davies, Maggie Meeks,
Coleen Caldwell, Melanie Welfare, and Judy Ormandy

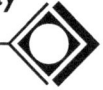

Introduction

In Aotearoa New Zealand (ANZ),[1] there has been a wealth of qualitative research on midwives and various aspects of midwifery practice (see for examples McAra Couper et al. 2014; Skinner and Maude 2016; Clemons et al. 2021). However, apart from a history of the leading obstetric hospital in the country (Bryder 2014), there has been virtually no ethnographic scholarship on obstetricians and obstetric practice in ANZ. This chapter presents a contribution to this field through the lens of a research project into "interprofessional education" (IPE) between final year midwifery students and trainee intern medical students on their obstetric rotations. This chapter has been written by two midwives (Lorna Davies and Melanie Welfare), a neonatal pediatrician (Maggie Meeks), two obstetricians (Coleen Caldwell and Judy Ormandy), and a sociologist/anthropologist (Rea Daellenbach). We are all involved in health-related professional education and have worked in our respective disciplinary fields for between 10 and 40 years. We have been brought together by our common interest in IPE. As we detail in this chapter, we have been working together on an action research project on developing education workshops for midwifery and medical students using simulations and debriefings. Our aim was that these workshops would foster more collegial interprofessional relationships between midwives and doctors, particularly in situations when women and babies require collaborative care in the context of Aotearoa New Zealand's unique maternity care system.

We held the first workshop in November 2019, but a follow-up workshop was interrupted by COVID-19, as lockdowns and other consequences of the pandemic prevented us from bringing further groups of students together until June 2021 (these two workshops are described below). This was an unfortunate and frustrating development, but it did mean that the members of the research team had more time to get to know each other, which inadvertently led to an unexpected development within the study. Through ad hoc conversations, we compared our own experiences to those that we witnessed or heard reported by the students in the cohorts involved in the IPE research project. We realized that there might be value in addressing these experiences in a more structured way. Consequently, we introduced a modification to the research design of the study using a collaborative autoethnographic (CAE) approach for our adjunct study. This approach enabled us to explore our own feelings about collaboration and communication among our respective professional positions, in the hope of gaining further insight into the experiences of interprofessional collaboration for the students in our research project.

"Autoethnography" is a qualitative research method in which a solo researcher uses autobiographical and ethnographic approaches to analyze personal experiences to understand their own cultural experiences (Ellis, Adams, and Bochner 2011). CAE uses the same elements, but in a collective and collaborative way that facilitates exploration of self within a group context. This form of social inquiry is emerging as a "pragmatic application of the autoethnographic approach" that allows the researchers to create a "meaningful understanding of sociocultural phenomena reflected in their autobiographical data" (Chang, Ngunjiri, and Hernandez 2013:21). We decided to record our discussions and together critically analyze our experiences within the multi-professional sphere of health care. We also had a sociologist (Rea Daellenbach) present in our group who was able to offer an external lens within this CAE theoretical context.

We shared memories and stories about our lives as nascent practitioners and found a surprising degree of common ground between our experiences as students and, later, as healthcare providers with recognized standings within our professions. We all acknowledged that lateral/horizontal violence[2] and incivility had detrimental effects for healthcare professionals and patients. We had all felt a degree of "impostor syndrome"[3] that seemed to occur as we realized the enormity of the responsibility that accompanies becoming a qualified healthcare practitioner

(Bell, Vest, and White 2021). We also agreed that it could be challenging to resist fear-based decision-making and negativity bias. There were also some very positive discussion points during the meetings, such as the sense of comfort that we drew from "knowing where we fit" within the hospital hierarchy. This concept might feel anachronistic to a student in the 2020s, but we agreed that the traditional hierarchy has been replaced by a risk discourse that imposes a new type of hierarchy, justified by biomedical science and based on specialized roles.

When we analyzed the transcribed data from our discussions, it became apparent that we were voicing many of the feelings and views described by the students in our primary study. In fact, many of the statements in our transcripts might have been made by the medical and midwifery students currently in healthcare education. From obstetric/midwifery and anthropological perspectives, we had at least as much in common with current students as we had differences. However, a significant theme from the CAE (collaborative autoethnographic) data hinged around the fact that out of the six researchers, four of us (Lorna Davies, Maggie Meeks, Melanie Welfare, and Coleen Caldwell) had been trained/educated in the United Kingdom, which added yet another dimension to our interpretations. It became apparent that our early exposure to practice within that healthcare system was very different to what we were introduced to when we came to ANZ and particularly within the domain of maternity care. There was consensus that there were, at times, levels of mutual distrust and incivility between the obstetricians and midwives that were unfamiliar to those of us from England and Scotland. Without an understanding of the history of the professionalization of obstetrics and midwifery in ANZ, this mutual distrust and incivility would be hard to comprehend.

We therefore begin the rest of this chapter by mapping the ways in which maternity services in ANZ have developed to provide a background for the some of the initial findings from this project. We explore the current interprofessional interfaces between midwives and obstetricians in ANZ, and outline some of the local historical factors that have contributed to the current situation. The next section outlines IPE (interprofessional education) and how we are adapting it to work for midwifery students and trainee intern biomedical students who undertake an obstetric rotation. The final section presents a discussion of what the students who participated in this project have shared with us, and what their findings indicate about the professional identities and approaches to the practices of midwives and obstetricians in maternity services.

Background and Context:
The Maternity Care System in Aotearoa New Zealand

The maternity care system in ANZ is unique. Universally accessible, government-funded maternity care is provided at no cost to citizens and residents and is based on continuity of care provided by a professional of the client's choice, with access to specialist biomedical care when required. Women/people can choose whether to have their pregnancy and birth care from either a community midwife, a doctor who is a general practitioner/family doctor (GP) with an obstetric qualification, or a private obstetrician (registered under the vocational scope of Obstetrics and Gynecology). This healthcare professional is then responsible for providing and coordinating maternity care during pregnancy, labor, and birth, and for four to six weeks after the baby is born. The Ministry of Health (2019) recorded that for almost all pregnant women/people (94.2%), this care is provided by a community midwife, while 5.6% registered with an obstetrician, and the remaining 0.2% accessed their primary maternity care from a GP. Private obstetricians may charge additional fees, which may partially account for the low rates of ob-provided care. Pregnant people can choose to give birth at home, at a birth center, or in a hospital, and community midwives, GPs, and private obstetricians need to have access to agreements with the birth centers and hospitals to be able to provide maternity care in these settings. Currently most child-bearers choose to give birth in hospitals (86.6%), while 3.4% birth at home, and 10% at a freestanding birth center (Ministry of Health 2019).

In ANZ, there are two types of midwives—"community" midwives and "core" midwives. The core midwives work on shifts in birth centers and hospitals, whereas the community midwives, who have offices in their respective communities, work on a caseload basis, taking on as many or as few clients as they wish and helping them to birth in any setting they choose. This system is flexible, as community and core midwives often change roles. For example, working on shifts as a core midwife is more conducive to raising small children, whereas community midwives are often on call 24/7, so tend to practice as such before they have children and after those children are grown up enough to no longer need their mothers to be available at the clear time intervals that shift work offers. This role-shifting works to ensure that all ANZ midwives share the same overall philosophy of care.

Birth centers are midwifery-led; women and their families come in with their community midwife and the centers employ core midwives to provide additional support. For example, when a community midwife is attending a woman who plans to give birth in a freestanding birth center, she will call the core midwife on shift at that birth center, who will then turn on all the lights and start filling up the labor and birthing tub. The core midwife knows where all the supplies are kept, and the two midwives work together in attending labors and deliveries in that birth center. In hospitals, there are core midwives, obstetricians, registrars (residents) training to become obstetricians, anesthetists, and resident doctors (meaning that they have completed their residencies). Many who birth in hospitals do not require any interventions that would necessitate biomedical consultation, and their care is provided by their community midwife with support from core midwives. If childbearers need care that is beyond the scope of a midwife or a GP, this care will be provided by the obstetric team based within the public healthcare system. In other words, for the most part, obstetricians only work with those women/people who have risks or complications that have been identified by their community midwife, placing significant emphasis on the interface between midwives and obstetricians, which shapes their professional identities, roles, and responsibilities, and interprofessional relationships. And again, 94% of ANZ childbearers choose community midwives as their primary caregivers.

Exploring the specific challenges and opportunities for IPE (interprofessional education) between ANZ medical and midwifery students requires an understanding of the country's maternity care system and how it has developed over the past decades. In addition to the description of this system provided above, two other key aspects of the ANZ maternity care system are, first, the pervasiveness of government influence over how services are organized; and second, that these services are provided free of charge, funded through general taxation. This system has emerged through a series of rounds of negotiations between the government, which funds healthcare services, and the healthcare professional groups, who seek to protect their autonomy and financial positions.

In 1980, senior obstetricians sought to change the scope of midwifery to an advanced nursing qualification to integrate nurse-midwives into the obstetric teams. These changes aimed to base the national maternity services firmly on what Robbie Davis-Floyd (2001, 2018, 2022) defines as the "technocratic model of birth" (described in the Introduction to this volume). While many obstetricians personally had a humanistic approach to patient care, they used the promise of technocratic progress to promote their bid to radically restructure the maternity services in Aotearoa New Zealand.

These obstetricians' initiatives had intended and unintended consequences. They changed the role of GPs to only providing non-complex maternity care, and led to the closings of many small birthing centers around the country. Also, most significantly in terms of maternity services in New Zealand today, these initiatives incited a backlash from some women and midwives (Daellenbach 1999). They rejected the technocratic depersonalization of hospital-based maternity care with its focus on risk assessment and the routinized management of labor and birth. Instead, they wanted protection of a person's right to control what was done to them in childbirth. They also wanted to retain the continuity of care throughout pregnancy and birth that they had been accustomed to receiving from a GP of their choice. Throughout the 1980s, maternity consumer groups, such as the Home Birth Association and midwifery collectives on the one hand, and senior obstetricians on the other, were engaged in debates through the media and politics about women's rights in childbirth.

Concerted political lobbying by midwives' and women's groups throughout the 1980s led to new legislation in 1990 that enabled direct-entry (non-nurse) midwives to offer the same kinds of caseload maternity services as GPs (see Hendry 2009). This legislation gave midwives and GPs the same remuneration and the same rights to prescribe medicines, order laboratory tests, make referrals to other healthcare professionals, and attend births in hospitals, birth centers, and homes. The legislation also enabled three-year midwifery-led education programs for student midwives to be set up within the polytechnic/university sector to prepare students for this new scope of midwifery practice and to increase their numbers to meet the growing demands for their care.

As more midwives graduated from these programs and went into community caseload practice, they distinguished themselves from doctors through articulating a midwifery professional framework of working "in partnership" with women/people, supporting informed decision-making, and providing culturally appropriate and safe care. This framework is explicitly based on what Davis-Floyd (2001, 2018, 2022; see also the Introduction to this volume) defines as a humanistic, and for some a holistic, model of maternity care. By 2000, most pregnant women/people were choosing community midwives and most GPs no longer offered maternity care. Community midwives continued to operate on a contract with the Ministry of Health that was similar to the contract that GPs had negotiated in 1938, and community midwives are paid for each client through a modular fee schedule. As previously noted, they are responsible for ensuring that their clients can access maternity care 24/7. Most community midwives work in small group practices with other midwives, and back each other up to be able to take time off call. As noted earlier, they exercise a great degree of autonomy over how many women/people they will provide care for and how this care will be provided.

Midwives can provide full maternity care for non-complex childbearers and undertake continual assessments throughout the pregnancy and childbirth journey to ensure that everything is normal. When midwives identify health concerns, they recommend that those clients consult with the appropriate professional. For obstetric conditions, midwives will make a referral for a consultation with an obstetrician. This means that obstetricians can focus on working with childbearers who need the level of specialist obstetric care that they can offer. It is an ideal model and generally works well, yet the ANZ cesarean birth rate in 2017 was 28% (Ministry of Health 2019). It is not known precisely why the cesarean birth rate in New Zealand is as high as it is; the reasons are probably multifaceted. Of note, the cesarean birth rate for Māori in 2018 was only 21.16% compared to the rate for people of European descent at 33.1%. Also, the cesarean rate for people from the most economically deprived quintile was 24.82%, whereas the rate for the least deprived quintile was 32.42%.

Obstetric and midwifery leaders recognize that these rates indicate that cesareans are being performed more often than necessary, and that this issue needs to be addressed. At a wider social level, many healthcare professionals and birthing families are risk averse; if cesareans are not done and there are poor outcomes as a result, then practitioners are legally considered to be negligent and both midwives and obs are blamed for not doing more. Also, ANZ obs have a preference for avoiding assisted births, particularly by forceps, because of the injuries they can cause to mother and baby; thus obs prefer to perform cesareans if technological birth assistance is needed.

Research on giving birth in ANZ indicates that many women/people who require both midwifery and obstetric care have good experiences. However, there are also tensions that need to be addressed. These studies also identify that some childbearers have the perception of conflict between the midwives and obs providing their care, and this leads to increased anxiety, distress, and trauma for such childbearers (Howarth et al. 2012; Currie and Barber 2016; Georges and Daellenbach 2019). Similarly, research with midwives suggests that they too have mixed experiences of referral and collaboration with obstetric teams (Skinner and Maude 2016; Crowther et al. 2019). In their recent study of more than 250 ANZ midwives, Janine Clemons and colleagues (2021) found that midwives experienced both "collegial relationships based on trust, respect and support" and interactions during which they felt "disrespected and judged" and that their professional opinions, which are based on their relationships with their clients and on the scientific evidence supporting normal physiologic birth, are not valued by obstetricians (Clemons et al. 2021:35).

There are several layers of complexity in establishing collaborative relationships between obstetricians and midwives. Often there are differences in philosophy, ideas about risk assessment and management (Skinner and Maude 2016), and definitions of "normal" (Davis and Walker 2009). As community midwives work with pregnant people on their entry into the maternity care system, the responsibility rests on these midwives to recommend consultations with or referrals to biomedical specialists. Obstetricians sometimes feel that such referrals do not happen in a timely or effective manner, and lead to adverse outcomes for childbearers and their babies. This causes concern, not only for the emotional toll it can exact on families and on all the healthcare professionals involved in their care, but also within the medicolegal context of blame. When this occurred historically in relation to GP practices, obstetricians were able to institute education programs for GPs. In contrast, midwifery education is not under obstetric jurisdiction. Instead, obstetricians try to address their concerns about "poor" midwifery practices by creating evidence-based guidelines—local and national—that outline assessment and decision pathways to manage various conditions that can arise in pregnancy and childbirth. While the New Zealand College of Midwives is increasingly involved in drafting these guidelines, many midwives feel that these guidelines reduce their autonomy and childbearers' choices. An additional complication for obstetricians in ANZ is that they need to attend to the education guidelines and statements from their collegial body, the Royal Australian and New Zealand College of Obstetricians and Gynecologists. However, as the Australian arm of this college has the majority of the membership and a very different maternity care system, some of these statements and guidelines do not fit well within the ANZ model of practice. In Australia, the multidisciplinary maternity team is under biomedical authority. In contrast, in Aotearoa New Zealand, midwives often view themselves as working collaboratively, rather than hierarchically, with obstetricians. Also, the guidelines generally specify what *should* happen to assess, categorize, and manage complexity in pregnancy, childbirth, and postnatally, rather than who is responsible for ensuring that it *does* happen. Overlapping scopes, knowledges, and skillsets mean that these factors need to be negotiated for each context.

Another issue that can make interprofessional communication difficult is that birthing people have an established relationship with their community midwife, but not with the obstetrician. Meeting in the context of referral or transfer of care can make it challenging for obstetricians to form partnerships with childbearers and to assess the effectiveness of their partnerships with their midwives. Sometimes midwives become advocates for clients to support them in their choices when obstetric interventions may be indicated; but conversely, obstetricians sometimes find that *they* need to be advocates when the relationship with the midwife has broken down—a rare occurrence. Obstetricians can feel constrained by the uncertainty and negotiation skills required in working with clients and midwives. As Clemons and colleagues (2021:36) explained, at the interface between midwives and obstetricians, "[d]etermining who is clinically responsible for a woman, the limits of each health professional's job autonomy, and when their decisions are honored or superseded by whom is complex and continually evolving."

Interprofessional Education (IPE)

Health care is a complex sociotechnical system, and evidence continues to accumulate that the highest standard of patient care requires the development of a healthcare culture based on teamwork (Braithwaite et al. 2009; Salas et al. 2018). Successful interprofessional (IP) teams understand where professional boundaries intersect and end, respect all members of the healthcare workforce, disrupt hierarchies, and activate all members of the healthcare team (McKimm 2010). More than 50 years ago, in 1969, a paper calling for more formal integration was published, entitled "Interprofessional Education (IPE) in the Health Sciences" (see Green 2014). Since then, IPE has been increasingly recognized as an important educational strategy. In 1987, the Centre for the Advancement of Interprofessional Education (CAIPE) was established in the United Kingdom. CAIPE began publishing the *Journal of Interprofessional Care* in 1992, and in 2002 provided the most commonly used definition of IPE (Barr et al. 2017:14), which is: "members or students of two or more professions learn with, from, and about each other to improve collaboration and the quality of care and services."

In ANZ, there are now several internationally recognized interprofessional courses aimed at improving clinical collaboration and practice; the PROMPT (Practical Obstetric Multi-Professional Training) course is one of these. PROMPT was developed in Bristol UK and is aimed particularly at obstetricians and midwives, and is also being extended to include staff from Emergency Departments, Neonatal Intensive Care, and Anesthesiology. The financial costs of running this type of training, which incorporates simulation based learning (SBL), can be considerable, which is why robust evaluation of effectiveness must be incorporated into the implementation strategy (Yau, Pizzo et al. 2016). PROMPT has been shown to reduce technical complications and to improve the safety, attitudes, and teamwork of staff (Shoushtarian et al. 2014; Crofts et al. 2016), which can ultimately be predicted to result in financial cost savings (Yau, Lenguerrand et al. 2021).

A recent review of 46 published IPE research studies provided evidence that this educational strategy is positively accepted by students and leads to improvements in attitudes and perceptions as well as in collaborative knowledge and skills (Reeves et al. 2016). The World Health Organization (WHO) has stated that the role of IPE is "to prepare all health professional students for deliberately working together with the common goal of building a safer and better healthcare" (Gilbert, Yan, and Hoffman 2010:196). Despite this positive statement, IPE has not been universally embedded into undergraduate healthcare professional training programs. The reasons for this lack of inclusion may include the existence of departmental and organizational barriers that make scheduling and the development of interprofessional faculty into challenges. There has also been debate about the optimal timing of an interprofessional intervention, with the suggestion that a professional identity should be developed prior to commencing IPE (Hudson et al. 2017). The alternative view is that taking IPE too late may allow unhelpful stereotypes to develop that can hinder the development of trusting collaborative relationships (Khalili, Hall, and DeLuca 2014). Recent evidence suggests that a professional and interprofessional identity can be developed in parallel, and that professional identity can be enriched by relevant IPE experiences when students feel enabled in the skills of communication and teamwork (Khalili, Orchard et al. 2013; Haugland, Brenna, and Aanes 2019).

Internationally, there is increasing interest in the use of IPE in the practice of midwifery, notably in the UK, the US, and Australia (Murray-Davis et al. 2011; Smith 2015: Avery et al. 2020; Burns et al. 2021), although this interest is less prevalent in ANZ, both within the continuing professional development space and within undergraduate midwifery programs. Midwives in this country have a very specific and unique role in the care of families who are undergoing the normal physiologic and emotional processes of pregnancy and birth. In most situations where the health of the pregnant person and fetus are uncomplicated, the midwife can take full responsibility for antenatal, perinatal, and postnatal care. This contrasts with the care of a medically unwell person (patient), for whom optimal care requires the coordinated practices of a variety of healthcare professionals, including doctors, nurses, physiotherapists, and dietitians. The capacity of midwives to collaborate with other healthcare professionals such as GPs, neonatal pediatricians, community nurses, and obstetricians has also been described as an essential skill to ensure the smooth transition of care when required (Skinner and Foureur 2010; Psaila et al. 2015). The increasing evidence that the management of pregnancy and birth is (unnecessarily) becoming more medically complex emphasizes the relevance of developing these collaborative skills for both obstetricians and midwives to ensure that pregnant people are fully informed and involved in what can be extremely complex decision-making when they require specialist care.

Collegial interprofessional relationships need to be stronger within health care in ANZ. There continue to be concerns raised about poor behavior and episodes of incivility both within and between professions. Some of these may be exacerbated by a lack of opportunity to socialize and a lack of understanding about professional roles. Within ANZ midwifery, there is also evidence for a perceived power imbalance and lack of trust and mutual acquaintanceship in midwives' collaborations with obstetricians (Skinner and Foureur 2010; Skinner and Maude 2016; Clemons et al. 2021). Midwives in ANZ who feel that they are constrained from working autonomously are highly susceptible to burnout and stress-related conditions in both hospital and community settings (Dixon et al. 2017). A UK study concluded that, although midwives are supportive of interprofessional learning for students, they are uncertain whether it will result in changes in practice (Murray-Davis et al. 2011). Further research into IPE specifically in the context of the ANZ maternity care setting is urgently needed to provide evidence of its long-term effectiveness in generating a strong foundation of mutual respect and collaboration with the development of a common professional or interprofessional language in maternity care.

An Action Research Interprofessional Education (IPE) Project

The aim of our action research study was to explore the area of IPE within the context of midwifery and medical education, and to develop an educational intervention from student feedback and observations by experienced clinical educators. As previously noted, the first cycle of our study was held in (pre-COVID) 2019, offering an opportunity for volunteer third-year midwifery and sixth-year trainee intern medical students (four midwifery students and five medical students) to socialize and ask questions about each other's profession and to participate in a collaborative simulation of an emergency scenario. This session validated the research team's expectation that the undergraduate students in these professions had little understanding of each other's knowledge and skillset and were not confident in how to work collaboratively, which is consistent with what has been found in research elsewhere (Murray-Davis et al. 2011; Burns et al. 2021). The feedback from the students was that they enjoyed the opportunity to find out more about each other. However, in the debriefing after the simulation, they discussed that they would have liked additional time before the clinical simulation to plan how they would work together before being placed in that situation.

The medical students expressed conflicting views on midwifery. On the one hand, they talked about how "lucky" midwives are to be able to work with "normal, healthy women" and "develop long-term relationships with women." On the other hand, they noted that they only saw "the bells going off" for the "risky," "high-acuity" hospital births, and that they were afraid of birth. However, they did not seem to realize that midwives and midwifery students would also have been present at those births (midwives are present at almost all ANZ births, even when they are cesarean births). The medical students stated that they struggled to understand how midwifery students could reconcile these kinds of births with a philosophy centered on supporting physiologic birth and did not appear to be swayed by the midwifery students' explanations. The discussion was left at the power of the firsthand experience of being present at a positive physiologic birth and witnessing the joy and empowerment for families that such a birth entails. For their part, the midwifery students tended to overestimate the trainee intern medical students' knowledge in relation to the emergency scenarios and their skills in employing interventions. In this interprofessional context, the midwifery students often stepped back in the hope that technocratic solutions, symbolized by the medical students, could resolve emergency situations. In the debriefing after the simulation, medical students talked about how this made them feel like they had an uncomfortable responsibility to step up, even though they felt that the midwifery students would have had greater knowledge and skills.

The next cycle, working with a different student cohort, took on board the feedback from the original groups, and introduced changes resulting from the evaluation from the research team. This session took place in June 2021 (between lockdowns) and was held with a volunteer student group of seven midwifery and seven medical students. This time, they were provided with details of the clinical scenario in advance and with clinical guidelines that enabled them to prepare themselves for the simulation. Prior to the clinical simulation, they were also given time in the small groups that would undertake the simulation together to discuss their knowledge and plan roles. An actor was brought in to play the laboring woman to increase authenticity, and the session was video recorded. In the initial socializing warm-up, similar assumptions about each other were displayed. The midwifery students asserted that, unlike doctors, "they worked in partnership with women," while the medical students expressed a mix of envy and incredulity that the midwifery students would want to become midwives within the ANZ context. These perceptions may reflect that in recent years, midwifery in ANZ has received significant media attention following a series of pay claims for both community-based and hospital-based midwives, which have highlighted the relatively poor remuneration for midwives in relation to the hours they work and the responsibilities they carry (Bealing 2020). The observation of our research team was that the small group activity of discussing and preplanning the simulation enabled the two groups to find out more about each other and was useful in promoting effective relationships, individual confidence, and mutual respect.

In the debriefing following the simulation, the students were much more positive about the experience than the first group had been. There were profound social and anthropological elements at play that permeated the sessions; these elements link back to the historical influences discussed earlier in this chapter. It appeared that the students began with a framing that assumed biomedical dominance in emergency situations. For example, one of the student midwives in the second-cycle planning session commented slightly sarcastically to a medical student: "You are going to be the doctor, so you take the lead." This comment may have been heard as a light-hearted aside, but it exemplified a perceived sense of hierarchy and what Elaine Burns and colleagues label the predominant "interprofessional conflict discourse" (2021:5). These researchers suggest that the challenge for IPE is to replace this conflict discourse with an "interprofessional collaboration discourse" (2021:5).

In the simulation, the students largely adopted what could be considered to be the expectations of their specific roles. For example, the midwifery students gravitated toward the woman and the baby, modelling the "partnership" relationship that underpins the midwifery philosophy in ANZ, whereas the medical students tended to focus on the clinical tasks and checking the guidelines. However, being able to discuss the simulation scenario in advance enabled one group to decide that a midwifery student who had more experience with these kinds of emergency situations than the trainee interns had would take the coordination role for the simulation of neonatal resuscitation. This enabled the trainee interns to spend some time communicating and sharing information with the woman actor, and it became difficult for the research team observers to distinguish between the two student groups—a most welcome turn of events!

In both rounds of the IPE, students discussed their clinical practice placement experiences. Both the trainee interns and the midwifery students noted observing positive collegial relationships as well as tensions and incivilities between midwives and doctors. The midwifery students talked about how, when needed, the midwives they worked with would seek out the obstetricians and obstetric registrars (residents) in the hospital whom they perceived as more supportive, and "would inwardly groan" when one turned up who, they felt, did not respect the midwife and client decision-making process. They also had witnessed unhelpful and damaging communications among healthcare professionals, such as midwives failing to involve the obstetric team at a point in labor when such intervention may have improved the outcome of the birth, or obstetricians appearing to not respect the advocacy role of the midwife in meeting the wishes of the woman in labor. The trainee interns talked about their personal experiences of some midwives who were rude and unwelcoming and the negative impacts that those kinds of behaviors had on them as students. The students felt that IPE offered opportunities to improve interprofessional collaborations, and that it needed to have happened earlier and more consistently within their respective education programs. In the second group, the students talked about how the IPE experience gave them a glimpse of the potential to be a "new generation" of maternity care professionals who could leave the "old" interprofessional tensions behind.

This IPE study provided us with insights into what could be achieved when students working toward registration in different, yet related, healthcare professions were able to communicate freely and work in a collaborative way within the simulated practice setting. It demonstrated to us that working together in a clinical simulation dealing with emergencies such as postpartum hemorrhage or neonatal life support was far more effective with the introduction of two simple interventions. These were: (1) the introduction of a "get to know you and your profession" activity, which allowed the students to question each other about their respective roles in a relaxed and respectful environment; and (2) a pre-briefing session outlining the scenario for the simulation and strategizing an approach to managing this emergency scenario. Our preliminary findings have led us to conclude that this approach can result in positive outcomes regarding building professional understandings of roles, and further research in the form of conducting more such IPEs is being planned.

In the CAE (collaborative autoethnographic) arm of the study, the research team acknowledged that a shared history had shaped us interprofessionally. As previously noted, there was consensus that there was a stronger sense of hierarchy in our incipient practitioner days, but that somehow it worked because those within this framework "knew their place." We did not view this in a negative way, but as a way in which we as students learned to understand the importance of boundaries—and about appropriate ways to move across them—within the complex world of maternity and health care.

As also previously noted, another influential concept that emerged from the discussions with and observations of the student groups was that of risk. This concept acted as a divider between the contemporaneous student group and the experienced research team members. Within the ideological paradigm of neoliberalism, risk has evolved to be viewed as something that is intolerable, spawning the belief that we can anticipate and control hazards and threats by implementing practices aimed at avoiding or mitigating any risk (Adams, Murphy, and Clark 2009). We have become a "risk-averse society that values control over and security from potential threats" (Jordan and Murphy 2009:181). Consequently, risk management has been incorporated into every corner of Western high-income countries, and particularly so in the fields of science and technology, including biomedicine and other healthcare fields (Sena 2014). In the context of maternity services in ANZ, the epistemology, the research evidence, and the practice guidelines related to risk are part of the obstetric knowledge system and are supported by the broader social moral responsibility to manage known risks. Regarding the concepts of risk aversion and risk management, the CAE group reflected how risk had insidiously become a dominant social concern. We identified how risk was of marginal significance as recently as the 1990s, when the focus was more on "standards of practice" and "healthcare consumer rights" in ANZ. As one of the team members noted, "I'm stunned how little attention anyone in the homebirth movement paid to risk." Conversely, the specter of risk was omnipresent in the student discussions and behaviors in the IPE sessions. This specter raises the question of how the best of the technocratic approach to childbirth can be combined with humanistic relationships and with a holistic understanding of childbirth and its deep significance in families' lives. (Again, see the Introduction to this volume for descriptions of the "technocratic, humanistic, and holistic models of birth and health care.")

Conclusion: The Importance of Teamwork and of Fostering Interprofessional Empathy

Developing a good model for interprofessional education for midwifery and medical students highlights the importance of ensuring that each profession has a clear sense of professional identity and familiarity with the professional skills and roles of others to negotiate, cooperate, and advocate as a team to achieve the best possible outcomes. In Aotearoa New Zealand, obstetrics and midwifery are in many respects now defined in relation to each other: midwives are experts in normal physiologic pregnancies and births and recommend referral to obs when they identify complications. Obstetricians are experts in complex care. While this appears to be an exemplary model, it is often undermined by past and current struggles, and, at times, irreconcilable approaches to childbirth. Too often these differences are not respected nor even discussed in decision-making, and this lack of discussion undermines the potential for creative and effective collaborations. The IPE research that we have conducted indicates that this lack is not an inevitable aspect of the interrelationships between obstetricians and midwives. More workshops that enable medical students, midwives, and other healthcare professionals to share their experiences of being human, uncertain, and self-doubting—the "impostor syndrome"—could foster a much-needed *interprofessional empathy*. In turn, this interprofessional empathy could lead to deeper understanding and respect for each other's professional contributions, generating the potential to enhance teamwork, to broaden the practice scope of each profession, and to replace interprofessional rivalries and resentments with interprofessional collaborations and trust.

Rea Daellenbach is a sociologist who teaches in midwifery and postgraduate health programs at Ara Institute of Canterbury in Christchurch, New Zealand. Her research interests include women's choices for childbirth and the professionalization of midwifery.

Lorna Davies is a midwife and academic who has worked in Aotearoa New Zealand for the past 17 years. She currently serves as an Associate Professor in the midwifery postgraduate program within Te Pukenga, New Zealand. Her specialist research area is sustainability and midwifery, including sustainable approaches to childbirth, self-care, and sustaining the midwifery profession in ANZ.

Maggie Meeks has a clinical role as a neonatal pediatrician at Christchurch Women's Hospital and educational roles in undergraduate and postgraduate simulation training. She is author of *Breech Birth, Woman Wise* ([1998] 2004). She has a particular interest in interprofessional simulation for developing teamwork.

Coleen Caldwell has a clinical role as a medical officer working in Gynecology at Christchurch Women's Hospital, and an educational role as a clinical lecturer in undergraduate and postgraduate education within the Department of Obstetrics and Gynaecology, University of Otago, Christchurch.

Melanie Welfare is a midwife and lecturer in the midwifery program at Ara Institute of Canterbury in Christchurch, New Zealand. She has conducted research on the sustainability of midwifery in New Zealand; her current research focus is on the use of virtual reality simulation in midwifery education.

Judy Ormandy graduated from Otago Medical School and completed her postgraduate obstetrics and gynecology training in Aotearoa New Zealand, the UK, and Papua New Guinea. She has a Masters in Clinical Education from the University of Auckland. She works as an obstetrician and gynecologist at Capital & Coast District Health Board and is a Senior Lecturer in Obstetrics and Gynecology at the University of Otago, Wellington.

Notes

1. "Aotearoa" is the Māori (the Indigenous people) name for this country. Loosely translated from the Māori, it means "land of the long white cloud." Placing "Aotearoa" before "New Zealand" signifies recognition of Māori settlement before British colonization. The Māori migrated from Polynesia around 1,000 years ago. They currently comprise 16.5% of ANZ's population.
2. Lateral or horizontal violence and workplace bullying are considered to be hostile and aggressive behaviors toward a co-worker or group. These are usually attitudinal, behavioral, or verbal and are generally directed against members of one's peer group (McKenna and Boyle 2016; Taylor 2016; Gamble Blakey et al 2018).
3. "Impostor syndrome" describes an experience where the person doubts their competence, skill, or accomplishments and has a fear of being exposed as a fraud (Sakulku and Alexander 2011).

References

Adams V, Murphy M, and Clark AE. 2009. "Anticipation: Technoscience, Life, Affect, Temporality." *Subjectivities* 28: 246–265.
Avery MD, Jennings JC, Germano E, et al. 2020. "Interprofessional Education between Midwifery Students and Obstetrics and Gynecology Residents: An American College of Nurse-Midwives and American College of Obstetricians and Gynecologists Collaboration." *Journal of Midwifery and Women's Health* 65(2): 257–264.

Barr H, Ford J, Gray R, et al. 2017. *Interprofessional Education Guidelines*. Fareham UK: Centre for the Advancement of Interprofessional Education (CAIPE).

Bealing M. 2020. "Sustainable Midwifery: Supporting Improved Wellbeing and Greater Equity." NZIER Report to New Zealand College of Midwives. https://nzier.org.nz/static/media/filer_public/61/26/61265ac7-06a6-43a5-af02-aa77 02f2bfe0/sustainable_midwifery_final_04032020.pdf.

Bell CM, Vest TA, White SJ. 2021. "Dealing with Doubt: Overcoming Impostor Syndrome in New Practitioners." *American Journal of Health System Pharmacy* 79(6): 421–423.

Braithwaite J, Runciman WB, Merry AF. 2009. "Towards Safer, Better Healthcare: Harnessing the Natural Properties of Complex Sociotechnical Systems." *BMJ Quality & Safety* 18: 37–41.

Bryder L. 2014. *The Rise and Fall of National Women's Hospital: A History*. Auckland, New Zealand: Auckland University Press.

Burns E, Duff M, Leggett J, Schmied V. 2021. "Emergency Scenarios in Maternity: An Exploratory Study of a Midwifery and Medical Student Simulation-Based Learning Collaboration." *Women and Birth* 34(6): 563–569.

Chang H, Ngunjiri FW, Hernandez K. 2013. *Collaborative Autoethnography*. Walnut Creek, CA: Left Coast Press.

Clemons J, Gilkison A, Mharapara TL, Dixon L, McAra-Couper J. 2021. "Midwifery Job Autonomy in New Zealand: I Do It All the Time." *Women and Birth* 34(1): 30–37.

Crofts JF, Lenguerrand E, Bentham E, et al. 2016. "Prevention of Brachial Plexus Injury—12 Years of Shoulder Dystocia Training: An Interrupted Time-Series Study." *British Journal of Obstetrics and Gynecology* 123: 111–118.

Crowther S, Deery R, Daellenbach R, et al. 2019. "Joys and Challenges of Relationships in Scotland and New Zealand Rural Midwifery: A Multicentre Study." *Women and Birth* 32: 39–49.

Currie J, Barber CC. 2016. "Pregnancy Gone Wrong: Women's Experiences of Care in Relation to Coping with a Medical Complication in Pregnancy." *New Zealand College of Midwives Journal* 52: 35–40.

Daellenbach R. 1999. *The Paradox of Success and the Challenge of Change: Home Birth Associations of Aotearoa New Zealand*. PhD dissertation. Christchurch, New Zealand: University of Canterbury. https://ir.canterbury.ac.nz/handle/10092/6525.

Davis-Floyd R. 2001. "The Technocratic, Humanistic, and Holistic Paradigms of Childbirth." *International Journal of Gynecology & Obstetrics* 75: S5–S23.

———. 2018. "The Technocratic, Humanistic, and Holistic Paradigms of Birth and Health Care." In *Ways of Knowing about Birth: Mothers, Midwives, Medicine, and Birth Activism*, Davis-Floyd R and Colleagues, 3–44. Long Grove IL: Waveland Press.

———. 2022. *Birth as an American Rite of Passage*, 3rd ed. Abingdon, Oxon: Routledge.

Dixon L, Guilliland K, Pallant J, et al. 2017. "The Emotional Wellbeing of New Zealand Midwives: Comparing Responses for Midwives in Caseloading and Shift Work Settings." *New Zealand College of Midwives Journal* 53: 5–14.

Ellis C, Adams TE, Bochner AP. 2011 "Autoethnography: An Overview." *Forum Qualitative Sozialforschung/ Forum Qualitative Social Research* 12(1): 1–10.

Gamble Blakey A, Anderson L, Smith-Han K. et al. 2018. "Time to Stop Making Things Worse: An Imperative Focus for Healthcare Student Bullying Research." *New Zealand Medical Journal* 131(479): 81–85.

Gilbert JH, Yan J, Hoffman SJ. 2010. "A WHO Report: Framework for Action on Interprofessional Education and Collaborative Practice. *Journal of Allied Health* 39 (Suppl 1): 196–197.

Georges E, Daellenbach R. 2019. "Divergent Meanings and Practices of Childbirth in Greece and New Zealand." In *Birth in Eight Cultures*, eds. Davis-Floyd R, Cheyney M, 121–154. Long Grove IL: Waveland Press.

Green C. 2014. "The Making of the Interprofessional Arena in the United Kingdom: A Social and Political History. *Journal of Interprofessional Care* 28(2): 116–122.

Haugland M, Brenna SJ, Aanes M. 2019. "Interprofessional Education as a Contributor to Professional and Interprofessional Identities." *Journal of Interprofessional Care* 30(4): 1–7.

Hendry C. 2009. "The New Zealand Maternity System: A Midwifery Renaissance." In *Birth Models That Work*, eds. Davis-Floyd R, Barclay S, Daviss BA, Tritten J, 55–88. Berkeley: University of California Press.

Hudson C, Gauvin S, Tabanfar R, et al. 2017. "Promotion of Role Clarification in the Health Care Team Challenge." *Journal of Interprofessional Care* 31(3): 401–403.

Jordan RG, Murphy PA. 2009. "Risk Assessment and Risk Distortion: Finding the Balance." *Journal of Midwifery & Women's Health* 54(3): 191–200.

Khalili H, Hall J, DeLuca S. 2014. "Historical Analysis of Professionalism in Western Societies: Implications for Interprofessional Education and Collaborative Practice." *Journal of Interprofessional Care* 28(2): 92–97.

Khalili H, Orchard C, Laschinger HK, Farah R. 2013. "An Interprofessional Socialization Framework for Developing an Interprofessional Identity among Health Professions Students." *Journal of Interprofessional Care* 27(6): 448–453.

McAra-Couper J, Gilkison A, Crowther S, et al. 2014. "Partnership and Reciprocity with Women Sustain Lead Maternity Carer Midwives in Practice." *New Zealand College of Midwives Journal* 49: 27–31.

McKenna L, Boyle M. 2016. "Midwifery Student Exposure to Workplace Violence in Clinical Settings: An Exploratory Study." *Nurse Education in Practice* 17: 123–127.

McKimm J, Sheehan D, Poole P, et al. 2010. "Interprofessional Learning in Medical Education in New Zealand." *New Zealand Medical Journal* 123(1320): 96–106.

Ministry of Health. 2019. *Report on Maternity 2017.* Wellington, New Zealand: Ministry of Health.

Murray-Davis B, Marshall M, Gordon F. 2011. "What Do Midwives Think about Interprofessional Working and Learning?" *Midwifery* 27(3): 376–381.

Psaila K, Schmied V, Fowler C, Kruske S. 2015. "Interprofessional Collaboration at Transition of Care: Perspectives of Child and Family Health Nurses and Midwives." *Journal of Clinical Nursing* 24(1–2): 160–172.

Reeves S, Fletcher S, Barr H, et al. 2016. "A BEME Systematic Review of the Effects of Interprofessional Education: BEME Guide No. 39." *Medical Teacher* 38(7): 656–668.

Sakulku J, Alexander J. 2011. "The Impostor Phenomenon." *International Journal of Behavioral Science* 6: 73–92.

Salas E, Reyes, D, McDaniel S. 2018. "The Science of Teamwork. Progress, Reflections and the Road Ahead." *American Psychologist Journal* 73: 593–600.

Sena B. 2014. "The Sociological Link between Risk and Responsibility: A Critical Review and a Theoretical Proposal." *International Social Science Journal* 65 (215–216): 79–91.

Shoushtarian M, Barnett M, McMahon F, et al. 2014. "Impact of Introducing Practical Obstetric Multiprofessional Training (PROMPT) into Maternity Units in Victoria, Australia." *British Journal of Obstetrics and Gynaecology* 121: 1710–1718.

Skinner J, Maude R. 2016. "The Tensions of Uncertainty: Midwives Managing Risk in and of Their Practice." *Midwifery* 38: 35–41.

Smith DC. 2015. "Midwife-Physician Collaboration: A Conceptual Framework for Interprofessional Collaborative Practice." *Journal of Midwifery and Women's Health* 60(2): 128–139.

Taylor R. 2016. "Nurses' Perceptions of Horizontal Violence." *Global Qualitative Nursing Research* 3: 1–9.

Yau CW, Pizzo E, Morris S, et al. 2016. "The Cost of Local, Multiprofessional Obstetric Emergencies Training." *Acta Obstetricia et Gynecologica Scandinavica* 95: 1111–1119.

Yau CW, Lenguerrand E, Morris S, et al. 2021. "A Model Based Cost-Utility Analysis of Multi-Professional Simulation Training in Obstetric Emergencies." *PLoS One* 16(3): e0249031.

CHAPTER 11

The Changing Face of Obstetric Practice in the United States as the Percent of Women in the Specialty Has Grown

Deborah McNabb

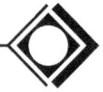

Introduction: The Feminization of Obstetrics

In this chapter about what one might call the "feminization of obstetrics," I will first address why this topic is important to me as a female obstetrician/gynecologist. Next, I will explore with my readers the reasons why female physicians might be better suited to providing empathic, patient-centered care to women, and in so doing, changing the face of the specialty. I will make the case for the value of the empathic patient-provider relationship with its power to decrease suffering and improve health for women. In the latter part of the chapter, I will present the challenges that female obstetricians continue to face, along with suggestions for alleviating those problems. These challenges are important because, if we decide that female obstetricians have made and are making valuable contributions to obstetrics, then the profession needs to address their concerns. Finally, we will look at some concerns about the specialty as women overtake the field, where we are today, and where our goals lie for obstetric health care going forward.

My belief going into this research was that the people who could best tell us whether or not female physicians have changed the face of obstetrics would be patients whose reproductive lifespans bridged the era between when the profession was male only, to now when women truly have a choice to see a female provider. I then thought that the next group whose insights would be valuable would be labor and delivery nurses whose careers bridged that same era. Finally, I thought that it would also be helpful to talk with female obstetric faculty members to learn if they perceived any differences as the obstetric residency classes moved from mostly male to now almost all female. I will share what I have learned from colleagues in these positions; however, my research has shown that the questions and answers are more complex than I had anticipated. As the reader knows, qualitative research is not only affected by the questions one chooses to ask, but also by what the participants choose, consciously or unconsciously, to answer.

Methods

I began this work from an autoethnographic standpoint and have included my experiences throughout. I then conducted interviews with three women obstetricians using open-ended questions. The first, Sue Davidson (her real name), was my co-resident, and after Fellowship training, she later became the Chief of Gynecologic Oncology at the Medical School-University of Colorado Denver. Next was a retired Maternal-Fetal Medicine faculty member and longtime ob/gyn residency program Director who wished to remain anonymous. The last physician, Leslie Cohan (her real name), has recently retired from an ob/gyn private practice. I then interviewed two retired labor and delivery room nurses, both of whom had worked in private and academic settings. One of them wished to remain anonymous, and one, Betsy Daviss, had also worked at a freestanding birth center. These interviews and my own experiences helped to guide further questions going into the extensive literature review that I carried out for the purposes of this chapter.

Feminism in the 1970s

> *"All the students said, 'Men who hate women go into ob/gyn.'"*
> —W. Lee McNabb, 1963 graduate, University of Texas
> Southwestern Medical School, Dallas, TX.

Feminism in the 1970s spawned organizations such as the Boston Women's Health Book Collective, which produced the well-known *Our Bodies, Ourselves* (1970), and the Federation of Feminist Women's Health Centers. Groups like these attempted to fill a gap in biomedicine regarding women's health with their focus on providing accessible information that would empower women to advocate for themselves within the authoritarian biomedical realm (Ruzek and Becker 1999), recognizing that the individual woman knew her own body. Feminist groups also became powerful advocates for women's health at the state and federal levels. In addition to general reproductive health information, this social movement had (and still has) a major focus on reproductive rights. Its members criticized the biomedical system for being oppressive because of authoritarian male physicians who tended to view women as beneath them, intellectually, socially, and regarding decision-making, and for medical research that did not address women's medical needs on par with those of men. Feminists viewed female physicians as simply a part of the male authoritarian biomedical model. One activist, Mary Roth Walsh, was quoted as saying that women were "likely to be co-opted into the medical establishment and, if anything, 'outman the men'" (Wilson 1987:286). They believed that change would come, not as more women entered medicine, but as female patients became more educated about their health needs, more empowered to advocate for themselves in health care, and better able to pressure physicians to change their practices (Lorber 2000).

Feminism and Women's Healthcare Activism in the 1980s and 1990s

Grass-roots feminist groups became less active when institutions, motivated by profits, began to purposely address women's needs. For example, when I started my private practice in the late 1980s, the hospital where I admitted my patients constructed a large "Women's Wing." The CEO said that women typically guided their families' decisions when it came to choosing hospitals, so if the hospital served women's needs well, profits would increase over the entire institution.

In the 1990s in the United States, women's healthcare activism led to the National Institutes of Health's (1991) "Women's Health Initiative," which, for the first time, began to study problems such as cardiovascular disease in women. Breast cancer, a disease previously not discussed in polite company, became less stigmatized as more activists spoke out and advocated for those afflicted with it.

My Biomedical Training

When I told my friends that I had decided to apply to medical school, they were disappointed in me, thinking that I had "sold out" to the biomedical field, which did not respond to women's healthcare needs as it should. I, however, believed that I could make the biggest difference *within* the profession by providing the care that women deserved and by advocating for them as well, bringing their voices to the front of the conversations. In retrospect, I can see that both my friends and I were partly correct.

When I entered medical school in 1980, my class was less than one-third female. At the time, that seemed like a very large step forward because it meant that more women were being admitted to medical schools. I told myself that a new day was dawning. However, I quickly learned that it would take far more than 30% of women in a medical school class to change the male-oriented culture of biomedicine. We were going to need over 50%, which we now have in medical schools today (American Association of Medical Colleges 2020). When I began residency training in 1984, I was excited because my residency class was the first at that institution to be majority female—four women and two men. Once again, a new day was dawning!

Moving forward to 1988, although my home city of San Antonio, Texas, is now the seventh largest in the country, I was one of fewer than ten women practicing ob/gyn in the community. When I went into the surgeon's lounge to grab a sandwich between surgical cases, I was almost always the only woman in the room. At that point, the reality finally sunk in. There would be no quick fixes, nor would there be a paradigm shift toward a more humane standard of care, probably for decades to come. Since the 1970s, I had hoped that as women entered ob/gyn in larger numbers, the specialty would transform into what our patients really needed, but that remained to be seen.

Obstetrics and Gynecology Residency Programs: An Insider's Look

> "I don't care how many nurses you have to sleep with, but just do what you have to do so that the nurses will get you what you need."
> —Chair of the Obstetrics/Gynecology Department
> at an academic medical school, speaking to male
> residents in 1983, anonymous source.

In this section, I first want to share an insider's look into obstetrics and gynecology residency programs. Every obstetrician/gynecologist (ob/gyn) must finish training with proficiency in several surgical procedures, similar to every other surgical specialty. For this reason, the number of residents must be limited to ensure that every trainee has the number of surgical cases necessary to achieve that competency. However, ob/gyn programs differ from other surgical specialties because of the obstetric component, which does indeed bring the most joy to the profession. Yet when a public program limits the number of residents to ensure surgical competence, there are never enough residents to cover the busy obstetric services. The physical demands of an ob/gyn residency are, therefore, brutal. Due to the exhaustion, a resident might find herself sitting in a chair across from a patient, feeling like she, the resident, was more miserable than the patient in front of her. In that setting, I, along with my co-residents, were at risk of losing our capacity for empathy and our reserve of the milk of human kindness. As a retired anonymous female Maternal-Fetal Medicine faculty and ob/gyn residency program director put it: "When I arrived, I learned that the medical students thought that the female residents were more toxic than the male residents."

Prior to the mid-1980s, at least, the entire US maternity care system was based on a male authoritarian model with almost all male faculty. Women were just beginning to enter the specialty in that era, and most of us believed that to survive and be successful, we had to be even tougher than our male co-residents. In addition to fitting into the biomedical culture, female residents found it harder to be taken seriously by other hospital staff. It was common knowledge that "If a female surgeon in the operating room behaves in the same respectful but authoritative manner as a male surgeon, she is regarded as a 'bitch'" (Susan Davidson, retired Chief of Gynecologic Oncology, Medical School-University of Colorado Denver). The common response to the lack of respect, unfortunately, was for women physicians to be even more authoritarian and tough with the staff in the clinic or hospital setting. So yes, at least in training, women were typically co-opted into the male model. Occasionally, they were also co-opted into the male model of relating to patients. As an example, two women in my residency program were known as the "Doberman Sisters." And yet, as an anonymous retired nurse whose career spanned antepartum care, labor and delivery, and teaching at a nursing school described:

> I observed a contrast between the older, more authoritarian male physicians and the younger female obstetricians who had a kinder, more cooperative demeanor and related to their patients with a woman-to-woman connection. I think that the older male obstetricians saw these young women as a threat.

Will Women Be Able to Make Humanistic Changes in Obstetric Practice?

Happily, as soon as I entered private practice, I encountered hospital staff who fostered a collegial atmosphere. I was no longer having to "make it in a man's world," because the only people I needed to please were my patients, and I quickly found that missing reservoir of the milk of human kindness and joy in my connections with patients. Could women who trained during a time when faculty, and the profession as a whole, were dominated by men, be able to approach patient care differently than that of their colleagues and teachers? Would it take, instead, ever larger numbers of women in ob/gyn residency programs, or increasing numbers of female faculty members, or even increasing numbers of post-residency female ob/gyns in the community to drive that change?

As I did, in 1982 Elianne Riska (2001:179) asked, "Will women physicians be able to 'humanize' [biomedicine]?" Some feminist scholars argued that women were, essentially, different from men. They believed that as women entered medicine in ever larger numbers, they would bring more empathy and more caring approaches with them, and that sexism on the part of physicians toward female patients would cease to exist. The follow-up question was: Will women change medicine or will medicine change women? But then in 2000, Judith Lorber (2001:13) again asked, looking back, "Has [the] presence [of women in medicine] made a difference in women's health care, or have they assimilated men's biases and perspectives?" And here I am, more than 20 years later, asking the same questions. To best serve women's reproductive health care needs, this is important information to have for the training of future physicians.

Nevertheless, I do want to state that there are many good men in ob/gyn—men who do an excellent job of treating women with respect and empathy, as well as being excellent practitioners. I was a woman who had male gynecologists when there was no other option, and I was, mostly, happy with the care that I received. I trained at a time when there were no female ob/gyn faculty members at my institutions, but most of the male faculty had a high level of respect for our patients and were committed to providing what was considered to be the best obstetric care at that point in time. Perhaps I had excellent faculty in my residency program because it was a relatively new medical center, and the founding Chair and many of the faculty had trained in New York City, so they might have been more enlightened than others in less progressive regions about feminists' criticisms of the profession and responded accordingly. Also, when I changed my private practice to gynecology only, I tended to recommend a male colleague with whom I had trained to my patients when they became pregnant. I told them, "He's just like me except he has a mustache!" They were universally happy that they had chosen him as their obstetrician.

Humanizing Biomedicine and Introducing the Ethics of Care into Obstetric Practice

Since the 1960s at least, those who study the biomedical profession have been talking about the significance of the patient-physician relationship and its fundamental importance in healing. Initially, it was a group of theologians who raised the concern that biomedicine had become so technology-oriented that the distance between patient and provider was growing ever wider (Fox 1985). They were then joined by philosophers and others interested in making biomedicine more humane and centered on the patient-physician relationship, as opposed to centering primarily on algorithms, lab work, and imaging studies (Fox 1985; Ramsey 2002; Carson 2011). This movement began the field of Medical Humanities, closely followed by Bioethics. Now "Medical Humanities" is more commonly called "Health Humanities" to turn the focus of education toward nurses and other medical staff, in addition to physicians. Areas of study within the Health Humanities, such as literature and medicine, as well as philosophy, bioethics, history, religion, anthropology, and sociology, have been found to be beneficial in efforts to increase empathic capacity in students (Trautman 1982; Hunter 1987; Murray 1987; Marshall 1992; Barnard 1998; Charon 2001; Jones 2013).

Jumping forward to the early 1980s, we began to see an interest among child psychologists in the development of the moral imagination of not just boys, but also girls, and later, to consider what impacts these traits found in women might have in improving patient health. Though the concept of care ethics has valid critiques, I think that it is important to recognize as we look at larger numbers of women physicians entering ob/gyn. A novel (at that time) moral theory known as "the ethics of care" came to prominence in the 1980s through the work of psychologist Carol Gilligan (1982) and writings from philosopher Nel Noddings (1984). Care ethics holds that, as human beings, relationships are of primary importance to us; thus the practice of reciprocal caring is universally basic to humanity. These relationships can be dyadic, or between large groups, or even human to animal. The mechanism in these relationships of care is imagined to be that the "one caring" perceives the needs of the "one cared for" through the latter's perspective, and then attempts, when possible, to help alleviate those needs. In biomedical maternity care, this would mean that the obstetrician's focus would be *not* on what *she* thinks the patient needs, but on what the *patient* feels that they need. Since relationships are universally important, there are times in life when everyone needs care, as well as times when we are all called upon to provide care.

As in almost every aspect of life at the time, the standard of moral development was male, and females were evaluated against a male standard. Gilligan's mentor in the Psychology Department at Harvard, Lawrence Kohlberg, had noted from his studies that in boys, moral development led to principled thinking, prioritizing universal values such as autonomy, independence, and justice. In contrast, Gilligan's work led her to conclude that female moral development was not inferior to the male model, but was instead "a different voice," focused more on the contexts of relationships and caring rather than on universal principles such as rights and justice.

I also believe that, in addition to girls and women being trained to be caregivers, they have also been silenced in society, just as people of color and LGBTQQIA+ (lesbian, gay, bisexual, transgender, queer, questioning, intersex, asexual) folks are often silenced because their perspectives are less valued. Those who are silenced tend to be good listeners and observers, sometimes in the interest of survival. If this is true, then we would expect to see that differences in women and men would narrow over time as our society progresses. As Gilligan (2011) later said, "Within a *patriarchal* framework, care is a feminine ethic. Within a *democratic* framework, care is a human ethic" (italics in original). Further, as with any other supposed male versus female distinction, I assume a range of abilities between the sexes with regard to perceiving the needs of the other through the other's eyes, willingness to help the other, and then taking that action. It follows that throughout history, there have been men who excelled as caregivers and women who fell short at that capability and vice versa. However, since women began entering ob/gyn residencies in larger numbers in the late 1970s, for the purposes of this chapter, I will assume that, at least at that point in time, care ethics was a concept that mostly applied to girls and women.

The Importance of the Capacity to Empathize with the Patient

According to Francis Peabody (1927), "One of the essential qualities of the clinician is interest in humanity, for the secret of the care of the patient is in caring for the patient." Essential for care ethics is the capacity to empathize, because that is the factor involved in understanding the cared-for person's point of view and needs. If the physician can learn to see a situation from the patient's point of view, and if the physician places a high value on the welfare of patients who are different from her, she achieves the capacity for empathy (Riess 2017). Frans Derksen, Jozien Bensing, and Antoine Lagro-Janssen (2012) describe empathy as having three components, including: (1) an affective attitude; (2) a cognitive competency; and (3) a behavior. It follows that a high capacity for empathy is necessary for a strong patient-provider connection. To be clear, empathy does *not* mean that the obstetrician feels what the patient feels. Rather, empathy is the ability to *imagine* and *understand* what the pregnant person in front of her may be experiencing; that is, to imagine and understand their journey, their desires, their fears, and their pain. As healthcare providers, we know that a strong connection with a patient furthers that patient's wellbeing and decreases their suffering for a variety of reasons. Anyone, especially a person in the vulnerable role of a patient, feels confirmed and valued when they feel heard, when the provider listens attentively and demonstrates understanding and compassion (Zachariae et al. 2003). The empathic connection generates trust, so the patient is more likely to divulge information that would lead to a more accurate assessment of their problem, and they also are more likely to try to follow the provider's recommendations (Vermeire et al. 2001). If an ob/gyn needs a more self-centered motive to pursue this strong connection with her patient, we also know that, should the physician commit a medical error, the patient who feels a strong sense of empathy and relationship with that physician is more likely to give them the benefit of the doubt and less likely to bring a lawsuit (Beckman et al.1994). And studies (although complex) demonstrate that, rather than empathy contributing to burnout among physicians, a strong patient-provider connection leads to more satisfaction in the practice of biomedicine (Hojat Vergare, Isenberg et al. 2015; Hunt et al. 2017; Morgan et al. 2021).

Mohammadreza Hojat and colleagues (2001) at the Jefferson Medical College in Philadelphia, Pennsylvania, developed the Jefferson Scale of Physician Empathy (JSPE), still widely used today. The first large study using this validated instrument was with physicians and their diabetic patients in Parma, Italy. In this study, high scores by physicians on the JSPE were significantly correlated with better outcomes for their patients, measured by the incidence of acute metabolic complications requiring hospitalization (Del Canale et al. 2012). Similar findings have been seen in the United States in many areas of medicine with different types of patient groups. Unfortunately, these days when physicians have more severe time constraints and are focused on their computers, entering a never-ending amount of data, it is all too easy to look at the screen, neglecting to focus on the patient, which leads to the risk of neglecting the close "reading" of the patient. Empathy and the empathic connection suffer without that focus on the patient, so their health care is impaired; therefore, strategies to turn our attention back to our patients are critical. As William Osler put it in 1899 in his "Address to the

Students of the Albany Medical College": "Care more for the individual patient than for the special features of the disease . . . Put yourself in [their] place . . . The kindly word, the cheerful greeting, the sympathetic look—these the patient understands."

The American Association of Medical Colleges (2019) has named empathy an essential learning objective. Empathetic skills can be taught and improved upon, even if one must start at a fairly rudimentary level. However, if a student comes to training already having a deep capacity for empathy, she has an easier time absorbing these lessons. Both male and female students show significant declines in empathy scores in the third year of medical school, and even further erosion in residency. The difference is that women's scores decrease less sharply than men's (Chen et al. 2012), and women start out with significantly higher scores than men, so the female trainees' nadirs in empathy scores are comparable to the men's highest scores (Hojat, Vergare, Maxwell, et al. 2009).

Hojat and colleagues have demonstrated not only that female students and physicians scored higher on the JSPE but also that trainees in "patient-oriented" specialties, such as primary care and ob/gyn, scored higher than trainees in technology-oriented specialties such as orthopedic surgery, radiology, and anesthesiology (Hojat et al. 2002a). In their next study that year (Hojat et al. 2002b), they looked at empathic capacity, studying more than 700 physicians of all ages in an academic medical center, and confirming that women consistently scored higher than men. Significant gender differences were found in responses to statements such as, "I believe that empathy is an important therapeutic factor in medical treatment" and "I consider understanding my patients' body language as important as verbal communication in caregiver-patient relationships" (Hojat et al. 2002b:S59). They also found that "gender differences [were] more pronounced on the 'perspective taking' aspect of physician empathy" (Hojat et al. 2002b: S60). In addition, this study reconfirmed that, when controlling for gender, physicians in people-oriented specialties consistently outscored those in technology-oriented fields. A notable difference in one type of specialty versus another was found in this statement: "An important component of the relationship with my patients is my understanding of the emotional status of themselves and their families" (quoted in Hojat et al. 2002b:S60).

These findings have been duplicated in meta-analyses (Roter, Hall, and Aoki 2002), as well as with other methods of scaling empathy, such as the Empathic Communication Coding System (ECCS) (Bylund and Makoul 2002). A 2012 longitudinal study with more than 1,100 medical student participants again showed that women and physicians in people-oriented specialties had higher empathic scores on the JSPE (Chen et al. 2012).

The Partnership Model of Communication

"Patient outcomes depend on a partnership model of communication."
—Committee on Patient Safety and Quality Improvement.
"Effective Patient-Physician Communication." American
College of Obstetricians and Gynecologists, February 2014

Prior to the major studies on physician empathy, there had been a large body of information gathered on gender differences in communication skills within biomedicine. For at least three decades and continuing, Debra L. Roter and Judith A. Hall (2014) have studied, along with colleagues across the United States and internationally, the dynamics and importance of physician communication to patient-centered medicine. They have looked at physicians of different genders, races/ethnicities, and social backgrounds, along with physicians in different countries. They have also studied patient groups with these different characteristics, as well as patients with different types of illnesses and even normal pregnancies. Among other things, they have found that both physicians and patients are experts with different areas of expertise. Physicians are experts in the technical and cognitive ways that are emphasized in their training. Patients are experts in their history and their experiences of illness, personality, lifestyle, life setting, values, and expectations (Roter, Frankel et al. 2006). The lesson here is that the patient-provider relationship depends on both partners in the dyad to further the goal of improving health and decreasing suffering.

In the early 1990s, Debra Roter, Mack Lipkin, Jr., and Audrey Korsgaard (1991) analyzed audiotapes of more than 500 patients with chronic diseases and their primary care physicians, comparing male and female physicians. They found that male physicians spent an average of 20.3 minutes per patient visit, while female physicians spent significantly more time at 22.9 minutes. Both patients and physicians talked more in the history-gathering segment when the physicians were women, with female physicians talking 40% more and their patients talking nearly 60% more. I see this finding as particularly important because, in most encounters, the patients will give you their own diagnosis when you take their history. All the physician needs to do is ask questions, listen carefully, ask follow-up questions, and read the patient's body language. What is gained in this approach, which only requires a couple of minutes more, is that the provider is able to narrow down the range of possible diagnoses and can then pursue more targeted testing—all of that plus a better patient-physician connection to boot! Why *do* patients talk more with female physicians? It might have something to do with what are called "partnership statements."

In the early 1990s, investigators evaluated female and male first-year residents up to faculty physicians in Internal Medicine on partnership statements and "back-channel responses," among other categories, in the setting of routine medical visits with patients (Hall, Irish et al. 1994). "Partnership talk" was defined as "requests for the other's opinion" or "requests for understanding." This describes a true partnership in which the perspectives of both patients and physicians are seen as valuable. Examples of "back-channel" responses by physicians were "mmhmm," "yeah," "okay," and "right!" as well as nodding as the patient spoke. These responses indicated that the physician was paying attention and was ready to hear more from the patient. As in the previous study, female physicians spent more time with patients, both the physicians and patients spoke more in these encounters—and further, female physicians and their patients split the talking time in half at a far higher rate than did male physicians with their patients. "Friendliness ratings" were the highest in same-sex communications, which adds to the argument that female obstetricians may be best-suited to care for pregnant people. To me, this also says that our society would benefit from having more female than male physicians in general, because in the latest data from 2016, women constituted a significant majority of all patient visits in primary care settings (Centers for Disease Control 2019). The two studies noted above found that female patients spoke more when the physician was female. In addition to the patient's assumption that the female physician might be more welcoming in receiving patient input, perhaps the patients are less intimidated by female physicians, and/or female physicians have encouraged that input in both verbal and nonverbal ways.

Of even greater concern was a 1993 study in which the researcher reviewed videotapes of physician-patient interviews and found that male physicians overwhelmingly used "explicit commands" for their directives, while female physicians "minimize[d] distinctions between themselves and their patients" in their directives, by saying things like, 'Let's do such and such'" (West 1993:61). During this same period of time, it was also found that women did not express a preference for female physicians *except* when choosing their ob/gyns (Elstad 1994). When this study was published in 1994, female ob/gyns were just becoming available in larger numbers, and women were beginning to have a choice in their provider's gender. Additionally, researchers found that female physicians, as opposed to male physicians, were also more willing to allow their patients to see them as imperfect, as they would consult references or other physicians *during* their patient visits (Shapiro 1990). Just as important as all the studies noted above is that female physicians engaged in more psychosocial and emotional talk, which then encouraged their patients to reveal problems in those areas because they felt more comfortable, instead of having to initiate such conversations uninvited (Roter et al. 1991).

These types of communication are important to all ob/gyn patient interactions. First, women suffer higher rates of depression and anxiety than men, though thankfully, women are more likely to raise this problem with their healthcare provider(s) (Addis and Mahalik 2003; Kuehner 2017). Teenagers get depressed, have difficulties with body image, and so forth. Working moms do far more housework and childcare than their male partners; hence ob/gyns see depression in this patient population. Perimenopausal women not only struggle with physical symptoms, but also with the existential issues of growing older in a society that values younger women. Postpartum depression (PPD) is quite common and can be fatal. Obstetricians are now supposed to screen postpartum patients for PPD, but it can't be known for certain what happens in each office. If the physician walks into the room with an open question such as, "How's it going?" or "How are you doing?" or even a directive question like, "Are you getting enough sleep?" that obstetrician is nearly guaranteed a longer patient visit than the time allotted, so some physicians will simply not pursue this type of information. These psychosocial and emotional conversations are essential to patient care, but they take empathy and a willingness to put the patient's needs before one's own—character traits that I believe are found more often in female physicians. Again, I cannot overemphasize how the time pressures placed on ob/gyns currently in practice affect their willingness and ability to extend visit lengths. There is no getting around the fact that an adequate amount of time is essential if a patient and physician are going to establish a solid connection built on communication and empathy, so that the patient's primary concerns can be addressed and their health improved.

Judith Lorber's (2000) literature review confirmed what had been noted previously: that women physicians seemed to be less intimidating to patients so that patients spoke out more freely; women doctors talked more to their patients and allowed their patients to talk more to them, especially about psychosocial issues; and women's nonverbal communication styles were superior to those of male physicians.

One of the available models to improve trainee communication is the "Five Step Patient-Centered Interviewing" technique (Fortin 2012).

Briefly, this technique involves: (1) setting the stage by welcoming the patient, introducing yourself, using the patient's name, and sitting down; (2) asking about the patient's chief concerns and summarizing them back to the patient so that the patient knows they have been heard, while also mentioning any time constraints beforehand; (3) helping the patient to express herself by using open-ended questions, listening carefully, and attending to nonverbal cues; (4) focusing on the symptom story within the patient's personal context and eliciting and responding to the emotional content in the story; and (5) checking the accuracy of your summary of the problems with the patient.

According to Betsy Daviss, a retired labor and delivery nurse whose career spanned different academic and private hospitals: "When I began my career in 1976, I thought that the female obstetricians were better at listening and picking up nonverbal cues from patients. But, as I went through the decades, the male trainees became more and more empathic. By that point, a physician's empathy was more a product of a personality trait than it was gender-related."

Physicians' communication skills are very important, but, again, there are two people in this dyadic connection. In a meta-analysis published in 2002, the researchers moved away from a "physician-centric" focus and began to look at the communication behaviors of patients to see if there were differences in how patients spoke to female or male physicians (Hall and Roter 2002).

In the studies reviewed, there were more than 1,500 patients and 250 physicians, all in primary care. Based on the studies cited previously, I can say that the findings were predictable. Patients spent more time talking to and gave more information to female physicians. Interestingly, both female and male patients interrupted female physicians more often. Several reasons could account for this phenomenon. One reason could be a relative lack of respect that would typically be given to male physicians because female physicians were more likely to be younger than male physicians, and it may be that there were some unfounded suspicions on the part of patients that the expertise of female physicians was less than that of male physicians. On the other hand, these interruptions could be reflective of trust in the physician so that patients feel more comfortable asserting their needs, questions, and opinions.

A meta-analysis carried out by Debra Roter, Judith Hall, and Yutaka Aoki (2004) summarized all of the findings previously noted. After evaluating 24 qualifying studies in primary care settings and two additional studies in obstetrics and gynecology, they learned that, when comparing female to male physicians, women spent more time with their patients (except in one of the ob/gyn studies); engaged in more partnership building by eliciting more patient input (and patients were also more likely to engage in partnership building with them); spent more time on emotional and psychosocial talk, looking at the broader contexts of their patients' lives; split the dialogue with patients on a more even basis; used more nonverbal clues to let the patient know that they were paying close attention; received more disclosures from patients, who were also more assertive with the female physicians; observed and recorded more diagnoses of psychosocial problems; and, again, were more comfortable allowing patients to see them as imperfect. The best observed patient-physician connections were in female-to-female dyads. In all the included studies, the differences noted between female and male physicians were small yet nevertheless statistically significant. As a male physician who was quoted in Lewin (2001) stated, "I think it's similar to certain fields where women have to work harder to prove themselves. Men in this field have to be more sensitive."

It is important to recognize that almost all of the studies cited above were carried out in primary care settings. In the few studies directly focused on obstetrics and gynecology, men performed better than they had in primary care at spending more time with patients, demonstrating more empathy, and placing a high priority on patient-centered behaviors (Roter, Geller, et al. 1999; van Dulmen 2000). Perhaps ob/gyn is a specialty where men have modeled female physicians' behavior to attract patients, or perhaps men with these kinds of traits self-select for ob/gyn. Further, these improved capacities in male obstetricians might simply be due to the effects of a younger generation in a society that has made progress with respect to women. Though it might be easier, clearly, one does not have to be a woman to empathize with female patients. When I began my career, I had never had a baby, experienced postpartum depression, or knew what the perimenopausal experience felt like, and I was fortunate to never have had to experience a reproductive system malignancy. But I believed, and my patients confirmed, that my empathic, communicative, and patient-centered skills were on target. I also believe that men, particularly men in this current generation, can be expected to achieve that same level of competence.

By now in this chapter, I have confirmed that, because of societal norms regarding womanhood, women have, in general, been more empathic and better at patient-centered communication than men. With all the other characteristics of an excellent physician being equal (which they are), it would seem that female physicians should be preferred over male physicians. Is that the case?

Examples of Gender Expectations

> *"All I'm asking is for a little respect."*
> —Otis Redding. "Respect." Song popularized by Aretha Franklin.

Here's an everyday example of gender expectations of which I've even found myself to be guilty. You see a woman at a grocery store with her child in the shopping cart seat, and you barely notice her. But, when you see a man with *his* child in the shopping cart, you're likely to think, "Wow! What a great guy to be doing the grocery shopping while caring for his child!" Sad but true. The expectations of the female gender in our society are that women are to display gentleness, empathy, nurturance, and better skills in listening, open communication, and caretaking. If men show these same characteristics, we find them remarkable, but for women who meet this standard, they are not particularly remarkable because they are simply behaving the way they are supposed to behave. This standard applies to female physicians, in that if patients' expectations are not met, the disappointment is greater than with the lower expectations of male physicians (Roter and Hall 2004; Mast, Hall, and Roter 2007; Blanch-Hartigan et al. 2010; Hall, Blanch-Hartigan, and Roter 2011; Hall, Gulbrandsen, and Dahl 2014), whereas if their expectations of the female physicians *are* met, the female providers get no extra credit (Roter and Hall 2014).

Roter and Hall (1998) concluded that the stereotypical male characteristics of competence, authority, expertise, independence, and self-confidence are essential to patient care when combined with the equally essential stereotypical female characteristics of warmth, sensitivity, a caring attitude, a relationship orientation, and interpersonal responsiveness. Thus, the characteristics that have always been considered to be female capabilities are now being recognized as essential to a high standard of biomedical practice. Of note, both the Institute of Medicine and the Patient Protection and Affordable Care Act frequently mention the importance of patient-centered care, which "also connotes an emotional connection such that the patient doesn't just feel cared for, but also cared about" (Roter and Hall 2014:273).

After gaining a full understanding of the importance of empathy to women's health, the evidence that female physicians perform at a higher level compared to male physicians when it comes to empathy, communication, and patient-centered behavior, and the reality that female physicians get little credit for these behaviors, it's time to turn to the quality of health care provided by female physicians. Do the behaviors of female physicians with regards to empathy, communication, and patient-centered care affect the quality of their medical care?

Not only has it been demonstrated repeatedly that in primary care settings, female physicians are more likely to provide preventive health counseling and screening for diseases for both male and female patients (Henderson and Weisman 2001), there is also data showing that female physicians achieve better patient outcomes in a variety of diseases in different settings (Henderson and Weisman 2001; Berthold and Gouni-Berthold 2008; Gouni-Berthold and Berthold 2011). These differences were thought to be due to better physician-patient communication, spending more time with patients, and emphasizing more preventive measures. Lower pregnancy rates in teenagers in a primary care setting were also seen when physicians were younger and/or female, and when nurses (the vast majority of whom are female) had more time to spend with patients (Hippisley-Cox, Allen, and Pringle 2000).

In addition to female physicians' communication styles, the difference could also be that female physicians reported less difficulty in discussing sexual problems, sexually transmitted disease prevention, and condom use. Additionally, in a study of more than 1.5 million elderly hospitalized patients, the patients of female internists had significantly lower mortality and 30-day readmission rates than those of the male internists (Tsugawa and Jena 2017).

Do Women Prefer Female Ob/Gyns?

> *A female obstetrician responding to an older male physician who said*
> *that he was shocked that patients preferred female obstetricians:*
> *"Too many years of patriarchy and cold speculums!"*[1]
> —Leslie Cohan, recently retired ob/gyn

Several studies support the validity of this claim that women prefer female ob/gyns. In a survey completed by 200 women attending an ob/gyn clinic, though nearly half of the respondents did not express a preference, the overwhelming majority of those who did express a preference wanted a female ob/gyn (Baskett 2002). A literature review (J. Marshall 2004) indicated that patients placed more importance on experience, reputation, interpersonal and communication styles, technical expertise, bedside manner, and competence than on physician gender, but when it came to choosing an obstetrician/gynecologist, the importance of the statement, "Doctor is female" rose remarkably. In a 2020 survey across the United States with more than 1,000 respondents designed to gauge their physician preferences, 51% of women said that it didn't matter with non-ob/gyn physicians, but when it came to ob/gyn physicians, everything else being equal, a full 66% of women preferred a female obstetrician (Tam and Hill 2020). I agree with some important points that Candace West (1993) made regarding physicians' gender. She reminded us that gender is a social construct, that we only need to mention it because the stereotypical characteristics of females and males have been "baked into" our society, and that, hopefully, a day will come when gender distinctions carry no significance.

The Particular Challenges Faced by Female Ob/Gyns

> Burnout:
> *"Disconnection from ourselves*
> *Loss of soul*
> *Emotional exhaustion*
> *Always on duty—somewhere."*
> —Fronek and Brubacker, "Burnout Woman-Style: The Female
> Face of Burnout in Obstetrics and Gynecology" (2019:466–468)

Moving on from patient preferences, I now address the particular challenges that female obstetricians face. The first is burnout, described in various ways, including those mentioned in the quotation at the beginning of this section. Burnout includes signs and symptoms of emotional exhaustion, depersonalization, and a diminished sense of meaning in one's work.

Female physician burnout rates are increasing in the United States at almost twice the rate of male physicians. Women are also disproportionately affected by anxiety/depression, which increases the risk of burnout. Over 71% of female physicians "report a considerable gap between their actual lives and their ideal lives" (Fronek and Brubacker 2019:468) as opposed to less than half of male physicians reporting that concern. It is extremely important to address burnout in physicians, not only because keeping women in the physician workforce is important to women's health in general, but also because burnout can be associated with suicidal ideations.

Several factors may contribute to the disproportionate burden of burnout experienced by female obstetricians. First, when female physicians are compared to the general female population, they take longer to conceive a child, require infertility treatment more often, have higher-risk pregnancies, and more miscarriages (Rangel et al. 2021). Pregnancy risks correlate with burnout symptoms. Next, female physicians receive less respect in the professional environment than male physicians do. While female physicians are frequently mistaken for nurses, this almost never happens to male physicians. Further, I have reviewed the increasing difficulty in providing good patient care due to time constraints. As previously noted, whereas male physicians may respond to time pressures by limiting psychosocial conversations, female physicians tend to extend the patient encounter time to include those types of conversations. If a female obstetrician/gynecologist spends an extra two-to-three minutes with each patient, that extra time can lengthen her working day by 30 minutes to an hour, with more electronic medical records (EMR) homework later (West 1993). To adjust to the patient visit time constraints, female physicians tend to schedule fewer patients in a day or work part-time; however, female part-time physicians spend even longer amounts of time on each patient visit!

Women physicians have higher expectations of themselves than male physicians do, so they tend to fall into self-blame more easily. An example of these higher expectations is that women physicians report that they would like to have more than one-third more time to spend with patients, while male physicians say that they would like to have one-fifth more time (Fronek and Brubaker 2019). Another factor has to do with conflict resolution, which is necessary in any profession. In childhood, boys can play rough, so they develop skills in tolerating conflict and conflict resolution. When girls play, they tend to value the relationship over resolving the conflict; therefore, girls don't get that practice early on. As previously noted, girls are also socialized to show tenderness, kindness, and sharing, and are not supposed to show aggression. When women are as assertive as male physicians, they tend to be described as "bossy" or "shrill," which, as I know from my own experience, is somewhat exhausting to endure time and time again.

Most likely, though, the primary causes of female obstetrician burnout are their added responsibilities on the home front. Certainly, the reasons why there was not as much burnout among obstetricians in the past included the lack of interference in patient care by insurance companies, fewer time restrictions on patient visits, and the fact that there were no such things as electronic medical records. But undoubtedly, another major factor was that, back then, obstetricians were men, and they all had wives! Women are always working, even at home, where they are more responsible for child care, elder care, and housework. To this day, only half of male physicians' spouses work outside of the home, while almost all female physicians' spouses do (Fronek and Brubaker 2019). In this study, only 5% of women's spouses performed "most or all duties at home," whereas more than 80% of men's spouses did so. Female physicians who had a supportive partner had a 40% less risk of burnout. Among surgeons, two-thirds of women "had experienced a work-home conflict in the previous three weeks" (Fronek and Brubaker 2019:469). However much a "work-life balance" is discussed in the literature as necessary to prevent burnout, it is quite rare to read a commentary that includes a critique of female obstetricians' partners. Fronek and Brubaker (2019) report various strategies used to combat female ob/gyn burnout, such as mindfulness, cognitive behavioral therapy, self-care, exercise, developing resilience, paying attention to meaningful events, reframing problems as "life lessons," and participating in support groups. For more such suggestions, see the chapter by Robbie Davis-Floyd (2023) in Volume II of this series, also briefly described in the Introduction to this volume). While these interventions are undoubtedly helpful, they all have one thing in common—they throw the responsibility back on the individual woman rather than addressing systemic social issues. My advice to young female obstetricians is that, especially if you want to have children, finding that partner who will carry at least half of the burden on the home front is critical and can be lifesaving.

With electronic medical records, it is now common for physicians to catch up on documentation at home. But for female ob/gyns, that "homework" typically does not start until the children have gone to bed, entailing less sleep. As the ob/gyn workforce becomes dominated by women, burnout, which Davis-Floyd (2023) would call "Substage" or "losing it," becomes an ever more critical issue. Social and institutional supports are essential. Physicians should have more reasonable time allotments for patients, more control over their work environments, and a decrease in electronic medical record responsibilities.

Are Female Obstetricians Benefiting from the Large Growth in Their Numbers?

> *"Gender stereotypes can contribute to falling salaries*
> *as female share increases."*
> —Pelley and Carnes, "When a Specialty Becomes
> 'Women's Work': Trends in and Implications of
> Specialty Gender Segregation in Medicine." (2020:1503)

As of 2018, over 80% of ob/gyn residents were women and nearly 60% of ob/gyn practitioners were female. Are female obstetricians benefiting from this growth in their numbers? Unfortunately, I am not optimistic.

Gender segregation is normative in the US workforce. Over 40% of men work in occupations where more than three-quarters of the workers are male, whereas only 6% of women work in those jobs (Pelley and Carnes 2020). The same patterns are seen in biomedicine. Despite the increasing numbers of female physicians, from less than 10% in 1970 to about half of trainees now, there has been no decrease in gender segregation. Pediatrics, psychiatry, and now ob/gyn are predominantly female specialties, while orthopedics and neurosurgery residents are predominately male, with only small changes since 1980, except for ob/gyn (Pelley and Carnes 2020). When a specialty reaches the level of just under half females, that is known as the "tipping point" where men's participation in the specialty begins to decrease. Pediatrics and ob/gyn are past this tipping point, but gender equity in these fields, in terms of prestige and pay, is not even close to the fields of orthopedics and neurosurgery.

Looking at reimbursements and salaries, I find that there are parallels between the worlds outside and inside of biomedicine. At every level of skill, female-predominant occupations (>75% female) earn less than gender-integrated occupations (25–75% female), which earn less than male-predominant occupations. When the numbers of women go up in a particular occupation, the earnings and prestige go down, because traits associated with women (warmth, kindness, helpfulness) are lower status than those associated with men (strong, independent, competitive). In the world of today's biomedicine, procedures are reimbursed at a much higher rate than spending time with patients and using one's cognitive faculties. This must change if we are to improve health care. We need our brightest and most empathic physicians providing direct patient care in primary care specialties like family medicine, internal medicine, pediatrics, and ob/gyn, instead of our best physicians following a purely surgical track for a better income. Early on in this chapter, I raised the question of what the field of ob/gyn would look like once we had larger numbers of female faculty at academic medical centers. That question is important, because it is at those upper faculty echelons where decisions are made about how obstetricians are trained, what subject areas are emphasized or de-emphasized, where money for research projects goes, which public policies the profession should support or oppose, standards of care, and how physicians in that specialty will be evaluated. Unfortunately, since I began training more than four decades ago, female ob/gyns have not reached those upper echelons in significant numbers. (There may be a component of women's choice here, because some female ob/gyns may not want to work in a male-dominated environment.) While we do have more female faculty in the United States now, they tend to be in the lower-ranked positions. In ob/gyn academic medicine, women are paid less than men (on average 36,000 USD per year less than men, correcting for typical variables that affect pay) and are promoted less and at slower rates, so women in senior faculty positions are still at unacceptably low numbers (Hughes and Bernstein 2018).

By 2017, nearly 60% of practicing ob/gyns were female, so it is time to look forward as we continue to witness the feminization of obstetrics (Orvos 2017). I see both potential advantages and disadvantages of the feminization of the biomedical workforce in general, and the field of obstetrics and gynecology in particular, as the physician workforce begins to mirror the gender (im)balance in our society (Levinson and Lurie 2004). Women excel at patient-centered care, so patient-physician relationships are expected to improve, and with that, improved quality of medical care. We now recognize that multidisciplinary team approaches to patient care in chronic disease management are associated with improved outcomes, and women are well-suited to this style of patient care. Studies of leadership styles indicate that women empower other team members to develop their potential and mentor team members, in what is called "transformative leadership" (Roesner 1990).

Women are also more likely to serve uninsured patients and to advocate for single-payer national health insurance (Crandall 1997; McCormick et al. 2004). Further, we need primary care practitioners more than any other specialties in medicine, and women tend to enter primary care fields, including ob/gyn, in greater numbers. Women do work fewer hours and take time off for raising children, but they tend to retire later than men, so those deficits in the workforce get made up over time (Batchelor 1990).

Women are also changing the profession to accommodate physicians who are also working parents as they attempt to balance career and family responsibilities. These changes, along with shared home responsibilities becoming more common as our society progresses, will benefit women, and also men and children. Women's skills in negotiating, teamwork, and leadership still need to be developed so that female ob/gyns don't have to "settle" for less money or worse working conditions.

The three biggest contributions that I think female obstetricians have made, and continue to make, to women's health care are women-modeled empathy, strong communication skills, and patient-centered behavior—all of which have now become the standard of care. Women have set the standard in direct patient care because, in my experience, their medical skills are as good as, if not better than, those of male physicians; women physicians are superior to male physicians in the "art" of medicine; and women use their voices, platforms, and power to advocate vigorously for their patients. Though it has taken decades to make this progress, I believe that female physicians' contributions to obstetrics and gynecology have been remarkable and deserve to be fostered, supported, and valued.

Deborah McNabb is a retired ob/gyn who had a solo private practice in San Antonio, Texas. She is now a PhD Candidate in Bioethics and Health Humanities at the University of Texas Medical Branch in Galveston, Texas. Her research focuses on the power of empathy to reduce stigma experienced by marginalized patient groups, particularly those who are seeking or who have had abortions. She is also interested in the value of using patient narratives to augment the capacity for empathy in trainees.

Note

1. "Speculums" are instruments used to open the vagina for exams. "Cold speculums" refers to the long-term usage of metal speculums during routine vaginal exams. Considerate ob/gyns would warm up these metal speculums with hot water; inconsiderate ones would not. Yet for years now, disposable plastic speculums (which, obviously, do not get cold) have been used instead of metal ones.

References

Addis ME, Mahalik JR. 2003. "Men, Masculinity, and the Contexts of Help Seeking." *American Psychologist* 58 (1): 5–14.

American Association of Medical Colleges. 2019. "Association of American Medical Colleges Medical School Objectives Project." Retrieved 5 August 2022 from http//www.aamc.org/meded/msop/msop1.pdf.

———. 2020. "More Students Are Entering Medical School." *AAMC.org*, 16 December. https://www.aamc.org/news-insights/more-students-are-entering-medical-school.

Barnard D. 1998. "The Coevolution of Bioethics and the Medical Humanities with Palliative Care, 1967–97." *Journal of Palliative Medicine* 1(2):187–193.

Baskett TF. 2002. "What Women Want: Don't Call Us Clients, and We Prefer Female Doctors." *Women's Health* 24(7): 572–574.

Batchelor AJ. 1990. "Senior Women Physicians: The Question of Retirement." *New York State Journal of Medicine* 90: 292–294.

Beckman HB, Markakis KM, Suchman AL, et. al. 1994. "The Doctor-Patient Relationship and Malpractice: Lessons from Plaintiff Depositions." *Archives of Internal Medicine* 154: 1365–1370.

Berthold HK, Gouni-Berthold I. 2008. "Physician Gender Is Associated with the Quality of Type 2 Diabetes Care." *Journal of Internal Medicine* 264: 340–350.

Blanch-Hartigan D, Hall JA, Roter DL, et. al. 2010. "Gender Bias in Patients' Perceptions of Patient-Centered Behaviors." *Patient Education and Counseling* 80(3): 315–320.

Boston Women's Health Book Collective 1970. *Our Bodies, Ourselves*. New York: Simon and Schuster.

Bylund CL, Makoul G. 2002. "Empathic Communication and Gender in the Physician-Patient Encounter." *Patient Education and Counseling* 48: 207–216.

Carson RA. 2011. "On Metaphysical Concentration: Language and Meaning in Patient-Physician Relations." *Journal of Medicine and Philosophy* 36(4): 385–93.

Centers for Disease Control and Prevention (CDC). 2019. "Data from the National Ambulatory Medical Care Survey, 2016." *NCHS Data Brief No. 331*. Retrieved 1 January 2022 from https://www.cdc.gov/nchs/data/databriefs/db331-h.pdf.

Charon, R. 2001. "Narrative Medicine: A Model for Empathy, Reflection, and Trust." *Journal of the American Medical Association* 286(15): 1897–1902.

Chen DCR, Kirshenbaum DS, Yan J, et al. 2012. "Characterizing Changes in Student Empathy throughout Medical School." *Medical Teacher* 34(4): 305–511.

Crandall SJ, Volk RJ, Cacy D. 1997. "A Longitudinal Investigation of Medical Student Attitudes towards the Medically Indigent." *Teaching and Learning in Medicine* 9: 254–260.

Davis-Floyd R. 2023. "Open and Closed Knowledge Systems, the 4 Stages of Cognition, and the Cultural Management of Birth." In *Cognition, Risk, and Responsibility in Obstetrics: Anthropological Analyses and Critiques of Obstetricians' Practices*, eds. Davis-Floyd R, Premkumar A, Chapter 1. New York: Berghahn Books.

Del Canale S, Louis DZ, Vittorio M, et. al. 2012. "Physician Empathy and Disease Complications: An Empirical Study of Primary Care Physicians and Their Diabetic Patients in Parma, Italy." *Academic Medicine* 86: 1243–1249.

Derksen F, Bensing J, Lagro-Janssen A. 2012. "Effectiveness of Empathy in General Practice: A Systematic Review." *British Journal of General Practice* 63(606): e76–84.

Elstad JI. 1994. "Women's Priorities Regarding Physician Behavior and Their Preference for a Female Physician." *Women's Health* 21: 1–19.

Fortin AH, Dwamena FC, Frankel RM, Smith RC. 2012. *Smith's Patient-Centered Interviewing: An Evidence-Based Method*, 3rd edn. New York NY: McGraw Hill.

Fox DM. 1985. "Who We Are: The Political Origins of the Medical Humanities." *Theoretical Medicine* 6 (3): 327–341.

Fronek H, Brubaker L. 2019. "Burnout Woman-Style: The Female Face of Burnout in Obstetrics and Gynecology." *Clinical Obstetrics and Gynecology* 62(3): 466–479.

Gilligan C. 1982. *In a Different Voice*. Cambridge MA: Harvard University Press.

———. 2011. "Looking Back to Look Forward: Revisiting *In a Different Voice*." *Classics@Journal*. Retrieved 12 December 2022 from https://classics-at.chs.harvard.edu/classics9-carol-gilligan-looking-back-to-look-forward-revisiting-in-a-different-voice/.

Gouni-Berthold I, Berthold HK. 2011. "Role of Physician Gender in the Quality of Care of Cardiometabolic Diseases." *Current Pharmaceutical Design* 17: 3690–3698.

Hall JA, Blanch-Hartigan D, Roter DL. 2011. "Patients' Satisfaction with Male Versus Female Physicians: A Meta-Analysis." *Medical Care* 49(7): 611–617.

Hall JA, Gulbrandsen P, Dahl FA. 2014. "Physician Gender, Physician Patient-Centered Behavior, and Patient Satisfaction: A Study in Three Practice Settings within a Hospital." *Patient Education and Counseling* 95(3): 313–318.

Hall JA, Irish JT, Roter DL, et. al. 1994. "Gender in Medical Encounters: An Analysis of Physician and Patient Communication in a Primary Care Setting." *Health Psychology* 13(5): 384–392.

Hall JA, Roter DL. 2002. "Do Patients Talk Differently to Male and Female Physicians? A Meta-Analytic Review." *Patient Education and Counseling* 48: 217–224.

Henderson JT, Weisman CS. 2001. "Physician Gender Effects on Preventive Screening and Counseling: An Analysis of Male and Female Patients' Health Care Experiences." *Medical Care* 39(12): 1281–1292.

Hippisley-Cox J, Allen J, Pringle M. 2000. "Association Between Teenage Pregnancy Rates and the Age and Sex of General Practitioners: Cross Sectional Survey in Trent 1994–1997." *British Medical Journal* 320: 842–845.

Hojat M, Gonnella JS, Nasca TJ, et al. 2002a. "Physician Empathy: Definition, Measurement and Relationship to Gender and Specialty." *American Journal of Psychiatry* 159(9): 1563–1569.

———. 2002b. "The Jefferson Scale of Physician Empathy: Further Psychometric Data and Differences by Gender and Specialty at Item Level." *Academic Medicine* 77(10): S58–60.

Hojat M, Mangione S, Nasca TG, et. al. 2001. "The Jefferson Scale of Physician Empathy: Development and Preliminary Psychometric Data." *Educational Psychology Measurements* 61: 349–365.

Hojat M, Vergare M, Isenberg G, et. al. 2015. "Underlying Construct of Empathy, Optimism, and Burnout in Medical Students." *International Journal of Medical Education* 6: 12–16.

Hojat M, Vergare MJ, Maxwell K, et. al. 2009. "The Devil Is in the Third Year: A Longitudinal Study of Erosion of Empathy in Medical School." *Academic Medicine* 84(9): 1182–1191.

Hughes F, Bernstein PS. 2018. "Sexism in Obstetrics and Gynecology: Not Just a 'Women's Issue.'" *Call to Action Supplement, American Journal of Obstetrics and Gynecology* 219(4): 364–366.

Hunt PA, Denieffe S, Gooney M. 2017. "Burnout and its Relationship to Empathy in Nursing." *Journal of Research in Nursing* 22 (1–2): 7–22.

Hunter K. 1987. "What We Do: The Humanities and the Interpretation of Medicine." *Theoretical Medicine* 8: 337–367.

Jones AH. 2013. "Why Teach Literature and Medicine? Answers from Three Decades." *Journal of Medical Humanities* 34 (4): 415–428.

Kuehner C. 2017. "Why is Depression More Common among Women than among Men?" *Lancet* 4(2): 146–158.

Levinson W, Lurie N. 2004. "When Most Doctors Are Women: What Lies Ahead?" *Annals of Internal Medicine* 141: 471–474.

Lewin T. 2001. "Women's Health Is No Longer a Man's World." *New York Times*, 7 February.

Lorber J. 2000. "What Impact Have Women Physicians Had on Women's Health?" *Journal of the American Medical Women's Association* 55(1): 13–15.

Marshall JF. 2004. "A Guest Editorial: What Do Women Want? What Do We Think Women Want?" *Obstetrical and Gynecological Survey* 59(7): 487–488.

Marshall PA. 1992. "Anthropology and Bioethics." *Medical Anthropology Quarterly* 6: 49–73.

Mast MS, Hall JA, Roter DL. 2007. "Disentangling Physician Sex and Physician Communication Style: Their Effects on Patient Satisfaction in a Virtual Medical Visit." *Patient Education and Counseling* 68: 16–22.

McCormick D, Himmelstein DU, Woolhandler S, et. al. 2004. "Single-Payer National Health Insurance: Physicians' Views." *Archives of Internal Medicine* 164: 300–304.

Morgan DS, Blanch-Hartigan D, Aleksanyan T, et al. 2021. "Empathy, Friend or Foe? Untangling the Relationship between Empathy and Burnout in Helping Professions." *Journal of Social Psychology* Nov 25: 1–20.

Murray TH. 1987. "Medical Ethics, Moral Philosophy and Moral Tradition." *Social Science and Medicine* 25: 637–644.

National Institutes of Health. 1991. "Women's Health Initiative." Retrieved 12 December 2022 from https://www.nhlbi.nih.gov/science/womens-health-initiativewhi.

Noddings N. 1984. *Caring: A Feminine Approach to Ethics and Moral Education.* Berkeley: University of California Press.

Osler W. 1899. "Address to the Students of the Albany Medical College." *Albany Medical Annals* 20.

Orvos JM. 2017. "ACOG Releases New Study on Ob/Gyn Workforce." *Contemporary OB/GYN* 62(7): 50–52.

Peabody F. 1927. "The Care of the Patient." *Journal of the American Medical Association* 88(12): 877–882.

Pelley E, Carnes M. 2020. "When a Specialty Becomes 'Women's Work': Trends in and Implications of Specialty Gender Segregation in Medicine." *Academic Medicine* 95(10): 1499–1506.

Ramsey P. 2002. *The Patient as Person: Exploration in Medical Ethics*, 2nd ed. New Haven CT: Yale University Press.

Rangel EL, Castillo-Angeles M, Easter SR, et al. 2021. "Incidence of Infertility and Pregnancy Complications in US Female Surgeons." *JAMA Surgery* 156(10): 905–915.

Riess H. 2017. "The Science of Empathy." *Journal of Patient Experience* 4(2): 74–77.

Riska E. 2001. "Towards Gender Balance: But Will Women Physicians Have an Impact on Medicine?" *Social Science and Medicine* 52: 179–187.

Roesner J. 1990. "Ways Women Lead." *Harvard Business Review* 68(6): 119–125.

Roter DL, Frankel RM, Hall JA, et. al. 2006. "The Expression of Emotion through Nonverbal Behavior in Medical Visits: Mechanisms and Outcomes." *Journal of General Internal Medicine* 21: S28–34.

Roter DL, Hall JA. 1998. "Why Physician Gender Matters in Shaping the Physician-Patient Relationship." *Journal of Women's Health* 7(9): 1093–1097.

———. 2004. "Physician Gender and Patient-Centered Communication: A Critical Review of Empirical Research." *Annual Review of Public Health* 25: 497–519.

———. 2014. "Women Doctors Don't Get the Credit They Deserve." *Journal of General Internal Medicine* 30(3): 273–274.

Roter DL, Hall JA, Aoki Y. 2002. "Physician Gender Effects in Medical Communication: A Meta-Analytic Review." *Journal of the American Medical Association* 288: 756–840.

Roter DL, Geller G, Bernhardt BA, et. al. 1999. "Effects of Obstetrician Gender on Communication and Patient Satisfaction." *Obstetrics and Gynecology* 93(5, pt 1): 635–641.

Roter DL, Lipkin, Jr. M, Korsgaard A. 1991. "Sex Differences in Patients' and Physicians' Communication during Primary Care Visits." *Medical Care* 29(11): 1083–1093.

Ruzek CB, Becker J. 1999. "The Women's Health Movement in the United States: From Grassroots Activism to Professional Agendas." *Journal of the American Medical Women's Association* 54(1): 4–8.

Shapiro J. 1990. "Patterns of Psychosocial Performance in the Doctor-Patient Encounter: A Study of Family Practice Residents." *Social Science and Medicine* 31: 1035–1041.

Tam TY, Hill AM. 2020. "Female Patient Preferences Regarding Physician Gender: A National Survey." *Minerva Ginecologia* 72(1): 25–29.

Trautmann J. 1982. "The Wonders of Literature in Medical Education." *Mobius* 2(3): 22–31.

Tsugawa T, Jena A. 2017. "Comparison of Hospital Mortality and Readmission Rates for Medicare Patients Treated by Male and Female Physicians." *Journal of the American Medical Association Internal Medicine* 177(2): 206–213.

Van Dulmen AN, Bensing JM. 2000. "Gender Differences in Gynecologist Communication." *Women's Health* 30: 49–61.

Vermeire E, Hearnshaw H, Van Royen P, et al. 2001. "Patient Adherence to Treatment: Three Decades of Research. A Comprehensive Review." *Journal of Clinical Pharmacological Therapy* 26: 331–342.

West C. 1993. "Reconceptualizing Gender in Physician-Patient Relationships." *Social Science and Medicine* 36(1): 57–66.

Wilson MP. 1987. "Making a Difference—Women, Medicine, and the Twenty-First Century." *Yale Journal of Biology and Medicine* 60: 273–288.

Zachariae R, Pedersen CG, Jensen A, et al. 2003. "Association of Perceived Physician Communication Style with Patient Satisfaction, Distress, Cancer-Related Self-Efficacy, and Perceived Control over the Disease." *British Journal of Cancer* 88: 658–665.

The Ethnographic Challenges of Gaining Access to Obstetricians for Surveys, Interviews, and Observations

The Ethnographic Challenges of Gaining Access to Obstetricians for Surveys, Interviews, and Observations

Robbie Davis-Floyd and Ashish Premkumar

Part 3 of this volume contains only this chapter; we had to give it a section of its own because it doesn't fit with the topics discussed in the preceding chapters, which focused on the possibilities for the humanization and de-colonization of obstetrics. In this chapter, we focus on a new, important, and intriguing subject: the ethnographic challenges faced by social scientists who seek to study the generally closed fields of maternity care wards and obstetricians' ideologies and practices. For example, it can be quite difficult to obtain permission to conduct ethnographic fieldwork in hospitals that includes observing obstetricians' behaviors during births. Obs are often resistant to observers, to being observed, and to sitting down for interviews. Here we recall Stuart Shapin's chapter on "How to Be Antiscientific" (2001:101), in which he stated:

> [M]embers of a family are permitted to say things about family affairs that outsiders are not allowed to say. It is not just a matter of truth or accuracy; it is a matter of decorum. Certain kinds of description will be heard as unwarranted criticism if they come from those thought to lack the moral or intellectual rights to make them.

And this is the case in the (usually) Stage 1, silo-oriented obstetric profession. So how did our chapter authors manage? What barriers did they encounter, and how did they overcome them? To answer these questions, we series editors—Robbie and Ashish—asked the chapter authors of Volumes II and III, who are mostly social scientists, how they met the ethnographic challenges of finding and interviewing obstetricians and observing their practice behaviors; most of them responded (see below). We didn't ask the authors of the chapters in Volume I (Davis-Floyd and Premkumar 2023a) to respond to our questions, as they are all obstetricians and/or perinatologists with easy access to their colleagues and to facilities, and their chapters are primarily autoethnographic. In what follows, we won't provide specific references in the reference section to the chapters we discuss, but only the chapter titles, as all the specific chapters we mention below can easily be referenced via referencing their appearances in Volumes II and III of this series (Davis-Floyd and Premkumar 2023b, 2023c).

Reponses from the Chapter Authors of Volume II

Cognition, Risk, and Responsibility in Obstetrics: Anthropological Analyses and Critiques of Obstetricians' Practices

Series editor Robbie Davis-Floyd, author of Volume II, Chapter 1 on "Open and Closed Knowledge Systems, the 4 Stages of Cognition, and the Obstetric Management of Birth," did not interview obstetricians specifically for that chapter, but rather based a great deal of it on her extensive past experiences of interviewing obs. Robbie made her first attempts to access obs for the writing of her article "Obstetric Training as a Rite of Passage" in 1987 by cold-calling 30 obs' offices seeking to make interview appointments; it took her months to make those appointments with the only 13 obs who agreed to the interviews.

In dramatic contrast, Robbie found it very easy to access obs after she was invited to speak at a conference of the American Holistic Medical Association (AHMA) in the early 1990s. Surrounded by doctors who had made a paradigm shift to holistic practice, amazed to see them dancing during the ballroom dinner while singing "I've got the healin' spirit, way down deep in my so-oul!" and eager to learn why, she whipped out the tape recorder she used to always carry (this was long before smartphones) and began to interview these physicians, some of whom were ob/gyns. She attended and gave talks at these AHMA conferences for the next four years,[1] interviewing more holistic physicians each time, for a total of 20—seemingly a small number, but the most she could do, as it was hard to find times for interviews during these action-packed conferences. This process culminated in her lead authorship of *From Doctor to Healer: The Transformative Journey* (1998). Her co-author was Gloria St.

John, a psychologist who had been running support groups for holistic physicians in San Francisco to help them deal with the ostracisms and persecutions they were experiencing, and who formally interviewed 20 of them. (Thus their book is based on 40 in-person interviews and 60 stories emailed to Robbie from holistic obs who wished to be included.) In general, as Robbie and other authors have found, Stage 4, open-minded (see Introduction) humanistic and holistic obs are easier to gain access to than technocratic obstetricians, as those who have made a paradigm shift are usually very eager to talk about it.

Later, together with her colleague Eugenia (Nia) Georges, Robbie traveled throughout Brazil giving talks and interviewing 32 humanistic and holistic obstetricians, who called themselves "the good guys and girls" (the "bad guys and girls" being the ones who did too many cesareans) (see their chapter in this volume). Finding them was also easy because they were all members of ReHuNa (Network for the Humanization of Birth), an activist group working to humanize Brazilian birth (thus to find one was to find all), and because all of them had read Robbie's books and had heard her speak at conferences all over Brazil. They said that her book *Birth as an American Rite of Passage* ([1992] 2003) had shown them *that* they needed to change and *why*, and that the book *From Doctor to Healer* had shown them *how* to change, as that book lays out various paths that they could follow. We include this information not to aggrandize Robbie, but to show that *social science works can make large differences in practitioners' ideologies and care*, as sociologist Beverley Chalmers did for the maternity care practitioners in the countries in which she worked (see her chapter in this volume and below).

Regarding Volume II, Chapter 2, "From 'Mastership' to Active Management of Labor: The Culture of Irish Obstetrics and Obstetricians," by Margaret Dunlea, Martina Hynan, Jo Murphy-Lawless, Magdalena Ohaja, Malgorzata Stach, and Jeannine Webster, one of these authors, Margaret Dunlea, carried out direct interviews with obstetricians as part of her PhD fieldwork. In addition to submitting the always-required detailed application to her university's ethics committee, with whom she then met, she also submitted applications to and met with the ethics committees of the hospitals where she planned to collect data. Access to the obstetricians formed part of the ethics approval application process and thus was unproblematic for Margaret.

Eugenia (Nia) Georges, medical anthropologist and author of Volume II, Chapter 3 titled "Becoming an Obstetrician in Greece: Medical Training, Informal Scripts, and the Routinization of Cesarean Births," relied on the networks she had built over many years of conducting research on birth in Greece; she told us:

Studying maternity care in the public sector requires relationships built on trust. For this reason, I have always initiated each project by depending on respected and trusted individuals who were willing to introduce me and my project to the hospital directors, obstetricians, and midwives key to my research. For the current project, I relied on these previously established contacts to develop a snowball sample of the obstetricians and midwives who are attempting to address the issues central to my chapter: Greece's high cesarean rate (65%) and the exponential increase in late preterm deliveries over the last few years. With the help of my research assistant, who is doing her residency in ob/gyn, I also generated a snowball sample of other current residents to interview about their training. While this strategy has worked well for me, an abiding challenge is scheduling (and rescheduling) interviews due to the busy and unpredictable work lives of my interlocutors.

This "abiding challenge" was also faced by many other chapter authors, as they describe below.

Michelle Sadler, a medical anthropologist, and Gonzalo Leiva, a practicing midwife, authors of Volume II, Chapter 4 on "Physiologic Birth Entails Economic Damage: Financial Incentives for the Performance of Cesareans in Chile," explained that:

Within the context of a project funded by the Ministry of Health, we got access to three big public maternities. The respective Health Services and Women's Health Directors of each institution opened the ground to interview the staff. We extended the invitation to participate to all ob/gyns, and a few accepted. In private hospitals, because none of them accepted to be part in the study as a whole, we did snowball sampling starting from medical staff we knew (midwives and ob/gyns) and asking them to contact colleagues. In both health sectors, the ob/gyns with a more humanistic approach towards childbirth were much easier to engage than those with a more technocratic one. But, because the aim of the study was to get a full range of approaches, we kept looking and insisting until we interviewed some ob/gyns with a fully technocratic approach.

Due to the difficulties in scheduling interviews, in some cases we had several short encounters (of around 20–25 minutes each) with one ob/gyn during their lunch or other breaks. In public maternities, most interviews were carried out during their work shifts, and for that reason, many of the interviews were interrupted one or more times with cases they had to attend. It could take up to a full shift to complete an interview, but we would do it while carrying out observations.

Regarding the flow of the conversations, most of the ob/gyns talked from a third-person standpoint, describing how things were done by others and not engaging in describing their own practices. We knew that some of the doctors interviewed had very high rates of interventions and of cesareans, yet nonetheless, most of them were describing the benefits of vaginal birth and the harms of cesarean births. So, as a strategy, when we were not getting information on their own beliefs and practices regarding childbirth (further than textbook "medical" information), we asked about their *colleagues'* practices and approaches towards childbirth. And in that way, we were able to get a full range of positions/views. In a few interviews, the doctors opened up in very profound ways, talking in depth about the vices of the system and giving thorough examples. In these cases, after long encounters, we scheduled further meetings to continue the interviews.

When COVID struck, we were beginning to carry out more interviews with ob/gyns to complement and deepen the previous fieldwork. The contact process this time was much easier, in part because we could carry out the interviews by Zoom, which allows a greater flexibility in schedules/places. Some interviews were conducted late at night when they were in their homes, for example after their children had gone to sleep.

This was also the case for other ethnographers who conducted their research during the pandemic; Zoom interviews allow for a scheduling flexibility that in-person interviews do not. But they also, to some extent, remove the possibility of affective connections between the interviewers and the interlocutors. Regarding the role of emotions in fieldwork, which, interestingly, none of our chapter authors addressed, we add here some words of wisdom from the authors of *Pregnancy and Birth in Russia*, sociologists Anna Temkina, Anastasia Novkunskaya, and Daria Litvina (2022:16), who pointed out that:

> Interaction between scholars and research participants/interlocutors is a bilateral process that reveals new knowledge both for the researcher and for the interlocutor as the researcher guides the latter through sequential reflection . . . Many researchers see huge analytical potential in the emotional responses that we see, feel, or produce in the field: "The greatest source of analytic value occurs during what we call the emotional overlap, or those moments during fieldwork when the emotions of both the informant and the ethnog-

rapher are shared" (Feldman and Mandache 2019:229). Whenever we ignore or exclude those moments from analysis as "biases," we impoverish our dataset and ourselves.

We (Robbie and Ashish) heartily agree, and ask other ethnographers to also consider, work with, and write about the roles of emotions in their fieldwork (see, for example, Arditti et al. 2010).

Obstetrician Nicholas Rubashkin, who is also a PhD student in Global Health Sciences and author of Volume II, Chapter 6 on "Scoring Women, Calculating Risk: The MFMU VBAC Calculator" responded that because he is an ob/gyn himself, as expected, he had few issues with getting access to maternity care sites and to other obs. Yet he did confront a different kind of major challenge, which for him was in learning to "make the familiar strange"—a term he picked up during his academic studies. He said:

I found that in my early interviews with ob/gyns, the transcripts read like pat discussions of risks and benefits. I think as ob/gyns we get really used to repeating the standard of care over and over in our discussions with each other and in our oral board examinations, such that in research interviews we have really prepared ways of saying things. So initially in my interviews, I was challenged to push people beyond the typical standard-of-care discussion. I asked ob/gyns to talk about controversial TOLAC/VBAC [trial of labor after cesarean/vaginal birth after cesarean] cases—complications that they had experienced themselves. For more established physicians, I asked how their approach to TOLAC/VBAC had evolved over time, which was also helpful for generating discussion. Ob/gyn trainees were great to interview because they were much more open about their ethical struggles.

Also, it was super important for me to triangulate with multiple sources. I was studying the VBAC calculator, and I recorded prenatal visits where providers introduced the calculator to their pregnant patients. These recordings really helped me to understand how providers *actually* talked about risk and benefits and technologies with patients, which was different than with me as a colleague/interviewer. My colleagues didn't feel comfortable having me sit in the room and take notes during VBAC consultations—that felt too embarrassing to them, as if I were going to correct their VBAC counseling or something. But they were open to me leaving a recorder in the room.

Finally, my interviews with women were revealing too in terms of how they remembered their ob/gyn's talking about the calculator. Also, interviewing women outside clinical settings and over the course of the entire pregnancy really helped me to get rich data. Many ob/gyns had the experience that presenting the VBAC calculator to women was easy and uncontroversial . . . BUT, outside the clinic, women had a lot to say about the calculator that they never would have said to their providers.

Anthropologist Lydia Zacher Dixon, co-author of Volume II, Chapter 7 "On Risk and Responsibility: Contextualizing Practice among Mexican Obstetricians," was initially able to observe and interview obstetricians through her connections with the CASA School of Professional Midwives in San Miguel, Guanajuato, Mexico—one of the few schools in Mexico that trains professional midwives (see Mills and Davis-Floyd 2009 for a description). An obstetrician who had long worked with the CASA Hospital and School was on staff as an ob at the local general hospital. He connected Lydia with the doctor in charge of hospital training and research, and through that contact, she was able to submit her proposal. Once this doctor had the staff review it, they approved Lydia's research project: "Then, once I arrived in Mexico, I met with him to get my proper paperwork, badge, etc. He announced to the obs that I would be there to observe, though I repeated my consent process with each ob prior to observing with them or interviewing them, to make sure that I had their individual consent."

Lydia's chapter co-author, Vania Smith-Oka, told us that her process of gaining access was similar to Lydia's:

> I've worked at a few different hospitals, and in some cases I received approval by the *Jefe de Enseñanza* (Research/Teaching Director) of the hospital; in others I simply received permission from the Hospital Director, and in others I have gone through the hospital's ethics boards. Once I was given permission, I would be provided with papers to show the hospital's approval of my presence (a badge, letter). Usually, one of the directors would then introduce me and my research to others; this would often include a tour of the hospital to get a sense of the place and the people. In any of these examples, I would always have IRB [Institutional Review Board] approval from my home institution, which would include the consent process as part of the conversation.

According to Katherine McCabe, author of Volume II, Chapter 9 on "The Limitations of Understanding Structural Inequality: Obstetricians Accounts of Caring for Substance-Using Patients in the United

States," she employed a purposive and snowball sampling strategy to access biomedical providers. McCabe sampled from five maternity care hospitals in the Chicago area by sending out 116 email solicitations to obs and neonatologists with publicly accessible email addresses. The original solicitation invited them to participate in an interview about their observations and experiences in working with substance using patients. McCabe's email recruitment resulted in 21 participants agreeing to meet for an interview; the fact that only 21 responded out of the 116 contacted again reveals how difficult it can be to reach obs and other biomedical practitioners, and the importance of *perseverance* and *patience* with the process. McCabe subsequently recruited an additional 9 participants via snowball sampling, for a total of 30 interviews, of which 13 were with obs. She noted that some of the more interesting challenges in the research process played out in the interviews themselves, as these interviews were loosely structured to capture the provision of care for substance using patients, including questions regarding how substance use was determined, drug screening and testing practices, hospital procedures and treatment protocols, professionals' attitudes toward substance using patients, medical interventions for maternal substance use, and child welfare involvement. McCabe stated:

> As an outsider (a medical sociologist with an interest in reproductive justice), I was able to ask questions about concepts, language, and practices that may have been taken for granted by providers. For example, I would ask providers to define terms like "clinically-indicated," particularly as it relates to toxicology screening, and this often rendered really interesting results—namely, it revealed a slippage in clinical and diagnostic norms in the provision of care for suspected substance users. As a sociologist, I was also able to position myself as having an interest in social inequality and racial disparities. I found that asking openly about racial and class inequalities was surprisingly productive: providers were often explicitly aware of racial profiling in drug testing practices, and some even admitted to profiling.
>
> This runs counter to so much work that emphasizes the implicit, unconscious nature of racial disparities in maternal care. I think that being positioned as an outsider, and specifically as a sociologist who studies inequality, may explain the types of conversations that arose that highlighted structural inequality as a causal factor in shaping maternal health for substance-using women (the topic of the chapter). On the flip side, I am unsure how deeply embedded these forms of structural causal thinking are in the clinical culture,

as I did not do an ethnography and must rely on what emerged from the interviews.

Community health specialist Melissa Goldin Evans, author of Volume II, Chapter 10 on "Contraceptive Provision by Obstetricians/Gynecologists in the United States: Biases, Misperceptions and Barriers to an Essential Reproductive Health Service," was an intern with the Louisiana Public Health Institute during her graduate program around 2013, helping them to collect information about interpregnancy care delivery and services in the Greater New Orleans area by conducting semi-structured interviews with ob/gyn providers (mostly obstetricians) and patients: "We gained access to providers for interviews via existing relationships, and then it was a snowball sampling technique to reach other providers and patients. We never observed them."

Responses from the Chapter Authors of Volume III

Obstetric Violence and Systemic Disparities: Can Obstetrics Be Humanized and De-Colonized?

For sociologist Lauren Diamond-Brown's chapter in this present volume on "'Selfish Mothers,' 'Misinformed' Childbearers, and 'Control Freaks': Gendered Tropes in US Obstetricians' Justifications for Delegitimizing Patient Autonomy in Childbirth," Lauren said that she had hoped to observe in the labor and delivery unit of a particular hospital and used an interesting set of techniques that may be of help to others:

> In my first round of interviews, I made that clear to every ob I met in hopes that one would facilitate my entry. I found one willing ob who had a background in anthropology, and we went back and forth a bit, but when he realized he'd have to be on the IRB of the hospital with me for approval, it was too much for him. After a year and a half of failed attempts at access, my dissertation chair suggested I stick to interviews and change my research questions. Finding obstetricians willing to be interviewed was also a challenge. It took a couple of years to get up to 50, and I lost track of how many I actually asked, so I don't have a response rate to share. It was certainly low.
> In each state in which I conducted interviews, I made an Excel spreadsheet of all the hospitals in the state, then researched the practices that had privileges in that hospital and organized the spreadsheet by practice, then I would list the doctors individually and start trying to find their individual contact info. Even that was

difficult, as doctors do not list their emails. In some cases, I tried cold-calling the office directly, which worked more often in smaller private practices. If obs worked in a teaching hospital, I could usually find their emails on their academic affiliate websites with some digging around. When I found a few emails from doctors in the same system, I could guess the logarithm for their emails using their names.

Once I actually secured an agreement to interview, I had to work within their very tight schedules. Luckily, at the time I was childless and in grad school and had tremendous flexibility. For the out-of-state interviews, it was a bit more challenging because I only had a specific window of time—especially in California where I went for just two weeks and traveled by car all over the state. I tried as best as I could to cluster the interviews in regions but did many long days of driving for just one interview.

These sorts of dedication and perseverance are usually necessary, as illustrated in the responses below from other chapter authors.

Medical anthropologists Annie Preaux and Arachu Castro, the authors of "Obstetricians and the Delivery of Obstetric Violence: An Ethnographic Account from the Dominican Republic" in this present volume, interviewed doctors and nurses in three public hospitals. Arachu explained:

I first talked to the director of each hospital, and I then requested formal authorization from the Ministry of Public Health and National Health Services. It was granted quickly, as I have worked there many times over the years. In the meantime, we gathered the lists of the entire staff by position (R1 [R is an abbreviation for "resident" physician], R2, R3, R4, ob/gyns, other specialists, nurses, nurse assistants, administrators). In one of the hospitals, the director invited us to present the study to the entire staff. The director of each hospital identified someone who reserved a room for us to use for the interviews and who would introduce us to doctors, nurses, and administrators.

Medical anthropologist Sarah Williams, author of the chapter in this volume on "'Bad Pelvises': Mexican Obstetricians and the Re-Affirmation of Race in Labor and Delivery," achieved access to ob/gyns initially through homebirth midwives. The midwives she was working with connected her to the obs whom they commonly used as backup or worked together with at particular home births. Those obs were happy to be interviewed (as, again, most humanistic obs are), to host Sarah in their birth centers and offices, and to introduce her to colleagues. Sarah also met obs who were hostile to midwifery at the grand opening of a hospital in the town where she was conducting fieldwork. She said that she introduced herself without going into too much detail about her work, and that they were generally "pretty happy to chat with an anthropologist." She attempted to formally arrange to interview clinical staff through a Health Jurisdicción in Cancún, Quintana Roo, Mexico, but was completely stymied by management, as six months previously, a doctor had given an interview to a journalism student that was later aired on the radio and was quite critical of the healthcare system and staff. Sarah's requests kept "disappearing" before the director could review them, so "I gave it up and stuck to interviewing doctors without asking permission from their employers or soliciting interviews through the Jurisdicción. My approach was basically limited to word-of-mouth and snowball recruitment."

When Anna Ozhiganova, co-author of the chapter in this present volume on "The Inconsistent Path of Obstetricians to the Humanization of Childbirth in Post-Soviet Russian Maternity Care," first started to study midwifery and obstetrics, she was interested almost exclusively in the practice of home birth, which is illegal in Russia. For this reason, she could not use any official channels to find interlocutors, and so resorted only to informal methods. Once her interest turned to obstetric practices, she found her first ob interlocutors in private childbirth preparation centers where homebirth midwives and doctors worked. She also turned for help to her friends and acquaintances working in the biomedical sphere. Thus, among her interlocutors there were two categories of ob/gyns: (1) those who advocated for the humanization of childbirth, some of whom even cooperated with homebirth midwives; (2) those who had a negative attitude toward home birth and were not particularly interested in any innovations. However, according to Ozhiganova, Russian maternity hospitals are becoming more open, and doctors are more willing to make contact with outsiders; for example, they hold open conferences, meetings, and hospital tours for pregnant women and their families. Ozhiganova also used this option to come into hospitals and meet obstetricians. Moreover, she told us that Russian obstetricians themselves have begun to take an interest in social science studies of obstetrics: "They willingly participated in social science events, which, for example, I conducted at my Institute, and even invited me to give lectures at the maternity hospital. A great help in finding doctors for interviews was also provided by doulas, who act as universal mediators between differing social worlds."

Ozhiganova found that it is not easy to record in-depth, semi-structured interviews with doctors, as they usually expect more standardized questions and tend to give short answers (as Nick Rubashkin also found); she continued that, as noted above, "Of course, it is much easier to communicate with doctors who themselves are in search of new approaches: they are more open, less mistrustful, they have something to say." Ozhiganova found that all the obs she approached were afraid of disclosing their identities for fear of Russian government reprisals, so often for the purpose of anonymity, "I do not even indicate the cities in which they work nor the names of their medical institutions."

Anna Temkina, chapter co-author with Anna Ozhiganova, explained that:

> Once, a decade ago, one hospital midwife attended my class on Gender Studies, and later, after we met at a university conference, she told me that she was interested in any changes and innovations in Russian maternity care; we began to work together. At that time, I already studied patient behavior, and we decided that it would be very interesting to explore the positions of obs and midwives in the new commercial departments (where services are paid privately instead of by the government). She helped me in her maternity hospital, and through her, I also found other obstetricians and midwives in other commercial departments of other hospitals. Later, I presented my results at various conferences, which increased my networks among obs and other maternity care attendants. After one particular presentation, I received a request to present my results at a large maternity hospital; thereafter I was invited to do ethnographic research there. I did not have many difficulties in access, though every time, trust must be established and reestablished.

This continual establishment of *trust*, like that of *respect*, was a trope that ran throughout the responses of our chapter authors to our question about how they gained access to obs, as did the trope of easier access to humanistic obs, which often occurred via midwives and doulas.

For her chapter in this volume on "Censusing the Quechua: Peruvian State *Obstetras* in Light of Historic Sterilizations, Contemporary Accusations, and Biopolitical Statecraft Obligations," anthropologist Rebecca Irons obtained ethics clearance from the Peruvian Ministry of Health before interviewing and working with obstetricians. For Rebecca, it was a fairly straightforward process; she thinks that this may have been partly due to a process of decentralization in Peruvian biomedical care, meaning that local branches of the Ministry of Health had ultimate say over who could gain access. As the area where Irons worked was "rural, scarcely researched, and still coming out of post-conflict Shining Path issues with both access and willingness for people to travel there, they were quite keen to get more health data, so were very accommodating." In reciprocity, Irons presented findings from her PhD research back to that Ministry, just as Anna Temkina had done for the staff of the large Russian maternity hospital where she had worked. We emphasize *the importance of presenting the results of social science research to practitioners* whenever possible. Even though that entails the risk that they may not appreciate what you say, with possible negative repercussions for you as the researcher, it also entails the possible benefits of generating positive changes.

The process for social scientist Genevieve Ritchie-Ewing, author of the chapter in this volume on "Implicit Racial Bias in Obstetrics: How US Obstetricians View and Treat Pregnant Women of Color," was much more trying. She termed her experiences in finding obstetricians willing to participate in a social science research study "difficult and frustrating." She began by contacting obstetrician's offices in her local area. She would have liked to visit these offices in person but concerns around COVID-19 prevented her from doing so; she was vaccinated, but her young child was not. Mostly her efforts were ignored, but she did receive a few responses:

> One obstetrician in particular, who runs a clinic for women of lower socioeconomic status in a predominantly Black community, wanted to speak with me personally about the project before he was willing to participate and forward the information to others. His main concern was that the clinic staff had worked very hard to build rapport with their patients. He understood the importance of the research, as it was similar to research he had done himself, but he wanted to make sure that the responses of the staff could not be connected back to the clinic. I acknowledged his concern and assured him that the survey was completely anonymous. He forwarded the survey link to his colleagues in the end, but as far as I can tell from the timing, no one from his clinic actually filled out the survey (including him).

Genevieve also contacted the medical schools in her state of Ohio, asking department chairs to forward the link to department faculty, but received no responses. Additionally, she contacted the American Board of Obstetricians and Gynecologists; they said to contact the American College of Obstetricians and Gynecologists (ACOG), which she did, still receiving no response. She sent listserv announcements to the American Anthropological Association (AAA) and to the Society for Medical Anthropology (SMA) and received a few responses from colleagues willing to help with her efforts. These colleagues had personal connections with obstetricians who they thought would be willing to help, and she did receive some responses from these colleagues' ob friends. Genevieve said:

> My overall sense from my own experience and from reading the experiences of others in this chapter is that unless a personal connection exists, obstetricians do not have much interest in social science research. They, therefore, aren't willing to devote time to filling out a survey or participating in an interview. Given the topic of this research, I suspect there also is concern about how they will look in their answers to a survey about how they view their patients of color.

Ultimately, Genevieve found only eight obstetricians willing to respond to her survey, possibly because it was too lengthy, containing 36 close-ended questions and ten open-ended questions. (In her various surveys of obs, Robbie has found that the shorter the list of questions, the more likely obs are willing to answer them.) And only five of these eight were willing to be interviewed; Genevieve conducted these five interviews online via Zoom, which, as noted above, has proven to be a highly useful interview tool for several of our chapter authors. Genevieve had hoped for dozens of responses so that she could draw generalizations, but in the end could only speak for those few ob respondents.

Beverley Chalmers, author of the Volume III chapter "Teaching Humanistic and Holistic Obstetrics: Triumphs and Failures," like others of our chapter authors as described above, also had a relatively easy time accessing obstetricians; she has much to say on the topic, all of which we include here because it is both fascinating and revelatory of the possibilities for collaborations among social scientists and biomedical practitioners, provided that those social scientists have sufficient knowledge, the needed credentials, and a respectful attitude:

> As a social scientist based in Departments or Schools of Psychology, I have worked closely with obstetricians all my 50 years of work life. Around the 1970s, I was first invited to consult with the Departments of Ob/Gyn and Neonatology at the (then) Baragwanath Hospital in Soweto, South Africa, on rooming-in NICU care for new mothers and their babies. This led to work in ob/gyn and resulted in me implementing very large surveys of mothers of four

cultural groups in South Africa on their birth experiences. My ob/
gyn and neonatology colleagues all assisted me enormously to conduct research with them and about their care at the time. At their
request, I was cross-appointed to the ob/gyn faculty as a Professor.
Perhaps my positions as a Full Professor in Psychology, with a PhD
in predicting obstetric outcomes on the basis of clinical and psychosocial variables, helped to establish my credentials and gave me
some credibility to discuss obstetric issues with them.

I also never approached the issues I was concerned about in a
confrontational "me vs. you," or "us vs. them," or "social scientist vs.
ob-gyn" manner, but always as a collaborative partner in care. As a
psychologist and not a doctor, midwife, or nurse, I was in no way
competing for client care and was seen as simply contributing to the
best possible care for mothers and their families. Also, at that time
there was considerable acceptance of the importance of psychosocial concerns in clinical care, due to my years of co-teaching with
obstetricians in medical schools and my (and others') contributions
of social science perspectives on perinatal care. In particular, appreciation of the importance of a social science perspective in obstetrics
was growing among obstetricians and other perinatal providers, due
to the remarkable annual "Priorities in Perinatal Care" conferences
that were organized in South Africa by the Department of Pediatrics for over a decade, from the early 1980s onwards. In addition,
at about the same time in South Africa, I was a founding member
and later National President of a multidisciplinary and multicultural
Association for Childbirth and Parenthood that facilitated and encouraged discussion of, and exposure to, clinical, psychosocial, and
cultural diversity issues in perinatal care across the country.

In the 1990s, after winning a University of the Witwatersrand
Fellowship that allowed me to spend a year working anywhere in
the world I wanted to, I began to work with UN health agencies,
and in particular WHO and UNICEF, primarily in the former Soviet Union (FSU) countries. In 1991, I worked as the acting head of
the Maternal Child Health Unit/Women's and Children's Health
Unit at WHO Copenhagen, and after my first few years as a volunteer, continued as a short-term consultant for these agencies and
others for about two decades. During this period, I was involved
in over 140 missions into the FSU countries, including the Russian
Federation, Lithuania, Latvia, Estonia, Hungary, Poland, Moldova,
Belarus, Georgia, Armenia, Azerbaijan, Tajikistan, Kyrgystan, Turk-
menistan, and Kazakhstan. I also drafted the course materials (with
input from other consultants, of course) for the "Effective Care in

Antenatal, Birth and Postpartum Care" course that we (WHO and UNICEF) ran throughout the FSU countries from 1998 to 2001. This course was extremely helpful in humanizing their practices and in strengthening perinatal care to be evidence-based, rather than simply based on experience and tradition.

I also shared in the launch of the Baby-friendly Hospital Initiative (BFHI) in 1993 in St. Petersburg and became a Master Trainer for WHO/UNICEF for all aspects of this program until 2002. These involvements meant that I would visit hospitals multiple times a year throughout the region as a WHO/UNICEF representative, providing advice and support for their efforts to strengthen maternal and newborn care. In each country, I was usually met by the chief of ob-gyn and (almost always) "his" seconds-in-command, and taken on ward rounds to view the care on offer. I was usually challenged on my knowledge of care and care practices for hours before being accepted by them as worthy of consideration. Having passed their "tests," I was, from then on, welcomed despite being a woman (an important consideration in this traditionally male-dominated culture) and not being a medical doctor. Later, this led to me being invited to consult with countries directly, without being appointed to the position through any allegiance to WHO or UNICEF (or other agencies such as *Médecins sans Frontières*, Save the Children, USAID, the Norwegian Board of Health, etc., for whom I also worked at times).

In all my interactions with ob/gyns, I found that, once I had established my knowledge credentials, and given that I was always respectful, I was welcomed, supported, assisted with my research needs, and my thoughts and suggestions given consideration and, most often, implemented in practice.

In Canada, where I have lived since late 1992, my perspective as a social scientist was also welcomed by clinical colleagues in ob-gyn and pediatrics. I was able to propose and implement the Public Health Agency of Canada's "Maternity Experiences Survey" as a direct response to my questioning why we relied totally on what doctors say about women's perinatal care (for examples, through clinical records, perinatal surveillance reporting, and databases), instead of asking women what *they* experienced or wanted. I always found my Canadian colleagues welcoming and respectful of my social science perspective, my decades of knowledge regarding large-scale surveys of women's experiences of perinatal care in South Africa among Black, White, Indian, and women of mixed cultural origin, and in many of the FSU countries (Russian Federation, Azerbaijan, Lithuania, Moldova), and my clear concern for mothers' perspectives on their care.

In essence, then, my interactions (teachings, research collaborations, clinical advice) with obstetricians were successful when:

1 My knowledge of the issues being addressed was solidly based on research;
2 My interactions with them were respectful;
3 My intentions were clearly for the betterment of their own clinical practices;
4 The results were clearly for the betterment of mothers, babies, and their families.

It is more than clear that Chalmers's contributions to the humanization and strengthening of evidence-based birth have been substantial (see her chapter in this volume for more examples), and we hope that other social scientists can learn from what she accomplished and how she accomplished it—which is why we have devoted so much space to her words—in which *respect* for the biomedical personnel with whom she worked stands out as salient, as it has for all other chapter authors.

Although Melissa (Missy) Cheyney is not a chapter author in this series, as Robbie's close friend and colleague, when she heard about this chapter, she wrote to tell us that when she wants to interview obs, her trick is finding out the time of their usual lunch hour and then showing up with lunch!

What we can conclude from these accounts about the research challenges presented by seeking to interview and observe obstetricians is that, unless, like Beverley Chalmers, Arachu Castro, Nicholas Rubashkin, and (sometimes) Robbie, you are already "in with the in-crowd," as the song goes, then those challenges can be extremely difficult to overcome. And, as for all chapter authors, respect, the establishment of trust, patience, perseverance, understanding, and doing your homework about the possibilities that may be available to you are essential ingredients of eventual success, as are Chalmer's four takeaway points above, which also include the importance of always treating one's interlocutors with respect.

And, as previously noted, various chapter authors found that doulas and midwives were good sources of contact information for obstetricians, as all of them must work with obs at some point, even if only during hospital transfers, and all doulas and midwives have relationships, however tentative and possibly fraught, with at least one or two obs. Thus, if researchers start with obs who support midwives and doulas, they can eventually get in touch with those who don't. Also much easier to access, as shown in the author responses above, are humanistic and holistic obstetricians, who, again, are usually quite happy to talk about the paradigm shifts and practice changes they have made and why they made them, as these tend to be constantly on their minds. And these obs always know technocratic colleagues with whom they can put the researcher in touch. Of course, personal introductions can make all the difference in whether a given obstetrician will agree to be interviewed and possibly observed, or not.

Long-term fieldwork is also quite helpful in establishing relationships of trust. Some of our authors carried out observations first, finding that proper comportment[2] during these observations led to a trust strong enough for richer interviews in which providers were much more open to answering questions in depth than they likely would have been had the researchers started out by doing the interviews first—although for some, that process worked in reverse. Some of our chapter authors found that interviewing obstetricians first, before observing them, was what established a relationship of trust and put the obs being observed at ease during the observations. And that can work in a feedback loop— initial interviews can be done, then observations, and then deeper, richer interviews as a result of the pre-established trust, then perhaps more observations, and so on. And Sadler and Leiva found that interviews could be conducted on the fly, during the process of observation.

In Conclusion: The Key Ingredients to Success

In conclusion, we hope that these insights into how they gained access to hospitals and to obstetricians provided by our chapter authors will be useful to others planning similar or related research projects. Remember the key ingredients to success: doing your preparatory homework, patience, perseverance, developing relationships of trust with your interlocutors, and always treating them with respect—no matter how appalled you may be by some of the obstetric practices you observe. The takeaway point is *to listen to obstetricians* to understand their perspectives, thought processes, burdens, stresses, and emotions.

Robbie Davis-Floyd, Adjunct Professor, Department of Anthropology, Rice University, Houston, Fellow of the Society for Applied Anthropology, and Senior Advisor to the Council on Anthropology and Reproduction (CAR) (if you wish to join the extremely helpful CAR listserv, contact Robbie), is a cultural/medical/reproductive anthropologist interested in transformational models of maternity care. She is also a Board member of the International MotherBaby Childbirth Organization (IMBCO), in which capacity she helped to wordsmith the *International Childbirth Initiative: 12 Steps to Safe and Respectful MotherBaby-Family Maternity Care* (www.ICIchildbirth.org). E-mail: davis-floyd@outlook.com.

Ashish Premkumar is an Assistant Professor of Obstetrics and Gynecology at the Pritzker School of Medicine at The University of Chicago and a doctoral candidate in the Department of Anthropology at The Graduate School at Northwestern University. He is a practicing maternal-fetal medicine subspecialist. His research focus is on the intersections of the social sciences and obstetric practices, particularly surrounding the issues of risk, stigma, and quality of health care during the perinatal opioid use disorder epidemic of the 21st century. E-mail: premkumara@bsd.uchicago.edu.

Notes

1. Interestingly, before these conferences, Robbie had been speaking and writing about only the "technocratic" and "holistic" models of birth (see Davis-Floyd [1992] 2003). Listening to multiple AHMA presentations, she realized that some of these doctors were not holistic at all—they did not speak of spirit and energy but only of compassionate care. Thus Robbie realized that they were *humanistic*, not holistic, enabling her to go beyond her previous dichotomy between the technocratic and holistic paradigms by including the "paradigm in the middle"—the humanistic model of care, which has since informed all of her writings and presentations (see the Introduction to this volume). When she first presented and delineated the three paradigms at a subsequent AHMA conference, several of the MDs in the audience came up to her exclaiming "Now we understand why we are so different from our supposedly holistic colleagues—they *say* they are holistic, but that is not how they practice!"

2. In an example of the difficulties of maintaining "proper comportment," Robbie once found herself standing in a tiny delivery room in a hospital in Brazil only a few inches behind the obstetrician who was attending the birth of a young woman. This woman, Carlotta, told Robbie that she had experienced no pain during labor until the ob reached for the scissors and cut a large and completely unnecessary episiotomy—the baby's head was gently crowning and receding, then crowning again—this process gives the perineum time to stretch. Robbie was so outraged that she had to hold her hands behind her back to keep her from grabbing the scissors out of his hand and throwing them across the room! In retrospect, she wishes that she had gently placed her hand on the ob's back and whispered to him that she would *really, really* love to see a birth without an episiotomy, and that if he would just wait for ten minutes, that would happen. He might have complied, or might have become quite irritated and done the episiotomy anyway, as these are performed on almost all birthing people in

Brazil—and indeed across Latin America—who do not have a cesarean: they get "the cut above," or "the cut below." Still, Robbie wishes she had tried, but it all happened so fast that she had no time to think of that option. On the brighter side, this was a Baby-Friendly hospital, so the baby was immediately passed to the mother; she was so fascinated with him that, as she told Robbie later, she barely even felt the repair stitching—which took longer than simply waiting would have done.

References

Arditti JA, Joest KS, Lamber-Shute J, Walker L. 2010. "The Role of Emotions in Fieldwork: A Self-Study of Family Research in a Corrections Setting." *The Qualitative Report* 15(6): 1387–1414.

Davis-Floyd R. 1987. "Obstetric Training as a Rite of Passage." *Medical Anthropology Quarterly* 1(3): 288–318.

———. 2001. "The Technocratic, Humanistic, and Holistic Paradigms of Childbirth." *International Journal of Gynecology & Obstetrics* 75, Supplement No. 1: S5–S23.

———. (1992) 2003. *Birth as an American Rite of Passage*, 2nd ed. Berkeley: University of California Press.

———. 2018. "The Technocratic, Humanistic, and Holistic Paradigms of Birth and Health Care." In *Ways of Knowing about Birth: Mothers, Midwives, Medicine, and Birth Activism*, Davis-Floyd R and Colleagues, 3–44. Long Grove IL: Waveland Press.

———. 2022. *Birth as an American Rite of Passage*, 3rd ed. Abingdon, Oxon: Routledge.

Davis-Floyd R, St John G. 1998. *From Doctor to Healer: The Transformative Journey.* New Brunswick NJ: Rutgers University Press.

Davis-Floyd R, Premkumar A, eds. 2023a. *Obstetricians Speak: On Training, Practice, Fear, and Transformation*. New York: Berghahn Books.

———. 2023b. *Cognition, Risk, and Responsibility in Obstetrics: Anthropological Analyses and Critiques of Obstetricians' Practices*. New York: Berghahn Books.

———. 2023c. *Obstetric Violence and Systemic Disparities: Can Obstetrics Be Humanized and De-Colonized?* New York: Berghahn Books.

Feldman LR, Mandache L-A. 2019. "Emotional Overlap and the Analytic Potential of Emotions in Anthropology." *Ethnography* 20(2): 227–244.

Mills L, Davis-Floyd R. 2009. "The CASA Hospital and Professional Midwifery School: An Education and Practice Model That Works." In *Birth Models That Work*, eds. Davis-Floyd R, Barclay L, Daviss BA, Tritten J, 305–336. Berkeley: University of California Press.

Shapin S. 2001. "How to be Antiscientific." In *The One Culture? A Conversation about Science*, eds. Labinger JA, Collins H, 99–115. Chicago: University of Chicago Press.

Temkina A, Novkunskaya A, Litvina D. 2022. *Pregnancy and Birth in Russia.* Abingdon, Oxon: Routledge.

Concepts, Conceptual Frameworks, and Lessons Learned

Robbie Davis-Floyd and Ashish Premkumar

In these Conclusions to Volume III of our three-volume series on *The Anthropology of Obstetrics and Obstetricians: The Practice, Maintenance, and Reproduction of a Biomedical Profession* (Davis-Floyd and Premkumar 2023a, 2023b, 2023c), we address the theoretical concepts and frameworks that our chapter authors found most useful and describe lessons learned from these chapters. Unless otherwise indicated, all direct quotes below are from the chapters themselves, and all italics are in the original chapters. We divide these Conclusions into Parts 1 and 2 of this volume. Part 3—the preceding chapter—describes the ethnographic challenges that our chapter authors faced in finding, surveying, interviewing, and observing obstetricians and is not addressed herein.

Part 1. Obstetric Violence and Systemic Racial, Ethnic, Gendered, and Socio-Structural Disparities in Obstetricians' Practices

In Chapter 1, medical anthropologists Annie Preaux and Arachu Castro addressed obstetric violence in the Dominican Republic. These authors used Jenna Murray de López's (2018:61) definition of "obstetric violence" as including "scolding, taunts, irony, insults, threats, humiliation, manipulation of information and denial of treatment; pain management during childbirth used as punishment; coercion to obtain 'consent' for invasive procedures, and even acts of deliberate harm." Annie and Arachu noted that Arachu Castro and Virginia Savage (2019:125–126) had created six typologies of obstetric violence: (1) verbal abuse; (2) poor rapport with women; (3) sociocultural discrimination; (4) physical abuse; (5) failure to meet professional standards of care; and (6) health system conditions. Annie and Arachu sought to understand these types of obstetric violence from the perspectives of those who perpetrate them.

Some of Preaux's and Castro's interlocutors preferred to euphemistically call obstetric violence "mistreatment." Annie and Arachu grouped these interlocutors' responses into four categories to explain why mistreatment occurs: (1) blaming women for being uncooperative; (2) blaming women for misinterpreting clinicians' actions as violence; (3) healthcare providers' lack of empathy, of humanization, people-centeredness, and sense of vocation; and (4) institutional factors, inclusive of "a lack of beds, blood donations, and running water." Another significant issue was the lack of care continuity, as women in the Dominican Republic see a different care provider almost every time they access the maternity care system, leading to inabilities to develop trusting relationships and the resultant withholding of certain intimate types of information, which can negatively affect their care. Additionally, Preaux and Castro noted that a woman's clinical history "may be incomplete or filled with predetermined values . . . that is, with values for vital signs and other health indicators that are written down in the clinical history but that are invented because they have not actually been taken. These factors may preclude the provision of high-quality follow-up care."

Citing Sara Cohen Shabot (2019), Annie and Arachu also highlighted the practice of "gaslighting"—"women being made to doubt their own experiences . . . by using psychological manipulation. As women doubt their own experiences and accept obstetric violence, clinicians continue working and mistreating women with impunity." Additionally, Preaux and Castor found helpful Pierre Bourdieu's concept of "habitus" and series co-editor Ashish Premkumar's (2023) definition of it as "a cognitive space where group perceptions live, a space that they inhabit." Accordingly, Preaux and Castro noted that: "In the Dominican public hospitals where we conducted our study, clinicians are trained and work within a context that condones and perpetuates obstetric violence and poor relationships between women and their clinicians as part of their habitus (Bourdieu 1977)." Again using the concept of habitus, Preaux and Castro also utilized various anthropological theories regarding ways in which clinicians can avoid obstetric violence:

> Paulo Freire's (1970) and Robbie Davis-Floyd's (2018b [see also the Introduction to this volume]) concepts of "humanization" can support the education and training of clinicians to match the ideals

and principles of humanized care . . . Tying in the concept of "habitus," Freire's framework is an opportunity to create a much-needed consciousness-raising process among providers that could expand the medical habitus and transform it from what Roberto Castro (2014) calls the "authoritative medical habitus" to a habitus that is humanized and patient-centered.

Utilizing Davis-Floyd's (2023) schema of the "4 Stages of Cognition," Annie and Arachu continued by noting that:

> many clinicians are relatively unaware of their own medical habitus . . . In Davis-Floyd's terms (see the Introduction to this volume), such "unaware" clinicians are Stage 1 naïve realists who believe that "our way is the only way"—or "the only way that matters" . . . Recognizing the issues that women face may be the first step for clinicians toward addressing obstetric violence in their own practices and within the systems in which they work and receive training.

Annie and Arachu concluded that "Only awareness of a problem can lead to finding solutions to address it," and importantly added that simply by dicussing obstetric violence with obstetricians and other hospital staff—some of whom said that they had never heard this term before—these anthropologists were able to raise that needed awareness. We can only hope that this awareness will lead at least to the mitigation of obstetrically violent practices in the Dominican Republic.

In Chapter 2 on "'Bad Pelvises': Mexican Obstetricians and the Re-Affirmation of Race in Labor and Delivery," medical anthropologist Sarah A. Williams made use of the concept of biomedicine's "hidden curriculum" as defined by Lydia Z. Dixon, Vania Smith-Oka, and Mounia El Kotni (2019:40):

> A large portion of knowledge can be transmitted in unintended ways, in what has been termed the "hidden curriculum" . . . defined as the gap between what people are *taught* (through direct means) and what they *learn* (through indirect means). In some cases what is transmitted is the opposite of what is intended. So, while clinicians might *speak about* patient-centeredness as an important goal, their *actions* might emphasize . . . [their] authority, or even attitudes of contempt for patients.

Williams traced "contemporary framings of Mexican women's pelvises as faulty back to the emergence of Mexican obstetrics and gynecology practice in the 1800s," and demonstrated their origins "in the race-making discourses of eugenics and *mestizaje*."

The trope of obstetric violence also runs throughout this chapter—the violence of performing unnecessary cesareans due to Mexican women's supposedly dysfunctional pelvises and of sterilizing them—most especially Indigenous women, whose genes are thought to be generally responsible for those "dysfunctional" pelvises in *mestiza* women—and the violence of eugenically based sterilizations of Indigenous women: "The justification and chain of events for birthing women, particularly Indigenous women, remains largely the same [as in the past]: deficient pelvis>>>surgical intervention required>>>sterilization."

Williams identified a serious and extremely racist global problem—the specter invoked by discourses of:

> Indigenous, Brown (hyper)fertility that must be controlled for Mexico to "modernize" . . . Continued calls by Global North governments and NGOs to limit fertility and control population growth in Global South countries reinforce the normalization of the idea that the world's problems—climate change, poverty, epidemics—can all be solved by eliminating future generations of Indigenous and Brown people, rather than through resource redistribution or decolonized relations.

To explain why the CB rate in Mexico has not gone down despite "increasing governmental policies designed to counteract and prevent unnecessary cesarean births," Sarah Williams pointed to, among other factors, the "obstetric dilemma" that Mexican obstetric trainees—like many obs elsewhere—almost never see normal physiologic births and thus cannot learn how to facilitate them. Williams also noted that an obstetrician, Jorge, described frustrations with the differences in care he was able to provide in public hospitals versus in his own private practice, where most of his clients were able to have successful home births without complications or interventions. Williams quoted Jorge as saying: "I was trained in the technocratic model, where we had to intervene as much as possible, and told that medicine had to make up for nature's faults." According to Williams: "Jorge's use of Davis-Floyd's term 'the technocratic model' indicates his familiarity with her work on 'the technocratic, humanistic, and holistic models of birth' . . . I mention this here as a demonstration of how anthropological work can impact practitioners by giving them terminology that is 'good to think with'" (Levi-Strauss 1962). Sarah also noted the "brain drain" of humanistic obs like Jorge, who, frustrated with their inabilities to create change in

Mexican public hospitals, often leave those hospitals for private practices, resulting in the loss of their potential contributions to humanizing
care in public hospitals.

Williams additionally found useful the work of Suellen Miller and
colleagues and that of Melissa Cheyney and Robbie Davis-Floyd:

> I, and the series editors Robbie Davis-Floyd and Ashish Premku-
> mar, argue that TLTL [too little too late] and TMTS [too much
> too soon] interventions [Miller et al. 2016] must give way to hu-
> manistic, RARTRW (the right amount at the right time in the right
> way) care [see Cheyney and Davis-Floyd 2020]. That is what [hu-
> manistic] obstetricians strive to achieve—but can only achieve it in
> private practices that generally cannot afford to provide free care
> for the poor. Thus, as Davis-Floyd (2018b) points out, humanism in
> maternity care, while not stratified by gender or ethnicity, is often
> economically stratified.

Williams concluded her chapter by noting that: "If Mexico's cesarean
rate is ever to be permanently and significantly lowered, obstetricians
and hospitals must account for the role of eugenics-based ideologies and
racist treatment of patients, and must adjust the hidden curriculum so
that obstetricians who wish to practice in more humanized ways are not
driven out of public practice."

In Lauren Diamond-Brown's chapter on "'Selfish Mothers,' 'Misinformed' Childbearers, and 'Control Freaks': Gendered Tropes in US
Obstetricians' Justifications for Delegitimizing Patient Autonomy in
Childbirth," Lauren noted that as some of her ob interlocutors "tried to
convince me of the illegitimacy of certain women's choices," they characterized certain women as "bad" women/mothers/patients by drawing
on the gender tropes of women as "overcontrolling," "naïve," "miseducated," "superficial," and/or "selfish"; these tropes "influence obstetricians' expectations for how to interact with patients."

When dividing her 50 ob interlocutors into two groups, Diamond-
Brown too found useful Davis-Floyd's "4 Stages of Cognition" schema
(described in the Introduction to this volume and in Davis-Floyd's
[2023] chapter in Volume II of this series): "the 22 members of Group
1 expressed narratives that reflect Stage 1 fundamentalist thinking, in
which they are convinced that their way is the only right way, whereas
the 28 members of Group 2 expressed narratives that fall somewhere
along a continuum of cognition from Stage 2 to Stage 4 (closed and
ethnocentric to open, fluid, and humanistic) thinking." Diamond-Brown
further noted that:

Scholars have focused on biomedical training as the primary agent of professional socialization for physicians, while missing the opportunity to examine *resocialization* throughout doctors' careers. Some of the ob interlocutors in Group 2 said that they "practice like a midwife"—meaning that they practice the Stage 4 humanistic and holistic midwifery model of care. For some, this was their training—showing what a difference the type of training can make in forming obstetric ideologies—whereas for others, it was exposure to a more humanistic model of birth later in their careers, often via watching midwives practice (see Davis-Floyd 2023).

Diamond-Brown also found theoretical grounding in "cultural health capital" theory, in which "[s]elf-efficacy, self-control, self-esteem, and health literacy are traits that have been identified as positive attributes" (Shim 2010:1). Yet, as Lauren illustrated, such traits were often interpreted as negative by the Group 1, Stage 1 ob interlocutors, who explicitly labeled the patients who came in with a birth plan as "problematic and irrelevant to their job of delivering a healthy baby": "By drawing on fetocentric thinking and broader cultural expectations that mothers should be selfless, they label the woman with a birth plan as a 'bad mother' with illegitimate demands."

Drawing on Brigitte Jordan's concept of "authoritative knowledge," Diamond-Brown noted that: "Part of dismissing women's choices in birth as irrelevant and illegitimate is to double down on paternalism and pronounce that biomedical professionals have exclusive ownership of the authoritative knowledge (Jordan 1997) to be used in labor and delivery." And in speaking of what Lauren termed "obstetric misogyny," she drew on the work of feminist philosopher Kate Manne (2018:33), who argued that rather than a general hatred of women, "misogyny—which can be perpetrated by both male and female obstetricians—is the act of putting a woman in her place when she deviates from socially acceptable gender norms."

Moving now to Genevieve Ritchie-Ewings's chapter on implicit racial bias among US obstetricians, we note that she found useful Kylea Liese and colleagues' (2021) UHDVA (unintentional harm, disrespect, violence, and abuse) iatrogenic spectrum, along with Melissa Cheyney's and Robbie Davis-Floyd's identification of the "obstetric paradox":

On one end of this spectrum is the *unintentional* harm originating from routine interventions that are meant to keep birth safe, but actually cause harm, in what Melissa Cheyney and Robbie Davis-Floyd (2019:8) term "the obstetric paradox." On the other side of the UHDVA spectrum lie *intentional* disrespect and discrimination, such as demeaning behaviors and insults to childbearers by health-care workers. In the United States, Black, Indigenous, and other People of Color experience intentional disrespect and abuse during pregnancy and childbirth more often than white women, due to the systemic racism in US society.

Ritchie-Ewing theoretically distinguished "explicit" and "implicit" racial bias:

> *Explicit bias* is bias of which people are aware, while *implicit bias* is unconscious bias. Expressions of explicit bias are strongly dis-couraged among healthcare providers, but implicit bias is harder to self-regulate . . . Implicit bias can influence nonverbal behaviors such as eye contact and posture, as well as how speech is delivered . . . higher levels of implicit bias among physicians adversely impact medical interactions.

In her quest to bring to light the implicit and explicit racial or ethnic biases among her ob interlocutors, Ritchie-Ewing learned that "Obstetri-cians, like other physicians, state a lack of preference for any race or eth-nicity, despite the abundance of research showing implicit bias among physicians similar to the implicit bias found in the general US popula-tion," and highlighted the limitations in medical school training in ad-dressing healthcare disparities. Ritchie-Ewing concluded her chapter by suggesting concrete changes in biomedical school curricula focused on ameliorating healthcare disparities and emphasizing humanistic training practices.

In Rebecca Iron's chapter on "Censusing the Quechua," she took a "nuanced approach to the complexities of obstetric violence and the *ob-stetras* who perpetuate it." Rebecca argued that: "a key role of Peruvian *obstetras* is to census and discipline the population as a form of stratified biopolitical statecraft (Bridges 2012) via administrative tasks and meet-ing quotas, resulting in dissatisfaction among *obstetras*, patient neglect, and obstetric violence." After explaining that all obstetricians in Peru are women, and that their services are thereby devalued by the biomedical establishment in that country, Rebecca demonstrated that *obstetras* of-ten feel that they must subtly coerce Indigenous Quechua women to use contraceptives to meet family planning quotas in order to keep their jobs. Given that many of the Peruvian *obstet*ras whom Rebecca stud-ied are Indigenous Quechua themselves, she pointed to Khiara Bridges's (2011:38–39) identification of the fact that biomedical practitioners often feel animosity toward patients of similar backgrounds, and thus wish to distance themselves from such patients, "such that they could not, or no longer, be considered abject forms of [themselves—the practitioners]." Irons continued:

> Indeed, in Peru, healthcare workers and other state employees, by virtue of their studies and their differential status, may place themselves "above" those with whom they grew up . . . Thus, practitioner behaviors may be classist if not racist, or both. These attitudes reflect a common phenomenon in Peru called *choleandao*: when one group of Peruvians looks down on another, who looks down upon another. Walter Pariona Cabrera (2017:41) asserts that in Ayacucho, *choleando* is quite prevalent, and that the healthcare practitioners' attitudes of looking down on their Indigenous patients (who may be similar to them in many ways) is *choleando*. Other Peruvians may look down on those same healthcare workers and so on.

We editors note that this is the same phenomenon addressed by Paolo Friere in his well-known book *Pedagogy of the Oppressed*, that it is a major cause of structural violence in hierarchical healthcare systems and elsewhere, and that this phenomenon is as dysfunctional now as it was when Friere originally published his book in 1970.

Part 2. Decolonizing and Humanizing Obstetric Training and Practice? Obstetricians, Midwives, and Their Battles against "The System"

Here we begin with Chapter 6 on "Decolonizing Medical Education in the UK," written by obstetrician Amali Lokugamage, medical doctor Tharanika Ahillan, and attorney SDC Pathberiya. These authors made use of an article by Sarah Wong, Faye Gishen, and Amali Lokugamage (2021), in which the term "decolonizing" is defined as broadly referring to a movement that:

1. Recognizes how forces of colonialism, empire, and discrimination have shaped the systems of the societies in which we live our day-to-day lives; and
2. Offers alternative ways of thinking about the world, re-centering perspectives of populations that have been historically oppressed and marginalized by these forces.

This chapter provided descriptions of the ways in which biomedical curriculum changes in the UK have been designed to address both of those issues. Citing Sara Stone, Samuel Myers, and Christopher Golden (2018:193), its authors described "a *planetary health* education curriculum," noting the global importance of an ecological approach to health and to life in general:

> As a result . . . biomedical educators have started to think of how a process of decolonization could produce doctors who can meet the complex needs of a diverse population, while recognizing the colonial influences that created the origins of biomedicine. The influence of biomedical education in propagating healthcare inequalities in the post-colonial hierarchy . . . is being realized.

As Lokugamage, Ahillan, and Pathberiya importantly reminded us, some of these colonial influences "that created the origins of biomedicine" include the horrendous experimental surgeries conducted on the unwilling bodies of Black slaves by J. Marion Sims, and the notorious Tuskegee experiment conducted on the bodies of unwitting Black men to explore the progressive courses of syphilis. Thus these authors stated that:

> Decolonizing the history of biomedicine promotes awareness and questions the traditional narratives and power imbalances to disrupt the prejudiced legacy of the colonization of medicine: these prejudices are not limited to racism, but also include classism, sexism, ableism, xenophobia, and gender discrimination . . . Re-framing, re-orienting, and reforming the profession require the reassessment of past biomedical colonial legacies.

In explaining why and how biomedical training curricula became colonized in the first place, these authors noted that historically: "Diversity in types of practitioners, such as midwives and folk healers, and schools of thought, such as Indigenous healing systems in the colonies, were excluded or oppressed. *Medical pluralism* was squeezed out of the growing biomedical power hierarchy"—and part of the de-colonizing movement is an effort to bring it back in. Important lessons that we volume editors (Ashish and Robbie) learned from this chapter are described by its authors in their Table 6.1, which provides a valuable comparison of the terms "unconscious bias," "cultural competence," "cultural humility," and "Cultural Safety" (which should always be capitalized, as these authors explained), as well as concepts such as "white fragility" and what these authors termed "privilege fragility," which our readers—and ourselves—would be well advised to consider.

In describing "the tensions between biomedical and traditional healing systems," Lokugamage, Ahillan, and Pathberiya cited Atwood Gaines and Robbie Davis-Floyd (2003:142) as stating that: "Like science, Western medicine was assumed to be acultural—beyond the influence of culture—while all other medical systems were assumed to be so culturally biased that they had little or no scientific relevance." Thus, as these authors noted, this attitude led "to the oppression of Indigenous medicines in favor of Western health practices. Eastern practices, such as those mentioned above [Ayurveda, Traditional Chinese Medicine] and other Indigenous healing systems, were regarded through the skeptical lens of a Western biomedical perspective, and their efficacy was rejected." Pointing to the lack of high-quality evidence for many biomedical practices, Lokugamage, Ahillan, and Pathberiya insisted that the decolonization of Western biomedicine must lead to a re-evaluation and a revaluation of such Indigenous healing systems, which have survived and even thrived in the contemporary world, yet remain labelled "alternative" or "complementary" to the still-hegemonic biomedical system. These authors pointed to "three scaffolding concepts of decolonizing the biomedical curriculum: epistemic pluralism, Cultural Safety, and critical consciousness" and explained these fully in their chapter, which is full of more rich theoretical concepts and lessons than we have space to address here. We do note an important lesson for practitioners described in this chapter:

> At an individual level, the process of providing Cultural Safety would essentially entail that a nurse, doctor, or student, as part their reflective practice prior to a patient encounter, quickly reflect on their privileged status and any potential power imbalances between themselves and the patient. This quick reflection should provide insight and situational awareness, aspiring to create a fairer clinical encounter.

We urge all such practitioners to apply this "quick reflection" in their practices to create "a fairer clinical encounter."

Moving now to Beverley Chalmers's chapter on her personal triumphs and failures in teaching humanistic and holistic obstetrics, we note that she began with a brief description of her 50 years of involvement in the education of obstetricians and Health Science students as a perinatal health psychologist, social scientist, and childbirth expert. Beverley defined "perinatal psychologists" as psychologists "trained in the essentials of clinical perinatal care, and in the multitude of psychosocial issues that accompany a family's transition to parenthood." (See also Hakan Çoker's (2023) chapter in Volume I of this series, in which he describes his team as including a "birth psychologist" and defines her roles in supporting both the birthing family and the other members of the birth team.) Chalmers insisted on the importance of interprofessional collaboration, including perinatal psychologists, noting that WHO "has taken up the challenge of directing attention to interprofessional models of education, practice, and policy across healthcare specializations, and has developed a framework within which to consider local initiatives for greater and more successful interprofessional practices." To that end, in 1984 in South Africa, she and a group of perinatal care professionals established the Association for Childbirth and Parenthood that emphasized shared knowledge, experiences, and practices across multiple groups (e.g., obstetrics, pediatrics, midwifery, nursing, childbirth education, and perinatal psychology). Providing an opportunity for multidisciplinary collaboration between childbirth educators and birth facilities led to improved relationships, less tension, and expansion to other sites across the country. Clearly, this is an excellent model of interprofessional collaboration; we strongly recommend its application in countries around the world. (See below for other examples of interprofessional collaboration models provided by our chapter authors).

Chalmers also described how she taught in multiple countries of the former USSR, introducing them to *Effective Care in Pregnancy and Childbirth* (Enkin, Keirse, and [Iain] Chalmers 1989) and to the concept of "evidence-based care" by having that book and hundreds of English-language articles translated into Russian and disseminating them widely. She explained: "Just as these concepts had been shocking in the West when first brought to attention—along with their support for a demedicalized, less interventionist approach to maternity care—so too were these ideas almost heretical in the face of traditional, highly medicalized and rigid approaches to care that characterized many aspects of Soviet obstetrics." Yet through her efforts and those of her collaborators, perinatal and maternal mortality in St. Petersburg improved over a five-year period without a concomitant increase in cesarean births; these results were conjoined with hospital visiting by family members, increased breastfeeding, and more favorable attitudes toward an increasing role for fathers in labor and delivery.

Chalmers taught other courses across Europe and the former Soviet countries developed by herself and/or in collaboration with WHO and UNICEF, including courses on the Baby-Friendly Hospital Initiative. These courses too resulted in decreases in interventions and improvements in breastfeeding, bonding, and maternal satisfaction, as detailed in this chapter and in Chalmers (2012). The longer-term effects of Chalmer's work are described by Russian authors Anna Temkina, Anastasia Novkunskaya, and Daria Litvina (2022) and in the following chapter by Anna Ozhiganova and Anna Temkina.

In her chapter, Chalmers asked the important question: "What succeeds and what fails in teaching obstetricians?" and responded by identifying five key factors for success: (1) noting and then taking advantage of a teachable moment; (2) combining clinical, technological, and humanistic care; (3) multidisciplinary teaching and participation; (4) a respectful approach to those taught, no matter how outdated or ill-advised their practices may be; and (5) teaching what's best for mothers, babies, and families based on scientific evidence.

In Chapter 8, co-authors Anna Ozhiganova and Anna Temkina described "The Inconsistent Path of Russian Obstetricians to the Humanization of Birth in Post-Soviet Maternity Care." They began with some anthropological concepts they found useful and with one of their own, "partial humanization":

> In this chapter, we consider the professional strategies of Russian obstetricians leading to the *partial humanization* of post-Soviet maternity care . . . The three paradigms of obstetric practice delineated by Robbie Davis-Floyd . . . the technocratic, humanistic, and holistic models . . . are applicable to Russian conditions, except that instead of the technocratic and holistic approaches, the concepts of "medicalized" and "natural" childbirth are used, and the State bureaucracy has an especially strong influence. The humanistic approach has been widely used by Russian perinatal specialists in recent years, and to them it means a model of care focused on the needs of women and newborns, and on shared decision-making between maternity care providers and childbearers.

Ozhiganova and Temkina conceptualized the post-Soviet system of maternity care "as a *hybrid* of the legacy of Soviet bureaucratic paternalism and neoliberalism," noting that "Bureaucratic paternalist and commercial principles in this new hybrid system coexist, often contradict each other, and lead to inconsistency in care, even where it has become more humanized." Citing the works of Michele Rivkin-Fish, these authors noted that:

> Soviet healthcare providers were responsible for fulfilling the interests of the State, not those of the individual patient. Providers often

felt helpless in the rigid State paternalistic hierarchies, since they lacked decision-making autonomy. They re-established their power in interactions with patients using crude and cruel techniques of domination—*khamstvo*. Patients remained docile, as obstetricians threatened any women whom they perceived as challenging their authority (Rivkin-Fish 2005a, 2005b).

Referring to the works of Beverley Chalmers and Brigitte Jordan, Ozhiganova and Temkina stated:

> Beverley Chalmers, who—as she describes in the preceding chapter in this volume—worked in the 1990s as a consultant for WHO/UNICEF on maternal and child health in Russia and other countries of Eastern Europe, noted that "Russian biomedical workers recognize that change is important and long overdue, and they are ready for a 'transition of authoritative knowledge'" (Chalmers 1997:275; Jordan 1997) . . . Chalmers saw factors that could lead to changes: the spread of evidence-based medicine; exposing the inadequacies and even harms of routine procedures that previously had been considered to be useful for women and newborns; and the influence of midwives, who represent alternative authoritative knowledges, but are also capable of compromising with the biomedical approach.

The humanistic changes in Russian maternity care described by Ozhiganova and Temkina include "the promotion of patient choice in both State and commercial services," in which, in what they termed "the commercialization of maternity care," the "paid services offer patients improved conditions (e.g., a remodeled room), and the possibility to choose an obstetrician and midwife." Thus these authors stated that:

> Marketization and the possibility of choice led to several significant shifts in the organization of maternity care: from a centralized system partly compensated by informal welfare payments to a less rigid market-driven system; from authoritarian State employees to market-driven providers; and from powerless obedient women to empowered consumers-clients.

These authors also pointed to a major change in Russian obs' behaviors that resulted from this commercialization:

> As we found in both of our research sites, providers—most especially obstetricians—have to perform a great deal of *emotional labor*—the

process of managing feelings and their expressions connected to work duties . . . to meet the demands of consumer-oriented women who expect polite service with a *smile*—which was almost never given during the Soviet *khamstvo*-style era . . . Providers maneuver between different emotional styles—*khamstvo* [extreme rudeness] and smiling—to meet patients demands and desires but also to make patients conform to institutional conditions.

This conformity was exemplified in women's expectations that their self-empowerment would consist of choosing their ob and midwife, "after that, they tend to *choose* to give over control of their birthing bodies to those practitioners."

In this chapter, co-author Anna Temkina built on the research that she and her colleagues carried out (Temkina, Novlunskaya, and Litvina 2022), during which they developed the term "manual management" to index the "individual, hands-on" work done by obstetricians and other physicians in the Hospital:

Working under rigid formal hierarchical rules and controls, maternity care providers—most especially obs—have to negotiate informally and to hybridize their daily work when clinical necessity does not fit into official rules, or rules do not exist, or they are outdated and unhelpful, or contradict each other; needed resources are lacking; or the trajectory of a patient is unclear; or inspection is expected, and so forth. . . . [Through manual management], providers must maintain the institutional order of the Hospital, meet women's expectations, and prevent their discontents, thereby preventing the dreaded government body inspections and the negative sanctions that may ensue.

And, as in many other countries, a primary obstacle to the humanization of birth in Russia "is that many ob/gyns do not understand the physiology of childbirth well and act in the ways they were taught, not relying on evidence-based medicine."

In one chapter section, co-author Anna Ozhiganova described the paradigm shift made by Dr. Olga Vladimirovna, who had visited the Netherlands, had seen how its excellent midwifery-based maternity care system worked, and had spoken with childbirth pioneer Michel Odent, after which she created a fully humanized maternity ward in an otherwise technomedical hospital. "Overall, the changes in obstetric practice [in this maternity ward] were aimed at abandoning obstetric iatrogenesis and implementing the principle of RARTRW care (the right amount

at the right time in the right way) (Cheyney and Davis-Floyd 2020)."
Sadly, yet not unsurprisingly, after four years this maternity ward closed
after Vladimirovna was fired by the Chief Physician, "who did not support Olga's changes." Yet Ozhiganova stressed that the full humanization
of this maternity unit showed that "obs *can* revise generally accepted
practices and become supporters of the humanistic approach"—as is
also shown in the following chapter.

In this following chapter on the "good guys and girls" of Brazil by
Robbie Davis-Floyd and Eugenia (Nia) Georges, we note that, in contrast to the "partial humanization" of Russian maternity care, the practices of the 32 ob interlocutors studied by Robbie and Nia are fully
humanized. In defining "humanization" and pinpointing its objectives,
Robbie and Nia noted that:

> Although a diverse project, humanization at its core is grounded in
> the principle that safe, respectful, and supportive maternity care,
> free of unnecessary medical interventions, is a *childbearer's human
> right*. To ensure that such unnecessary interventions are eliminated,
> the humanization movement also insists that care of mother and
> infant consist exclusively of "best practices" that are supported by
> up-to-date, evidence-based medicine . . . Thus, the objectives of
> humanization are simultaneously ethical (promoting the view of
> childbearers as persons with the right to respect and autonomy and
> of doctors as committed to protecting those rights) and instrumen-
> tal (improving the quality of care), and thereby improving both
> physical and psychological outcomes for mothers and babies.

In this chapter, Robbie and Nia traced "the transformative trajectories of these 32 interlocutors, who have been pioneers in radically
reshaping how women are cared for during childbirth," examining their
motives for making a paradigm shift. On the spectrum technocratic—
humanistic—holistic, which Robbie (Davis-Floyd 2022) has redefined
as "technocratic—superficially humanistic—deeply humanistic—holistic"
(see also the Introduction to this volume), all interlocutors placed themselves very much on the deeply humanistic side (centering the woman
and facilitating what Robbie calls the *deep physiology* of birth)—merging
into holism (perceiving the body as energy and birth as a spiritual process). Robbie and Nia examined the processes by which the obstetricians
they interviewed "managed to resocialize and recraft themselves into
different sorts of humanized practitioners." These authors also examined
the "tools and resources for self-transformation" that had served their ob
interlocutors well. Briefly, these included guidance from books and films,

guidance from midwives, learning to work with doulas, and the social movements and online networks that supported them and which they in turn supported. Although some "AHA! Moments" suddenly caused these obs to question their technocratic practices, "Changing deeply embodied knowledge and habits typically occurred 'step-by-step, step-by-step' . . . and could take years to complete."

Along these journeys, these increasingly humanistic obs were continually rewarded by their improved outcomes and the high satisfaction levels of their patients. Yet for many, there were also high prices to pay in the forms of ostracism, bullying, and outright persecutions by their city and state Stage 1, silo-oriented obstetric establishments, as Robbie and Nia described, and as one of their interlocutors, Ricardo Jones (2023), described for himself in his chapter in Volume I of this series (Davis-Floyd and Premkumar 2023a).

Robbie and Nia also presented the concept expressed by one of their interlocutors that "the obstetrician should be the hero of the hospital, swooping in to save the day when truly needed, while all the rest of the births should be attended by midwives who practice the midwifery model of care." Additionally, these authors noted that the members of the younger generation of these Brazilian "good guys and girls" rarely read articles or books as the older ones had done; rather, they bring their tablets to births and get on Facebook to ask the more experienced "good guys and girls" for advice when needed.

Robbie and Nia concluded their chapter with Ricardo Jones' (2012: 223) important synthesis of the characteristics of humanization as applied to childbirth, which include:

1. The protagonism it gives to women, without which we would be merely further entrenching the dependence of women on men imposed over millennia by patriarchy.
2. An integrative and interdisciplinary view of birth focused on a deep understanding of the characteristics of the biological process and its emotional, social, cultural, and spiritual aspects, which must all be equally valued and attended to.
3. A visceral connection with evidence-based medicine, making clear that the humanization of childbirth movement, which nowadays has spread all over the world, works under the aegis of reason.

Chapter 10 was "written by two midwives (Lorna Davies and Melanie Welfare), a neonatal pediatrician (Maggie Meeks), two obstetricians (Coleen Caldwell and Judy Ormandy), and a sociologist/anthropologist (Rea Daellenbach)." In this chapter, these authors addressed "Interprofessional Education for Medical and Midwifery Students in Aotearoa New Zealand" (ANZ; this country has been renamed as such to honor the Indigenous Māori). As they detailed in their chapter, these authors have been "developing education workshops for midwifery and medical students using simulations and debriefings." Their aim was to "foster more collegial interprofessional relationships between midwives and doctors, particularly in situations when women and babies require collaborative care in the context of Aotearoa New Zealand's unique maternity care system." To recap a bit, we note that in this system, a full 94% of ANZ childbearers choose midwives as their primary caregivers, and midwives are present at almost 100% of births, even when they are cesarean births. Midwives refer their clients to obstetricians when needed and interact with them frequently; thus there is a clear need for the collaborative care model proposed in this chapter. To that end, Daellenbach and colleagues developed interprofessional workshops for midwifery students and medical students who were in the process of doing obstetric rotations. In their first workshop, which they described in detail in their chapter, these authors noted a dichotomy in medical students' perceptions of midwives:

> One the one hand, they talked about how "lucky" midwives are to be able to work with "normal, healthy women" and "develop long-term relationships with women." On the other hand, they noted that they only saw "the bells going off" for the "risky," "high-acuity" hospital births, and that they were afraid of birth.

For their part, the midwifery students commonly overestimated the knowledge that medical students had about the management of labor, ceding to technocratic solutions during emergencies. Yet through the interprofessional workshops that these authors designed, both medical and midwifery students learned to respect each other's professions while still grappling with the tensions around the differing philosophies of each specialty. In the second workshop, the students talked about how the interprofessional education experience gave them a glimpse of the potential to be a "new generation" of maternity care professionals who could leave the "old" interprofessional tensions behind. We (Ashish and Robbie) celebrate that "new generation," and highlight these authors' concept of *interprofessional empathy*. We highly recommend the widespread application of interprofessional empathy and the development of interprofessional education in all countries and institutions where a variety of practitioners must collaborate in order to provide optimal maternity care, and refer our readers to James Ruiter and Carol Cameron

(2021), who describe the MORE[OB] model that was developed in Canada and is spreading to the United States to enhance interprofessional collaboration.

The trope of the importance of empathy was continued by obstetrician Deborah McNabb in her chapter on "The Changing Face of Obstetric Practice in the United States as the Percent of Women in the Specialty Has Grown." McMabb described "the feminization of obstetrics," and made the case "for the value of the empathic patient-provider relationship with its power to decrease suffering and improve health for women," insisting that while male obs can certainly be empathic with their patients, this is a skill primarily fostered in women from girlhood on. McNabb referred to the works of Carol Gilligan (1982) and Nel Noddings (2003) regarding "the ethics of care": "Care ethics holds that, as human beings, relationships are of primary importance, so that the practice of reciprocal caring is universally basic to humanity . . . As Gilligan (2011) later said, "Within a *patriarchal* framework, care is a feminine ethic. Within a *democratic* framework, care is a human ethic."

McNabb also described a study by Debra Roter and Judith Hall (1998), who found that when comparing female to male physicians:

> stereotypical male characteristics of competence, authority, expertise, independence, and self-confidence are essential to patient care when combined with the equally essential stereotypical female characteristics of warmth, sensitivity, a caring attitude, a relationship orientation, and interpersonal responsiveness. Thus, the characteristics that have always been considered as female capabilities are now being recognized as essential to a high standard of biomedical practice.

Additionally, McNabb addressed female obstetrician burnout, noting that a major cause was "their added responsibilities on the home front," and, by looking to the past, provided some future-oriented advice for female obs:

> undoubtedly, another major factor was that, back then, obstetricians were men, and they all had wives! Women are always working, even at home, where they are more responsible for childcare, elder care, and housework. To this day, only half of male physicians' spouses work outside of the home, while almost all female physicians' spouses do . . . only 5% of women's spouses performed "most or all duties at home," whereas more than 80% of men's spouses did so. Female physicians who had a supportive partner had a 40% less

risk of burnout . . . My advice to young female obstetricians is that, especially if you want to have children, finding that partner who will carry at least half of the burden on the home front is critical and can be life-saving.

Noting that "as the ob/gyn workforce becomes dominated by women, burnout . . . becomes an ever more critical issue," and that "social and institution supports are essential," McNabb also introduced the concept of "transformative leadership," asserting that:

> By 2017, nearly 60% of practicing ob/gyns were female, so it is time to look forward as we continue to witness the feminization of obstetrics . . . Women excel at patient-centered care, so patient-physician relationships are expected to improve, and with that, improved quality of medical care. . . Studies of leadership styles indicate that women empower other team members to develop their potential and mentor team members. This is called "transformative leadership."

McNabb enumerated: "The three biggest contributions that I think female obstetricians have made, and continue to make, to women's health care are: women-modeled empathy; strong communication skills; and patient-centered behavior," and stressed that all of these "have now become the standard of care," which McNabb interpreted as stemming from the growing numbers of female obstetricians (see Roter and Hall 2014). McNabb also made the extremely important point that "rather than empathy contributing to burnout among physicians, a strong patient-provider connection leads to more satisfaction in the practice of medicine"—meaning that *providers can nurture themselves by nurturing their patients.*

Having completed our overview of the theoretical frameworks and constructs found useful by the chapter authors in this volume, and of the lessons we have learned from them, we turn now to the Series Conclusions to this three-volume series on *The Anthropology of Obstetrics and Obstetricians: The Practice, Maintenance, and Reproduction of a Biomedical Profession.*

Robbie Davis-Floyd, Adjunct Professor, Department of Anthropology, Rice University, Houston, Fellow of the Society for Applied Anthropology, and Senior Advisor to the Council on Anthropology and Reproduction (CAR) (if you wish to join the extremely helpful CAR listserv, contact Robbie), is a cultural/medical/reproductive anthropologist interested in transformational models of maternity care. She is also a Board member of the International MotherBaby Childbirth Organization (IMBCO), in which capacity she helped to wordsmith the *International Childbirth Initiative: 12 Steps to Safe and Respectful MotherBaby-Family Maternity Care* (www.ICIchildbirth.org). E-mail: davis-floyd@outlook.com

Ashish Premkumar is an Assistant Professor of Obstetrics and Gynecology at the Pritzker School of Medicine at The University of Chicago and a doctoral candidate in the Department of Anthropology at The Graduate School at Northwestern University. He is a practicing maternal-fetal medicine subspecialist. His research focus is on the intersections of the social sciences and obstetric practices, particularly surrounding the issues of risk, stigma, and quality of health care during the perinatal opioid use disorder epidemic of the 21st century. E-mail: premkumara@bsd.uchicago.edu.

References

Bourdieu P. 1977. *Outline of a Theory of Practice*. Translated by R. Nice, *Cambridge Studies in Social and Cultural Anthropology*. Cambridge: Cambridge University Press.

Bridges K. 2011. "Pregnancy, Medicaid, State Regulation, and Legal Subjection." *Journal of Poverty* 16(3): 323–352.

———. 2012. *Reproducing Race: An Ethnography of Pregnancy as a Site of Racialization*. Berkeley: University of California Press.

Cabrera WP. 2017. *Hampiq: Salud y Enfermedad en Ayacucho* [Doctor: Health and Disease in Ayacucho]. Ayachucho, Peru: Universidad San Cristobol de Huamanga.

Castro A, Savage V. 2019. "Obstetric Violence as Reproductive Governance in the Dominican Republic." *Medical Anthropology* 38(2): 123–136.

Castro R. 2014. "Génesis y Práctica del Habitus Médico Autoritario en México" ["Genesis and Practice of the Authoritarian Medical Habitus in Mexico"] *Revista Mexicana de Sociología* 76(2): 167–197.

Chalmers B. 1997. "Changing Childbirth in Eastern Europe: Which Systems of Authoritative Knowledge Should Prevail?" In *Childbirth and Authoritative Knowledge: Cross-Cultural Perspectives*, eds. Davis-Floyd R, Sargent C, 263–286. Berkeley: University of California Press.

———. 2012. "Childbirth across Cultures: Research and Practice." *Birth* 39(4): 276–280.

Cheyney M, Davis-Floyd R. 2019. "Birth as Culturally Marked and Shaped." In *Birth in Eight Cultures*, eds. Davis-Floyd R, Cheyney M, 1–16. Long Grove IL: Waveland Press.

———. 2020. "Birth and the Big Bad Wolf: A Biocultural, Co-Evolutionary Perspective, Part 2." *International Journal of Childbirth* 10(2): 66–78.

Cohen Shabot S. 2019. "'Amigas, Sisters: We're Being Gaslighted': Obstetric Violence and Epistemic Injustice." In *Childbirth, Vulnerability and Law: Exploring Issues of Violence and Control*, eds. Pickles C, Herring J. Abingdon, Oxon: Routledge. https://www.taylorfrancis.com/chapters/edit/10.4324/9780429443718-2/amigas-sisters-re-being-gaslighted-sara-cohen-shabot.

Çoker H. 2023. "'Birth with No Regret' in Turkey: The Natural Birth of the 21st Century." In *Obstetricians Speak: On Training, Practice, Fear, and Transformation*, eds. Davis-Floyd R, Premkumar A. Chapter 10. New York: Berghahn Books.

Davis-Floyd R. 2001. "The Technocratic, Humanistic, and Holistic Paradigms of Childbirth." *International Journal of Gynecology & Obstetrics* 75, Supplement No. 1: S5–S23.

———. 2018b. "The Technocratic, Humanistic, and Holistic Paradigms of Birth and Health Care." In *Ways of Knowing about Birth: Mothers, Midwives, Medicine, and Birth Activism*, Davis-Floyd R and Colleagues, 3–44. Long Grove IL: Waveland Press,

———. 2022. *Birth as an American Rite of Passage*, 3rd ed. Abingdon, Oxon: Routledge.

———. 2023. "Open and Closed Knowledge Systems, the 4 Stages of Cognition, and the Obstetric Management of Birth." In *Cognition, Risk, and Responsibility in Obstetrics: Anthropological Analyses and Critiques of Obstetricians' Practices*, eds. Davis-Floyd R, Premkumar A. Chapter 1. New York: Berghahn Books.

Davis-Floyd R, Premkumar A., eds. 2023a. *Obstetricians Speak: On Training, Practice, Fear, and Transformation*. New York: Berghahn Books.

———, eds. 2023b. *Cognition, Risk, and Responsibility in Obstetrics: Anthropological Analyses and Critiques of Obstetricians' Practices*. New York: Berghahn Books.

———, eds. 2023c. *Obstetric Violence and Systemic Disparities: Can Obstetrics Be Humanized and Decolonized?* New York: Berghahn Books.

Dixon LZ, Smith-Oka V, El Kotni M. 2019. "Teaching about Childbirth in Mexico: Working across Birth Models." In *Birth in Eight Cultures*, eds. Davis-Floyd R, Cheyney M, 17–48. Long Grove IL: Waveland Press.

Enkin M, Keirse M, Chalmers I. 1989. *Effective Care in Pregnancy and Childbirth*. Oxford: Oxford University Press.

Freire P. 1970. *Pedagogy of the Oppressed*. New York: Seabury Press.

Gaines A, Davis-Floyd R. 2004. "Biomedicine." *Encyclopedia of Medical Anthropology*, eds. Ember C, Ember M, 95–108. New York: Kluwer Academic/Plenum Publishers.

Gilligan C. 1982. *In a Different Voice*. Cambridge MA: Harvard University Press.

———. 2011. "Looking Back to Look Forward: Revisiting *In a Different Voice*." Classics@Journal. Retrieved 12 December 2022 from https://classics-at.chs.harvard.edu/classics9-carol-gilligan-looking-back-to-look-forward-revisiting-in-a-different-voice/.

Jones R. 2012. *Entre as Orelhas—Histórias de Parto [Between the Ears: Birth Stories]*. Porto Alegre, Brazil: Editora Ideias a Granel.

———. 2023. "The Bullying and Persecution of a Humanistic/Holistic Obstetrician in Brazil: The Benefits and Costs of My Paradigm Shift." In *Obstetricians Speak: On Training, Practice, Fear, and Transformation*, eds. Davis-Floyd R, Premkumar A. Chapter 7. New York: Berghahn Books.

Jordan B. 1997. "Authoritative Knowledge and Its Construction." In *Childbirth and Authoritative Knowledge: Cross-Cultural Perspectives*, 55–79. Berkeley: University of California Press.

Levi-Strauss C. 1962. *Le Totémisme Aujourd'hui*. Paris: Universitaires de France.

Liese K, Davis-Floyd R, Stewart K, Cheyney M. 2021. "Obstetric Iatrogenesis in the United States: The Spectrum of Unintentional Harm, Disrespect, Violence, and Abuse." *Anthropology & Medicine* 28(2): 1–17.

Manne K. 2018. *Down Girl: The Logic of Misogyny*. New York: Oxford University Press.

Miller S, Abalos E, Chamillard M, *et al.* 2016. "Beyond Too Little, Too Late and Too Much, Too Soon: A Pathway Towards Evidence-Based, Respectful Maternity Care Worldwide." *Lancet* 388(10056): 2176–2192.

Murray de López J. 2018. "When the Scars Begin to Heal: Narratives of Obstetric Violence in Chiapas, Mexico." *International Journal of Health Governance* 23(1): 60–69.

Niles PM, Stoll K, Wang JJ, Black S, Vedam S. 2021. "'I Fought My Entire Way': Experiences of Declining Maternity Care Services in British Columbia." *PLoSOne* 16(6): eO25645.

Noddings N. 1984. *Caring: A Feminine Approach to Ethics and Moral Education*. Berkeley: University of California Press.

Premkumar A. 2023. "My Transformation from an Obstetrician to a Maternal-Fetal Medicine Subspecialist: Autoethnographic Thoughts on Situated Knowledges and Habitus." In *Obstetricians Speak: On Training, Practice, Fear, and Transformation*, eds. Davis-Floyd R, Premkumar A, Chapter 3. New York: Berghahn Books.

Rivkin-Fish M. 2005a. *Women's Health in Post-Soviet Russia: The Politics of Intervention*. Bloomington: Indiana University Press.

———. 2005b. "Gifts, Bribes, and Unofficial Payments: Towards an Anthropology of Corruption in Russia." In *Corruption: Anthropological Perspectives*, eds. Haller D, Shore C, 47–64. London: Pluto Press.

Roter DL, Hall JA. 1998. "Why Physician Gender Matters in Shaping the Physician-Patient Relationship." *Journal of Women's Health* 7(9): 1093–1097.

———. 2014. "Women Doctors Don't Get the Credit They Deserve." *Journal of General Internal Medicine* 30(3): 273–274.

Ruíter JA, Cameron C. 2021. "Birth Models that Nurture Cooperation between Traditionally Competitive Professionals: Pizza and Other Keys to Disarmament." In *Birthing Models on the Human Rights Frontier: Speaking Truth to Power*, eds. Daviss BA, Davis-Floyd R, 327–346. Abingdon, Oxon: Routledge.

Shim J. 2010. "Cultural Health Capital: A Theoretical Approach to Understanding Health Care Interactions and the Dynamics of Unequal Treatment." *Journal of Health and Social Behavior* 51(1): 1–15.

Stone SB, Myers SS, Golden CD. 2018. "Cross-Cutting Principles for Planetary Health Education." *Lancet Planetary Health* 2(5): e192–e193.

Temkina A, Novkunskaya A, Litvina D. 2022. *Pregnancy and Birth in Russia: The Struggle for "Good Care."* Abingdon, Oxon: Routledge.

Wong SHM, Gishen F, Lokugamage AU. 2021. "Decolonising the Medical Curriculum: Humanising Medicine through Epistemic Pluralism, Cultural Safety, and Critical Consciousness." *London Review of Education* 19(1).

Creating the Anthropology of Obstetrics and Obstetricians and Suggesting Directions for Future Research

Robbie Davis-Floyd and Ashish Premkumar

We begin these Series Conclusions by noting that we have divided them into two parts. Part 1 describes some brief reflections on the overall nature of this three-volume series and some futuristic ideas. Part 2 offers suggestions from our chapter authors for future research, as students and other researchers are always looking for new topics to study, and we aim to provide them with some good ones!

Part 1: Reflections on This Series

In our Series Overview in Volume I (Davis-Floyd and Premkumar 2023a), we asked the question, "Can a book create a field?" and answered that question with a resounding "Yes!" by pointing to the official creation of the field of the Anthropology of Reproduction by Faye Ginsburg and Rayna Rapp with their book *Creating the New World Order: The Global Politics of Reproduction* (1995). For us, the official creation of the field of the Anthropology of Obstetrics and Obstetricians has taken not one, but the three volumes that constitute this Book Series on *The Anthropology of Obstetrics and Obstetricians: The Practice, Maintenance, and Reproduction of a Biomedical Profession*. These three volumes, all co-edited by ourselves—Robbie Davis-Floyd and Ashish Premkumar—and published by Berghahn Books of New York, are:

- Volume I. *Obstetricians Speak: On Training, Practice, Fear, and Transformation*
- Volume II. *Cognition, Risk, and Responsibility in Obstetrics: Anthropological Analyses and Critiques of Obstetricians' Practices*
- Volume III. *Obstetric Violence and Systemic Disparities: Can Obstetrics Be Humanized and Decolonized?*

To the question in the title of Volume III, we respond that there is some hope for a more decolonized, non-racialized, socially unstratified, egalitarian, and humanistic future for birth—an achievement that would take a global paradigm shift that, as most of our chapters in this series make clear, would require midwives trained in the midwifery model of care to become the primary maternity care providers in all countries. Yet that shift is unlikely, because as William Arney (1982), Robbie Davis-Floyd ([1992] 2003, 2022), and others have shown, at least in high-resource countries where some childbearers actually have choices, the technocratic treatment of birth is often *consensually constructed* by the obstetricians (most of whom consider themselves the ultimate authorities on it) who practice it and by the childbearers who accept it and who believe that obstetricians are the most qualified maternity care providers. The key points of unity between most childbirth care receivers and hospital care providers are *fear* and *safety*. *Fear* of injury or death draws childbearers to hospitals and obs to the technocratic model, which for both provides a sense of *safety*. Yet "safety" is the disguise worn by technocratic obstetrics; in truth, it has long been shown that, when attended by skilled midwives, community births (meaning births at home or in freestanding birth centers) are just as safe as hospital births, and even safer, as they entail far fewer maternal and newborn morbidities. (For references to the multiple studies on this topic, see the chapter in Volume II by Amali Lokugamage and Claire Feeley [2023]). Regarding such morbidities, we point here, as we did in our Series Overview in Volume I (Davis-Floyd and Premkumar 2023a), to Peter Reynold's (1991) concept of the "1–2 Punch of mutilation and prosthesis." To recap, Punch 1: deconstruct/mutilate a natural process with technological interventions; Punch 2: reconstruct/prosthetize that process with more technology. As previously explained, Reynold's brilliant insight was that most often, Punch 2 is the point: we in technocratic societies tend to believe that by technologically intervening in natural processes, we have improved them—made them safer, more controllable. To figure out why this 1–2 Punch has become so prevalent, exemplifying the "obstetric paradox" referred to in multiple chapters (intervene to keep birth safe, thereby causing harm), ethnographic research on obstetricians has been needed, and the volumes in this series are filled with the results of such research.

However, technocratic solutions have issues that extend beyond iatrogenic harm: the rise and maintenance of entire healthcare systems that have environmental and thus planetary consequences. As Amali Lokugamage, Tharanika Ahillan, and SDC Pathberiya described in their chapter in this volume, from a global health perspective, climate change debates and associated civil protests resonate with Indigenous ideas of *planetary health*, which focus on the harmonious interconnections of the planet, the environment, and human beings. These authors stated that: "This shines the light of importance" on displaced Indigenous ideas, which must be "re-centered and foregrounded to highlight the importance of human health within planetary ecology." They emphasized Indigenous peoples' perspectives on health, noting that in "How Decolonizing Health Could Save the Planet," Rebekah Jaung (2019) explained that:

> Indigenous people have always had ecological perspectives on health, which have only recently entered "mainstream" health discourse. The scope now is planetary health—approaches which benefit all people and the natural environment. Ideas we have learned from Indigenous people include seeing climate breakdown as a symptom of non-reciprocal and exploitative relationships with land and acknowledging that such a relationship exists. Ways of honoring the land will not only restore it, [they] will lead to good health for the people who live on it. This is not just a nice sentiment but the approach on which cutting edge thinking on global climate action is structured.

Following this quotation, Lokumage, Ahillan, and Pathberiya went on to note that:

> Presently, there is a rising social tide of interest in climate change and health . . . These issues are likely to challenge the present and future generations of doctors. It is therefore important to incorporate non-biased critical thinking about these issues on global health and ecological public health, and to raise awareness of the emerging field of *planetary health* within the biomedical education curriculum. (Asakura et al. 2015) but this seems to have faded. The burden of disease the developing world is facing cannot be addressed solely by reductionist approaches. Holistic approaches are called for that recognize the fundamentally interdependent nature of health and

other societal, developmental, and ecosystem related factors in human communities.

A focus on planetary health—inclusive of economic and societal impacts—would lead us to consider novel interventions to ameliorate ongoing adverse maternity and other health outcomes. For example, hospitals are major sources of environmental pollution and non-recyclable waste. And it is important to understand that *11 billion USD per year* could be saved in the United States if only 10% more births took place in homes and freestanding birth centers (FBCs)—321 million USD per percentage point rise (Anderson, Daviss, and Johnson 2021). Surely such costs savings are options for other countries as well. Should childbearers around the world refuse unnecessary routinized technocratic interventions because they understand that these interfere with the normal physiology of birth, generate unnecessary costs, and use too many environmental resources, they would have to flee hospitals in droves in favor of community births—births at home and in FBCs—for which the world's community midwives, traditional and professional, are completely unprepared—which is why we need many more of them.

Should that highly unlikely scenario ever unfold, then to stay in business, maternity care hospitals and wards would have to offer deeply humanistic births, and not the superficially humanistic births now on offer in birthing centers in high-resource hospitals, for which the joke has long been that the in-hospital "ABC" (Alternative Birth Center) stands for "A Beautiful Cesarean." Or they could abandon any attempts to facilitate normal physiologic births in favor of leaving those in the capable hands of community midwives, whose outcomes in many countries have been shown to be excellent (again, as thoroughly demonstrated in the Volume II chapter on "Cognition, Risk, and Responsibility: Home Birth and Why Obstetricians Fear It" by Amali Lokugamage and Claire Feeley) and specialize only in the minority of births that can actually benefit from obstetricians' understandings of pathologies and how to deal with them using at least a superficially humanistic approach. Because epidurals generate the well-known "cascade of interventions," the vast majority of childbearers whose pregnancies and births are normal would have to accept the pains caused by contractions, using doula care and water immersion (where possible) for pain relief instead of epidurals and other types of analgesia. They might reinterpret this pain as Japanese women and midwives tend to do, perceiving it as *metamorphic*—as the character-forging process that turns a woman into a mother (Williamson and Matsuoka 2019).

But there is no such arising in high-resource countries, due to the above-mentioned consensus. And in low-resource countries, as the push for facility birth continues, fewer and fewer women have the choice to use their traditional community midwives, as those midwives are rapidly being phased out of practice or simply dying without transmitting their knowledge to younger generations. Despite the extremely poor conditions in under-resourced hospitals, described in various chapters in Volumes II and III, most laboring people would rather be in a biomedical clinic or hospital, no matter what quality of care is provided or isn't. On the parts of both patients and practitioners, fear, and perceptions of the hospital and its interventions as representing safety, drive the continued hegemony of the technocratic approach to birth.

Chapters in all three volumes have described the reasons why most obstetricians feel the need to over-intervene in birth, as summarized in our Conclusions to these volumes. Here we provide a brief summary of why obs over-perform cesarean births (CBs) that we have gleaned from the chapters that address high CB rates in Volumes II and III. As these chapters have shown, obstetricians' motivations for performing often-unnecessary CBs are complex and are often country-specific. Yet ultimately, these motivations can be summed up in four words: money, convenience, fear, and control. Even in countries where obs are paid the same for cesareans as for vaginal births, the time-saving nature of cesareans allows them to make more money by seeing more private patients in their offices. And scheduling CBs provides them with convenience. As for fear, obs fear litigation if something goes wrong and they don't perform a cesarean. And many obs with high CB rates have become de-skilled in attending vaginal births—most especially VBAC (vaginal birth after cesarean), breech, and twin births—so such obs have come to fear those as well. In fact, most technocratic obstetricians are afraid of vaginal births because all have seen terrible outcomes, which (understandably) lead them to practice defensively—which means performing unnecessary cesareans "just in case." Obstetricians have the kind of control over cesarean births that they can never have over vaginal births, and they tend to highly value that sense of control. Ironically, since obs with extremely high CB rates have become so entirely de-skilled in attending vaginal births, in their cases, CBs are actually the safer option for their patients. To put this more succinctly: the more you do cesareans, the more you become de-skilled in attending vaginal births, and the more cesareans you do!

Thus, despite the many reasons why cesarean birth rates should go down to the 15–20% rates recommended by WHO (2015), and also despite the multiple humanizing trends described in many of our chapters, we see no indications from our chapters or from our knowledge of global trends that they will. (Hence the importance of the "gentle" cesareans described by Caroline Chautems, Irene Maffi, and Alexandre Farin (2023) in their chapter in Volume II. If obs are going to perform cesareans anyway, at least they could do them in family-friendly ways.) Yet we do believe that these humanistic trends will continue to increase, because all birthing women want respectful and compassionate care, because such care is evidence-based, and because obstetricians and other practitioners themselves derive more satisfaction from birth attendance when they provide such care. As some of our chapter authors have pointed out, these humanizing trends—at least in higher-resource countries—have long included the presence of partners, and sometimes doulas, at births and more considerate treatment of laboring people. Increasingly, laboring people are allowed and even encouraged to use the "deeply humanistic" (see the Introduction to this volume) practices of moving freely during labor, eating and drinking at will, and laboring and birthing in the positions of their choice. And, as some of our chapters demonstrate, these deeply humanizing trends are also coming to include much-needed models of improved communication and collaboration between obstetricians and midwives.

Yet sadly, many of our chapters, especially those in Volume I, illustrate the ostracisms, bullyings, and persecutions from the Stage 1, silo-oriented, and fundamentalist members of their obstetric establishments suffered by deeply humanistic obs who do offer women the full range of truly informed choice. These chapters also provide descriptions of the many ways in which such obs have withstood such attacks. We point here specifically to Turkish ob Hakan Çoker's (2023) successes in turning such attacks into opportunities to further explain the evidence that supports his deeply humanistic model of "Birth with No Regret" to such obstetricians; his respectful, non-defensive attitude toward them caused many of them to secretly start attending his education courses and to change their practices accordingly over time. Models like Hakan's are still islands of humanism in an ocean of technocratic practices, yet they are growing in number, and at some magical tipping point, there may be enough of them to actually make such practices also normative for others. This growth is also illustrated in the chapter by Robbie Davis-Floyd and Eugenia Georges in this volume on the paradigm shifts made by increasing numbers of Brazilian obstetricians, some of whom are humanizing the practices of entire maternity wards in their respective hospitals. A contributor to this growth is the *International Childbirth Initiative*, as we further discuss below.

And then there is huge body of scientific evidence—cited and explained in many of our chapters—that supports the facilitation of normal physiologic birth. Biomedical obstetrics purports itself to be a science as well as an art, yet the vast majority of its routine procedures during labor and birth are very, very far from being evidence-based. Perhaps someday the actual evidence will win out, and normal physiologic births will be supported to unfold as nature has designed. Yet again, that is only likely to happen when professional midwives who practice the humanistic and holistic midwifery model of care become the primary first-line maternity care providers in all countries and are treated as respected colleagues by obs rather than being considered below them in the obstetric hierarchy. Robbie (Davis-Floyd 2022) has suggested that the proper ratio for birth attendance is 80% midwives and 20% obstetricians, for certainly obs are needed when actual (not imagined) pathologies are present. Thus it seems clear that fewer obs and more midwives will create a better and far more humanistic future for birth.

We now turn to the suggestions for future research provided by ourselves and our chapter authors. As previously noted, students and other researchers are always looking for something to study, so we hope to provide them with some viable ideas!

Part 2: Suggestions for Future Research

Some of these suggestions for future research from our chapter authors were either emailed to us directly and/or we extrapolated them from their chapters. We begin with Robbie's strong suggestion, repeated in many of her bios in these volumes, to research the processes of the implementation of the above-mentioned *International Childbirth Initiative* (ICI): *12 Steps to Safe and Respectful MotherBaby-Family Maternity Care*, as described in detail in André Lalonde's (2023) chapter in Volume I of this series, in Lalonde and colleagues (2019), and at the International Childbirth Initiative (ICI) website.[1] The ICI is a deeply humanistic template for optimal maternity care based on a series of foundational principles, on the scientific evidence on normal physiologic birth, on the proper management of true complications, and also on a "MotherBaby-Family"-centered model of care. The ICI has been endorsed by multiple international organizations, the names of which are displayed on its website. According to André Lalonde's (2023) chapter in Volume I, as of January 2022, the ICI's underlying philosophy and 12 Steps were implemented in hospitals and other birthing facilities in:

Austria, Brazil, Canada, Chile, Colombia, Fiji, India, Indonesia, Kenya, Mongolia, Papua New Guinea, the Philippines, the Solomon

Islands, Trinidad, Turkey, and the United States. Countries that are initiating implementation (applications in progress) include Argentina, Australia, Burkina Faso, China, the Czech Republic, Germany, Honduras, Mexico, Nigeria, and Uruguay.

And there will be many more to come! Research on the processes of implementation, any barriers to them, and possible solutions to those barriers is much needed.[2]

For those interested in narrative, Robbie's suggestion for future research is a comparison and analysis of the differences in the stories about birth told by obstetricians and midwives. In her experience, obs gathered in groups tend to tell stories about pathological births in which they saved, or failed to save, either the mother's or the baby's life. In contrast, in midwives' storytelling sessions, which are often structured into the programs of midwifery conferences, midwives of all ilks tend to tell profound stories of amazing births or funny stories in which the unexpected happened—such as one midwife arriving at the house of a pregnant friend just to check in with her, then suddenly having to attend a precipitous birth with only one glove and a shoestring! Another example of this kind of story comes from homebirth midwife Kate Bowland of Santa Cruz, California, in which, during a storytelling session at a conference, she described (and acted out) a home birth that had been going well until the pushing stage. The doula present suggested that they all do the "hula, hula, stomp, stomp," which consisted of swinging hula hoops around their waists, then stomping down hard with their feet several times. After three repetitions of this technique, the woman sank down on her knees and gave birth! Thus we can see that such stories can contain valuable information about how to facilitate normal physiologic birth.

The differences between the birth stories told by obs and midwives are immense and revelatory, and recording and analyzing them could reveal much about the differences in the ways in which obs and midwives conceptualize birth and how those conceptualizations affect their practices—all of which are contextualized by the location of care (e.g., hospital, home, FBC). Listening to midwives' stories is easy—just attend a conference into which a storytelling session is scheduled, or get a group of midwives in your locale together and ask them to tell birth stories, which they are always happy to do! Although such sessions are not structured into obstetric conferences, a researcher could attend such a conference, strike up several acquaintances with obs, then invite them all to dinner and ask them to tell birth stories over drinks (the more alcohol people consume, the more likely they are to tell stories!), then do it all again the next day.

And Robbie offers another suggestion: to think more about the differences between "superficial" and "deep" humanism—are practitioners aware of these differences? Do they think that their practices are fully humanized because they allow partners and doulas into the labor room? Deeply humanistic practice is so much more than that, as described in the Introductions to Volume II (Davis-Floyd and Premkumar 2023b) and to this volume, and in the Series Overview in Volume I (Davis-Floyd and Premkumar 2023a). Simply by asking obstetricians and other maternity care practitioners who believe that they are practicing humanistically (these are the easiest to interview, as they are usually quite happy to talk about their paradigm shifts) if they are aware of the differences between superficial and deep humanism, and then explaining those differences if needed, can generate that awareness and possibly further more deeply humanistic changes in their already humanistic practices. (As a reminder, Chapter 12 in this volume describes the methods that many of our chapter authors used to find, survey, interview, and observe obstetricians and other maternity care practitioners.)

In the third edition of *Birth as an American Rite of Passage* (Davis-Floyd 2022), which is based on interviews with 165 postpartum people, Robbie provides "An Argument for a Re-Classification of the 'Three Stages of Labor.'" Concerned about the number of unnecessary cesareans performed in the United States for "failure to progress," and about obstetricians' failures to understand the importance of recognizing the latent phase of labor, which can safely last for hours or days until active labor kicks in (see Lewis 2020; Mayo Clinic Staff 2020)—and during which laboring people should usually not be admitted to their hospital, where they are placed on a clock as soon as they enter—Robbie argues that:

> the widely accepted term "first stage of labor," which has long been defined as lasting through to "second stage"—pushing, should be categorically separated into two stages: the first stage being latent labor and lasting up to 5 cm, the second stage being active labor, starting at 6 cm and lasting up till pushing begins, the third stage being not just complete cervical dilation and effacement, but active pushing, following the urge to push until the baby is born, and the fourth stage being delivery of the placenta. Such a redefinition would clarify and re-name the latent stage as a clearly separate category from what I suggest calling "second stage" active labor, and make it less likely that the latent stage could be ignored under the technocratic model as it has been for so long. It would also stop practitioners from urging laboring people to push before they feel the actual urge to push, as care providers so often do.

And Robbie wonders here if any researchers might be willing to take this suggestion seriously, and to investigate what kinds of impacts it might have on lowering the cesarean rates in various countries. However, it seems that if the CB rate in a hospital gets lowered for one particular reason, such as not performing cesareans for failure to progress, it then rises for other reasons, so that ultimately, it stays the same. Why? This would indeed be a rich area for future research!

Not stopping here, Robbie also wonders why none of the childbearers she interviewed who chose to have epidurals understood their risks. Among many others, as Robbie explains and references in the new edition of her book *Birth as an American Rite of Passage* (2022), these risks include the fact that the medication in the epidural affects the baby and often makes newborns "floppy" at birth. Epidurals can also result in a temperature rise in the mother; often pediatricians don't know whether that rise reflects an infection-induced fever or is simply a result of the epidural. As a result, many newborns whose mothers have fevers at birth (10–15%) are given antibiotics,[3] which have been associated with alterations in babies' gut microbiomes (see Tapiainen et al. 2019). Most interlocutors stated unequivocally that they wanted no drugs for pain relief that would negatively affect their babies, yet, again, none of the interlocutors who chose epidurals understood these risks. Thus this too is a subject ripe for research. And of course, simply asking pregnant women about such understandings can generate their awareness of these risks, and perhaps cause them to act accordingly. Robbie firmly believes that it is a laboring person's right to choose an epidural; she just wants them to be fully informed of all the implications of that choice.

Series and volume co-editor Ashish Premkumar suggests these directions for future research:

> I would love to see more in terms of how providers linguistically "construct" risky pregnancies in the delivery room, particularly through participant observation. I think about practices that will preemptively call "arrest of descent" and recommend forceps with little to no indication. What is interpreted by the pregnant person as the indication? And how can risk become this force that becomes literally operationalized, dictated, and subsequently incorporated into future counseling for mode of delivery through the medical record?

And Ashish noted in his Volume I chapter (Premkumar 2023) that:

> While affective/emotional work is part and parcel of clinical work, the ability to effectively produce and maintain a particular affective

environment—one that emphasizes quietness, allowing simultaneously for the potential for calm to a patient, yet able to effectively allow for communication and coordination of multiple medical care teams—during difficult, and often traumatizing, situations is a hallmark of transitioning from an obstetrician/gynecologist to an MFM [maternal-fetal medicine specialist].

Thus, we suggest that more research is needed on this process of transitioning from an ob/gyn to an MFM, and on the affective/emotional labor that ob/gyns and MFMs must do. Correspondingly, Anna Temkina, co-author of the chapter in this volume on the partial humanization of Russian maternity care, suggested (via email) that a direction for future research could be: "Emotional styles and the emotional labor of professionals—how they study and learn appropriate emotional styles, and how these styles have been changed."

We also suggest research on the practitioners of other specialties related to obstetrics, such as pediatricians, neonatologists, anesthesiologists, labor and delivery nurses, and nurses who work in NICUs (although many such nurses have already engaged in much research, and one would need to review their work before proceeding). Additionally, we suggest research on the gynecological aspects of obstetricians' practices, which are not addressed in this series.

In his Volume I chapter (Moses 2023), abortion provider and obstetrician Scott Moses offered the following direction for future research:

> I am affected by the reality that the fetus I extract from the uterus will not become a child. Surprising even to myself, my emotional response is similar whether I remove a live fetus during an abortion or dead fetus after a miscarriage . . . In both cases, these losses are complex and difficult . . . I am changed as well . . . Both patient and provider (as well as the nurse, scrub tech, anesthesiologist and many other people involved in the experience) have distinct yet interconnected narratives [about their experiences with providing abortions] that warrant further investigation.

To this suggestion, Scott added that: "Publicly disclosing and revealing the narratives of abortion providers has a relatively short history; much remains to be discussed and processed."

In response to our call for suggestions for future research, Jesanna Cooper, author of a chapter in Volume I (Cooper 2023), briefly stated: "I think that the business side of cesarean section with regard to physician time commitment, call schedules, and allocating portions of a global fee need to be explored further. Researchers could study the effects of various call payment arrangements and call schedules on cesarean rates." And Michelle Sadler, co-author of a Volume II chapter, suggests research on several topics:

- The "feminization" of obstetrics: I'm not sure of what's going on in other countries, but at least in Chile and other South American countries, the university enrollment to study obstetrics/gynecology is rapidly changing from mainly male to female. In Chile, currently 75% of enrollees are women, whereas a couple of decades ago it was almost only men. Due to our ingrained cultural biases, the more Chilean obstetrics has been feminized, the less prestigious it has become.
- Sexism in medical education/hidden curriculum: not enough has been said! There is a lot to research to show how deeply sexist medical education is. It's easily blurred under pompous statements of gender equality approaches in health education, which are not translated in the actual programs. Toward that end, medical students who are also interested in medical anthropology could do ethnographies of the lectures they attend, perhaps in terms of contrasting what is explicitly said with the implicit biases that may be unconsciously embedded in those lectures. This research suggestion could also extend to critical examinations of clinical training as it occurs that identify the biases and the hidden curriculum that inform that training, and to the lived experiences of medical and midwifery students: embodiment approaches to understand better how deep the process of transformation is.

In their chapter in Volume II of this series, Vania Smith-Oka and Lydia Dixon (2023) suggested that "Continued research into the perspectives of the obstetricians and nurses working on the front lines is needed to develop further changes, as are re-socialization courses that train them in how to facilitate normal physiologic birth. By including their buy-in and input, they can be central to attempts to ensure much-needed systemic changes." Thus, researchers could study both Vania and Lydia's first suggestion, and could also investigate whether any such "re-socialization" courses exist, and if so, who teaches them and where, and what are the contents of these courses and whether or not they generate any actual practice changes in the practitioners who take such courses.

Jo Murphy-Lawless, co-author of a Volume II chapter (Dunlea et al. 2023), issued (via email) an urgent call for future research that resulted from the abrupt closure of the Albany midwifery practice, which had reached a homebirth rate of 43% in an all-risk London district and then was shut down despite its excellent outcomes. (For a description of the Albany practice in its heyday, see Reed and Walton 2009. For a presentation and analysis of its statistics, see Homer et al. 2017. For a description and analysis of the reasons why it was shut down, see Reed and Edwards, in press):

> We urgently require wide-ranging research on why well-structured midwifery initiatives have consistently been closed down: what were the organizational rationales proffered, what have been the elements in common of the power blocs that imposed these decisions, what have been the impacts on women and communities, what has been the impact on the midwifery profession?

We editors (Ashish and Robbie) reiterate this call, and extend it to suggesting research on the members of obstetric establishments who bully and persecute humanistic and holistic obstetricians, as described in the chapters of Volume I, in which several of our ob authors who made a paradigm shift from technocratic to deeply humanistic and/or holistic practice describe the ostracisms, bullyings, and persecutions they experienced. For example, Ágnes (Agi) Geréb of Hungary stated in her Volume I chapter (Geréb and Fábián 2023):

> Women wishing to give birth outside of hospitals are a fraction of a percent of pregnant women in Hungary. Such a small group, even with all their supporters, could not possibly pose a significant challenge to the biomedical establishment nor shake the foundations of their substantive economic interests. However, the political and medical authorities in Hungary perceive even the tiniest challenge as potentially lethal to them ... What could be the rationale of the political and medical authorities to engage in such oppressive practices?

And for another example, in Puerto Rico—an island on which there are only 24 midwives usually attending less than 1% of births—during the COVID-19 pandemic when home births were on the rise, the obstetricians there launched a vicious media campaign against those midwives and against home birth (Reyes 2021). Thus, it would be fascinating to interview obstetricians (and the members of obstetric organizations) who ostracize, bully, and sometimes actively persecute deeply humanistic obs and midwives to try to understand their rationales and motives for such punitive treatments. What are these powerful obstetricians so afraid of? Why can't they tolerate the existence of alternative practices and points of view?

To conduct this kind of important research could prove difficult: you would have to find obs and midwives who are currently being persecuted (of which there are plenty), then interview their persecutors—who may well not be willing to be interviewed unless you approach them correctly (again, see Chapter 12 of this volume). Alternatively, you could conduct such research from a historical perspective by studying cases of persecution that have already occurred, then interviewing the most important parties involved.

In an interesting take on this trope, Margaret Dunlea, co-author of the Volume II chapter on the culture of Irish obstetrics (Dunlea et al. 2023), offered via email the following suggestions:

> A research question could be: What are the determining factors around governance structures for the midwifery profession in state-run maternity services across the world? This brings us back to the vulnerability of newly developed midwifery-led services to budget withdrawal as a strategy to maintain obstetric dominance and undermine midwifery services.
>
> Another research question could be: How do we safeguard newly developed midwifery initiatives from being shut down or undermined by hegemonic groups, who are in the business of protecting their vested interests?

To these suggestions for future research, Robbie adds in her Volume II chapter (Davis-Floyd 2023):

> How fundamentalist or fanatical you are tends to depend on your level of socialization and embodied habituation into the areas in which your thinking becomes rigidified—the deeper the socialization and habituation, and the more rituals associated with them, the "truer believer" (Hoffer 1951) you are likely to be. The "true believer" phenomenon is fairly well understood, but *why some people become open and fluid thinkers is not*; thus, this is a subject ripe for further research.

In her chapter, Robbie also suggests that:

> If you are a social scientist, it might be well to consider what roles the social sciences might play in facilitating the expansion of Stage

4, globally humanistic thinking and related practices within health-care systems, as well as in policy . . . social scientists tend to be very good at describing, analyzing, and critiquing closed systems like that of technocratic obstetrics—not stopping at critiques, but moving forward to provide "thick" interpretations . . . of why such systems and their practitioners are as they are, think and act as they do. This approach might be further facilitated by increased interdisciplinary work, participation in public health education and events, and greater involvement in multidisciplinary policy and protocol development. Perhaps we anthropologists could also educate the public about the power of ritual both to stabilize us cognitively and to effect change. I ask, in what other ways could anthropology in particular, and social science in general, facilitate the kinds of Stage 4 systems that would make our world a safer place? And I encourage social scientists to respond.

Beverley Chalmers, author of the chapter in this volume on teaching humanistic and holistic obstetrics, offered (via email) multiple suggestions for future research:

1. Explore which/how many universities/Health Science schools in North America or elsewhere include courses in human behavioral science (or something similar) in medical students' undergraduate or graduate studies? How is this done? What works best?
2. Do any medical schools today include psychologists and social scientists in the teaching of humanistic/holistic perinatal care? If so, how do they do this: as separate courses or integrated into the mainstream teaching of ob/gyn? What could/should be done in this arena?
3. Do schools/departments of psychology in North America or elsewhere prepare perinatal psychologists for this profession? If so, what training are they/should they be given?
4. How do healthcare professionals (such as ob/gyns, pediatricians, midwives, perinatal nurses, and social workers) view the value of and the need for perinatal health professionals in hospital or community settings?
5. How many (and where are they?) perinatal healthcare settings regularly employ perinatal full-time (or part-time) psychologists in their healthcare services?
6. Which, and how many, medical schools prepare students for international/global perinatal health consulting, and how? What works best?

7. What on-site training opportunities are available for healthcare provider students to learn about global perinatal health? What are the outcomes of such opportunities for the students? And for the sites?

8. How are perinatal healthcare organizations structured? As silos? Or as integrated and multidisciplinary organizations? How often and where are the latter approaches being introduced? What are best practices in this regard?

Irene Maffi, co-author of the Volume II chapter on "gentle cesareans" (Chautems, Maffi, and Farin 2023), offered (via email) these suggestions for research topics:

1. The construction of knowledge (or ignorance) about endometriosis. At least in Switzerland, it is extremely difficult to find ob/gyns who are able to identify and cure endometriosis. Very few hospitals offer specialized services to women suffering from this pathology and the therapeutic itineraries of the latter are often very complex and painful.

2. The training and knowledge of ob/gyns about contraception. In many countries, they are the main providers of biomedical contraceptives but often have a superficial and short training about them. It would also be interesting to study whether the critiques of hormonal contraception that many women share in various countries affect ob/gyns.

In tandem, author of the Volume II chapter on contraceptive provision by US ob/gyns (Evans 2023), Melissa Goldin Evans offered (also via email) these suggestions for future research:

To better understand issues of access to long-acting reversible contraceptives (LARCs), more population-based research is needed at the clinical level. Same-day LARC provision depends in part on clinical protocols that allow for same-day insertions and have LARCs available on-site. The cost of storing LARCs on-site is often cited as a barrier to same-day insertion protocols. Yet it is difficult to measure clinical protocols at scale. One ob/gyn outpatient center in Hawaii successfully piloted a "buy and bill" program where it found stocking devices on-site, and then billing the patient's insurance for the cost of the device was cost-effective . . . Future interventions and research should test "buy and bill" programs at a state level to determine if a comprehensive increase in availability of same-day LARC insertions reduces barriers and increases uptake.

In her chapter in Volume II on cesarean births in Greece, author Eugenia (Nia) Georges (2023) noted that the Greek approach to biomedical training is divided into two segments: abstract theory and clinical practice. Thus Nia stated:

> In this chapter, I have suggested that this approach to biomedical training may be a vestige of the European training experienced in the last century by the influential pioneers in Greek obstetrics. However, further research would help to clarify why, given that many doctors since then were trained in the United States and elsewhere under different pedagogical approaches, the top-down Greek model [of education] remains robust.

If anyone out there wishes to do, or is doing, research in Greece, Nia's suggestion would be a viable approach.

In her chapter on racial and ethnic biases among US obs in this volume, Genevieve Ritchie-Ewing offered several directions for future research, stating that:

> In the United States, there is a "perfect storm" of mistrust and misunderstanding and personal and structural roadblocks that prevent many physicians and patients from building the patient/physician relationship necessary for reducing healthcare disparities. While . . . I cannot make general conclusions about US obstetricians from the impressions and experiences of the eight participants in this study, their responses do reveal several avenues for future research.

Given that Ritchie-Ewing was able to interview only eight obs, despite her multiple efforts to interview more, we suggest that racial and ethnic biases among obstetricians in multiple countries, and how they impact maternity care, remain strong subjects for future research. As Genevieve found, obstetricians are often reluctant to admit to having such biases, so observations of their practices would be a more fruitful way to identify these biases and their effects on maternity care.

In their chapter on interprofessional education (IPE) among midwifery and obstetric students in Aotearoa New Zealand (this volume), co-authors Rea Daellenbach, Lorna Davies, Maggie Meeks, Coleen Caldwell, Melanie Welfare, and Judy Ormandy suggested that "Further research into IPE specifically in the context of the ANZ maternity care setting is urgently needed to provide evidence of its long-term effectiveness in generating a strong foundation of mutual respect and collaboration with the development of a common professional or inter-professional language in maternity care." To their call for future research in their country, we add that interprofessional education should be provided for all obstetricians and midwives (among many others) in all countries where they work together, and that any such programs should be studied, analyzed, and evaluated for efficacy. We argue that it is essential for humanizing birth that obstetricians work to develop collegial relationships with midwives and to stop treating them as subordinates. Only when midwives—hospital- or community-based—have autonomy in their practices can they fully implement the midwifery model of care.

In their chapter in this volume on decolonizing medical education in the UK, co-authors Amali Lokugamage, Tharanika Ahillan, and SDC Pathberiya noted that "Research is urgently needed to understand why Black women are five times more likely and Asian women are twice as likely to die during pregnancy and childbirth compared to white women" in their country. (Yet in the United States, Asian women do not have higher mortality rates than white women [Singh 2021], so it would be helpful to research the reasons why their maternal mortality rates are high in the UK and low in the United States.) These authors strongly imply that researchers in many countries should investigate healthcare practitioners'—and mostly biomedical professors' and teachers'—levels of awareness about the colonialism inherent in biomedicine and any efforts they have made toward de-colonizing biomedical education. Simply by asking these questions, researchers can generate awareness in biomedical educators of this concept and of the importance of decolonizing their educational curricula, so that a new generation of doctors would grow up with this awareness and could work to decolonize their practices. Thus, such researchers should come to their interviews equipped with information on how to do so, in case their interlocutors ask for such information. We reiterate here the suggestion provided in the Conclusions to this volume from Lokugamage, Ahillan, and Pathberiya—that:

> At an individual level, the process of providing Cultural Safety would essentially entail that a nurse, doctor, or student, as part their reflective practice prior to a patient encounter, quickly reflect on their privileged status and any potential power imbalances between themselves and the patient. This quick reflection should provide

insight and situational awareness, aspiring to create a fairer clinical encounter.

And again, we urge all such practitioners to apply this "quick reflection" in their practices to create "a fairer clinical encounter," and suggest that their level of awareness of Cultural Safety (as described by Lokugamage, Ahillan, and Pathberiya, this volume) and whether or not they engage in "reflective practice" are subjects for future research. Again, simply asking these questions could make practitioners aware of these issues, and that awareness could lead to more reflective practices.

Conclusion: Possibilities for Humanized Maternity Care

No consensual verdict has appeared in the chapters in this present volume in answer to the question in its subtitle, "Can Obstetrics Be Humanized and De-Colonized?" The answers to this question that we—Robbie and Ashish—can come up with, based on the chapters in Part 2, are: "Yes, sometimes and in some places with some maternity care practitioners" and "No, at most times in most places among most practitioners." It is our hope that those dualities will eventually be transformed into "Yes, at all times and in all places with the support of all maternity care providers, including obstetricians." This entire series, many of our own written works, Ashish's practices as a perinatologist, and Robbie's activist work (see her bio below), are devoted to that goal.

Robbie Davis-Floyd, Adjunct Professor, Department of Anthropology, Rice University, Houston, Fellow of the Society for Applied Anthropology, and Senior Advisor to the Council on Anthropology and Reproduction, is a well-known medical/reproductive anthropologist and international speaker and researcher in transformational models in childbirth, midwifery, obstetrics, and reproduction. Over the course of her long anthropological career, which began in the early 1980s, she has taught at four universities (Trinity University in San Antonio, Texas; University of Texas Austin; Rice University Houston; and Case Western Reserve University in Cleveland, Ohio, where she served for a year as Visiting Professor), given more than 1,000 talks at universities and at birth, midwifery, and obstetric conferences around the world, and has received multiple grants and awards. For 15 years (1994–2009), she served on the Board of the North American Registry of Midwives

(NARM—the organization that maintains and administers certification for certified professional midwives [CPMs]). She is author of more than 80 journal articles and 24 encyclopedia entries, of *Birth as an American Rite of Passage* (1992, 2003, 2022) and of *Ways of Knowing about Birth* (2018); co-author of *From Doctor to Healer: The Transformative Journey* and of *Ritual: What It Is, How It Works, and Why* (2022); and lead or co-editor of 17 volumes, the latest of which are *Birth in Eight Cultures* (2019), co-edited with Melissa Cheyney; *Birthing Models on the Human Rights Frontier: Speaking Truth to Power* (2021), co-edited with Betty-Anne Daviss; *Sustainable Birth in Disruptive Times*, lead-edited by Kim Gutschow and co-edited with Betty-Anne Daviss (2021); and the solo-edited *Birthing Techno-Sapiens: Human-Technology Co-Evolution and the Future of Reproduction* (2021). In process are a collection on *Traditional Midwives: Cross-Cultural Perspectives*, to be co-edited with Pakistani anthropologist Inayat Ali and Canadian midwife Betty-Anne Daviss; and a textbook on the anthropology of reproduction, to be co-authored with Maya Unnithan and Marcia Inhorn. Robbie is also a Board member of the International MotherBaby Childbirth Organization (IMBCO), in which capacity she helped to wordsmith the *International Childbirth Initiative: 12 Steps to Safe and Respectful MotherBaby-Family Maternity Care* (www.ICIchildbirth.org). Researchers are needed to assess the ICI implementation process, to identify and analyze barriers to implementation, and to suggest ways of overcoming these barriers. If you are interested, please contact Robbie. E-mail: davis-floyd@outlook.com.

Ashish Premkumar is an Assistant Professor of Obstetrics and Gynecology at the Pritzker School of Medicine at The University of Chicago and a doctoral candidate in the Department of Anthropology at The Graduate School at Northwestern University. He is a practicing maternal-fetal medicine subspecialist. His research focus is on the intersections of the social sciences and obstetric practices, particularly surrounding the issues of risk, stigma, and quality of health care during the perinatal opioid use disorder epidemic of the 21st century. E-mail: premkumara@bsd.uchicago.edu.

Notes

1. International Childbirth Initiative. Landing page. Retrieved 12 December 2022 from www.icichildbirth.org.
2. If you are interested, please contact Robbie at davis-floyd@outlook.com; Debra Pascali Bonaro at debrapascalibonaro@gmail.com; and/or André Lalonde at alalonde1801@gmail.com.

3. Many hospitals are moving towards use of the Kaiser Early-Onset Sepsis calculator, which takes into consideration more variables that are associated with sepsis in the newborn. (See Kaiser Permanente. n.d. "Neonatal Early-Onset Sepsis Calculator." Retrieved 12 December 2022 from https://neonatalsepsiscalculator.kaiserpermanente.org/.)

References

Anderson DA, Daviss BA, Johnson KC. 2021. "What If Another 10% of Deliveries in the United States Took Place at Home or in a Birth Center? Safety, Economics, and Politics." In *Birthing Models on the Human Rights Frontier: Speaking Truth to Power*, eds. Daviss BA, Davis-Floyd R, 205-228. Abingdon, Oxon: Routledge.

Arney WR. 1982. *Power and the Profession of Obstetrics*. Chicago: University of Chicago Press.

Asakura T, Mallee H, Tomokawa S, et al. 2015. "The Ecosystem Approach to Health Is a Promising Strategy in International Development: Lessons from Japan and Laos." *Globalization and Health* 11(1): 3–10.

Chautems C, Maffi I, Farin A. 2023. "The Introduction of the 'Gentle Cesarean' in Swiss Hospitals: A Conversation with One of Its Pioneers." In *Cognition, Risk, and Responsibility: Anthropological Analyses and Critiques of Obstetricians' Practices*, eds. Davis-Floyd R, Premkumar A, Chapter 5. New York: Berghahn Books.

Çoker H. 2023. "'Birth with No Regret' in Turkey: The Natural Birth of the 21st Century." In *Obstetricians Speak: On Training, Practice, Fear, and Transformation*, eds. Davis-Floyd R, Premkumar A. Chapter 10. New York: Berghahn Books.

Cooper J. 2023. "An Awakening." In *Obstetricians Speak: On Training, Practice, Fear, and Transformation*, eds. Davis-Floyd R, Premkumar A, Chapter 5. New York: Berghahn Books.

Davis-Floyd R. (1992) 2003 . *Birth as an American Rite of Passage*, 2nd ed. Berkeley: University of California Press.

———. 2022. *Birth as an American Rite of Passage*, 3rd ed. Abingdon, Oxon: Routledge.

———. 2023. "Open and Closed Knowledge Systems, the 4 Stages of Cognition, and the Obstetric Management of Birth." In *Cognition, Risk, and Responsibility in Obstetrics: Anthropological Analyses and Critiques of Obstetricians' Practices*, eds. Davis-Floyd R, Premkumar A, Chapter 1. New York: Berghahn Books.

Davis-Floyd R, Premkumar A. 2023a. "The Anthropology of Obstetrics and Obstetricians: The Practice, Maintenance, and Reproduction of a Biomedical Profession." In *Obstetricians Speak: On Training, Practice, Fear, and Transformation*, eds. Davis-Floyd R, Premkumar A, Series Overview. New York: Berghahn Books.

———. 2023b. "Introduction to Volume I: Obstetricians Speak." In *Obstetricians Speak: On Training, Practice, Fear, and Transformation*, eds. Davis-Floyd R, Premkumar A, Introduction. New York: Berghahn Books.

Dunlea M, Hynan M, Murphy-Lawless J, et al. 2023. "From "Mastership" to Active Management of Labor: The Culture of Irish Obstetrics and Obstetricians." In *Cognition, Risk, and Responsibility in Obstetrics: Anthropological Analyses and*

Critiques of Obstetricians' Practices, eds. Davis-Floyd R, Premkumar A, Chapter 2. New York: Berghahn Books.

Evans MG. 2023. "Contraceptive Provision by Obstetricians/Gynecologists in the United States: Biases, Misperceptions and Barriers to an Essential Reproductive Health Service." In *Cognition, Risk, and Responsibility in Obstetrics: Anthropological Analyses and Critiques of Obstetricians' Practices*, eds. Davis-Floyd R, Premkumar A, Chapter 10. New York: Berghahn Books.

Georges E. 2020. "Becoming an Obstetrician in Greece: Medical Training, Informal Scripts, and the Routinization of Cesarean Births." In *Cognition, Risk, and Responsibility in Obstetrics: Anthropological Analyses and Critiques of Obstetricians' Practices*, eds. Davis-Floyd R, Premkumar A, Chapter 3. New York: Berghahn Books.

Geréb A, Fábián K. 2023. "Hungarian Birth Models Seen through the Prism of Prison: The Journey of Ágnes Geréb." In *Obstetricians Speak: On Training, Practice, Fear, and Transformation*, eds. Davis-Floyd R, Premkumar A, Chapter 8. New York: Berghahn Books.

Ginsburg F, Rapp R, eds. 1995. *Creating the New World Order: The Global Politics of Reproduction*. Berkeley: University of California Press.

Hoffer E. 1951. *The True Believer: Thoughts on the Nature of Mass Movements*. New York: Harper and Row, Perennial Classics.

Homer C, Leap M, Edwards N, Sandall J. 2017. "Midwifery Continuity of Carer in an Area of High Socio-Economic Disadvantage in London: A Retrospective Analysis of Albany Midwifery Practice Outcomes Using Routine Data (1997–2009)." *Midwifery* 48: 1–10.

Jaung R. 2019. "How Decolonising Health Could Save The Planet." *The Spinoff*, 16 April. Retrieved 12 December 2022 from https://thespinoff.co.nz/society/16-04-2019/how-decolonising-health-could-save-the-planet/.

Lalonde A. 2023. "How an Obstetrician Promoted Respectful Care in Canada and in the World." In *Obstetricians Speak: On Training, Fear, and Transformation*, eds. Davis-Floyd R, Premkumar A, Chapter 13. New York: Berghahn Books.

Lalonde A, Herschderfer K, Pascali Bonaro D, et al. 2019. "FIGO Statement: *The International Childbirth Initiative: 12 Steps to Safe and Respectful MotherBaby–Family Maternity Care*." *International Journal of Gynecology and Obstetrics* 146(1): 65–73.

Lewis R. 2020. "What to Expect when You're in the Latent (Early Phase) of Labor." *Healthine Parenthood*, 30 June. Retrieved 12 December 2022 from https://www.healthline.com/health/pregnancy/latent-phase-of-labor.

Lokugamage A, Feeley C. 2023. "Cognition, Risk, and Responsibility: Home Birth and Why Obstetricians Fear It." In *Cognition, Risk and Responsibility in Obstetrics: Anthropological Analyses and Critiques of Obstetricians Practices*, eds. Davis-Floyd R, Premkumar A, Chapter 11. New York: Berghahn Books.

Moses S. 2023. "On Becoming an Abortion Provider in the United States: An Autoethnographic Account." In *Obstetricians Speak: On Training, Practice, Fear, and Transformation*, eds. Davis-Floyd R, Premkumar A, Chapter 1. New York: Berghahn Books.

Mayo Clinic Staff. 2020. "Stages of Labor and Birth." *Mayo Clinic*, 13 January. Retrieved 12 December 2022 from https://www.mayoclinic.org/healthy-lifestyle/labor-and-delivery/in-depth/stages-of-labor/art-20046545.

Premkumar A. 2023. "My Transformation from an Obstetrician to a Maternal-Fetal Medicine Subspecialist: Autoethnographic Thoughts on Situated Knowledges and Habitus." In *Obstetricians Speak: On Training, Practice, Fear, and Transformation*, eds. Davis-Floyd R, Premkumar A, Chapter 3. New York: Berghahn Books.

Reed B, Edwards N. In press. *Closure*. London: Pinter and Martin.

Reed B, Walton C. 2009. "The Albany Midwifery Practice." In *Birth Models that Work*, eds. Davis-Floyd R, Barclay L, Daviss BA, Tritten J, 141–158. Berkeley CA: University of California Press.

Reyes E. 2021. "Born in Captivity: The Experiences of Puerto Rican Birth Workers and Their Clients in Quarantine." *Frontiers in Sociology* 6: 613831.

Reynolds PC. 1991. *Stealing Fire: The Mythology of the Technocracy*. Palo Alto CA: Iconic Anthropology Press.

Singh GK. 2021. "Trends and Social Inequalities in Maternal Mortality in the United States, 1969–2018." *International Journal of MCH and AIDS* 10(1): 29–42.

Smith-Oka V, Dizon LZ. 2023. "On Risk and Responsibility: Contextualizing Practice among Mexican Obstetricians." In *Cognition, Risk, and Responsibility in Obstetrics: Anthropological Analyses and Critiques of Obstetricians' Practices*, eds. Davis-Floyd R, Premkumar A, Chapter 7. New York: Berghahn Books.

Tapiainen T, Koivusaari P, Brinkac, L, et al. 2019. "Impact of Intrapartum and Postnatal Antibiotics on the Gut Microbiome and Emergence of Antimicrobial Resistance in Infants." *Scientific Reports* 9:10635 (2019).

World Health Organization (WHO). 2015. "WHO Statement on Cesarean Section Rates." WHO/RHR/15.02. Retrieved 25 December 2022 from https://www.who.int/publications/i/item/WHO-RHR-15.02.

Williamson E, Matsuoka E. 2019. "Comparing Childbirth in Brazil and Japan: Social Hierarchies, Cultural Values, and the Meaning of Place." In *Birth in Eight Cultures*, eds. Davis-Floyd R, Cheyney M, 89–128. Long Grove IL: Waveland Press.

Index